Pediatric Quality

Guest Editors

LEONARD G. FELD, MD, PhD, MMM, FAAP
SHABNAM JAIN, MD, FAAP

PEDIATRIC CLINICS OF NORTH AMERICA

www.pediatric.theclinics.com

August 2009 • Volume 56 • Number 4

SAUNDERS an imprint of ELSEVIER, Inc.

W.B. SAUNDERS COMPANY
A Division of Elsevier Inc.

1600 John F. Kennedy Boulevard • Suite 1800 • Philadelphia, Pennsylvania 19103-2899

http://www.theclinics.com

THE PEDIATRIC CLINICS OF NORTH AMERICA Volume 56, Number 4
August 2009 ISSN 0031-3955, ISBN-13: 978-1-4377-1256-8, ISBN-10: 1-4377-1256-8

Editor: Carla Holloway
Developmental Editor: Theresa Collier

The Pediatric Clinics of North America (ISSN 0031-3955) is published bimonthly by Elsevier Inc., 360 Park Avenue South, New York, NY 10010-1710. Months of publication are February, April, June, August, October, and December. Periodicals postage paid at New York, NY and additional mailing offices. Subscription prices are $162.00 per year (US individuals), $350.00 per year (US institutions), $220.00 per year (Canadian individuals), $466.00 per year (Canadian institutions), $262.00 per year (international individuals), $466.00 per year (international institutions), $81.00 per year (US students and residents), and $138.00 per year (international and Canadian residents and students). To receive students/resident rare, orders must be accompanied by name of affiliated institution, date of term, and the signature of program/residency coordinator on institution letterhead. Orders will be billed at individual rate until proof of status is received. Foreign air speed delivery is included in all *Clinics* subscription prices. All prices are subject to change without notice. **POSTMASTER:** Send address changes to *The Pediatric Clinics of North America*, Elsevier Journals Customer Service, 3251 Riverport Lane, Maryland Heights, MO 63043. **Customer Service: 1-800-654-2452 (US and Canada). From outside of the US and Canada: 1-314-447-8871. Fax: 1-314-447-8029. For print support, e-mail: JournalsCustomerService-usa@elsevier.com. For online support, e-mail: JournalsOnlineSupport-usa@elsevier.com.**

Reprints. For copies of 100 or more, of articles in this publication, please contact the Commercial Reprints Department, Elsevier Inc., 360 Park Avenue South, New York, NY 10010-1710. Tel.: 212-633-3812; Fax: 212-462-1935; E-mail: reprints@elsevier.com.

The Pediatric Clinics of North America is also published in Spanish by McGraw-Hill Inter-americana Editores S.A., Mexico City, Mexico; in Portuguese by Riechmann and Affonso Editores, Rua Comandante Coelho 1085, CEP 21250, Rio de Janeiro, Brazil; and in Greek by Althayia SA, Athens, Greece.

The Pediatric Clinics of North America is covered in *MEDLINE/PubMed (Index Medicus), Excerpta Medica, Current Contents, Current Contents/Clinical Medicine, Science Citation Index, ASCA, ISI/BIOMED*, and *BIOSIS*.

Printed and bound by CPI Group (UK) Ltd, Croydon, CR0 4YY

Transferred to Digital Print 2011

GOAL STATEMENT

The goal of the *Pediatric Clinics of North America* is to keep practicing physicians and residents up to date with current clinical practice in pediatrics by providing timely articles reviewing the state-of-the-art in patient care.

ACCREDITATION

The *Pediatric Clinics of North America* is planned and implemented in accordance with the Essential Areas and Policies of the Accreditation Council for Continuing Medical Education (ACCME) through the joint sponsorship of the University of Virginia School of Medicine and Elsevier. The University of Virginia School of Medicine is accredited by the ACCME to provide continuing medical education for physicians.

The University of Virginia School of Medicine designates this educational activity for a maximum of 15 *AMA PRA Category 1 Credits*™. Physicians should only claim credit commensurate with the extent of their participation in the activity.

The American Medical Association has determined that physicians not licensed in the US who participate in this CME activity are eligible for 15 *AMA PRA Category 1 Credits*™.

Credit can be earned by reading the text material, taking the CME examination online at http://www.theclinics.com/home/cme, and completing the evaluation. After taking the test, you will be required to review any and all incorrect answers. Following completion of the test and evaluation, your credit will be awarded and you may print your certificate.

FACULTY DISCLOSURE/CONFLICT OF INTEREST

The University of Virginia School of Medicine, as an ACCME accredited provider, endorses and strives to comply with the Accreditation Council for Continuing Medical Education (ACCME) Standards of Commercial Support, Commonwealth of Virginia statutes, University of Virginia policies and procedures, and associated federal and private regulations and guidelines on the need for disclosure and monitoring of proprietary and financial interests that may affect the scientific integrity and balance of content delivered in continuing medical education activities under our auspices.

The University of Virginia School of Medicine requires that all CME activities accredited through this institution be developed independently and be scientifically rigorous, balanced and objective in the presentation/discussion of its content, theories and practices.

All authors/editors participating in an accredited CME activity are expected to disclose to the readers relevant financial relationships with commercial entities occurring within the past 12 months (such as grants or research support, employee, consultant, stock holder, member of speakers bureau, etc.). The University of Virginia School of Medicine will employ appropriate mechanisms to resolve potential conflicts of interest to maintain the standards of fair and balanced education to the reader. Questions about specific strategies can be directed to the Office of Continuing Medical Education, University of Virginia School of Medicine, Charlottesville, Virginia.

The faculty and staff of the University of Virginia Office of Continuing Medical Education have no financial affiliations to disclose.

The authors/editors listed below have identified no financial or professional relationships for themselves or their spouse/partner:
Richard C. Antonelli, MD, MS; Maria T. Britto, MD, MPH; David G. Bundy, MD, MPH; Cheryl D. Courtlandt, MD, FAAP; Karen S. Cox, RN, PhD, FAAN; Mark A. Del Beccaro, MD; Megan Esporas, MPH; Gerry Fairbrother, PhD; David C. Goodman, MD, MS; James B. Hendricks, PhD; Carla Holloway (Acquisitions Editor); Charles J. Homer, MD, MPH; Daniel Hyman, MD, MMM; Shabnam Jain, MD (Guest Editor); Uma R. Kotagal, MBBS, MSc; Paul Kurtin, MD; Susan R. Lacey, PhD, RN, FAAN; Mariellen Lane, MD; Christine A. Limbers, MS; Keith E. Mandel, MD; Peter A. Margolis, MD, PhD; Sara Massie, MPH; Stephen E. Meuthing, MD; Paul V. Miles, MD; Daniel R. Neuspiel, MD, MPH; Laura Noonan, MD, FAAP; Lloyd P. Provost, MS; Greg Randolph, MD, MPH; Karen Rheuban, MD (Test Author); Ramesh C. Sachdeva, MD, PhD, JD, FAAP; Pamela J. Schoettker, MS; Joseph Schulman, MD, MS; Lisa A. Simpson, MD, BCh, MPH; F. Bruder Stapleton, MD; Erin Stucky, MD; Renée M. Turchi, MD, MPH; Kerry T. Van Voorhis, MD; Steven E. Wegner, JD, MD; Tina Schade Willis, MD; David D. Wirtschafter, MD; and Alan E. Zuckerman, MD.

The authors/editors listed below identified the following professional or financial affiliations for themselves or their spouse/partner:
Leonard G. Feld, MD, PhD, MMM, FAAP is a consultant for Bristol Myers Squibb.
Patrick J. Hagan, MHSA serves as a speaker for Joan Wellman and Associates.
Norman "Chip" Harbaugh, Jr., MD owns stock in Kids Time Pediatrics and 187 Healthcare, and serves on the Advisory Committee for Kids First Alliance.
Richard Lander serves on the Advisory Committee for Merck, Sanofi, Wyeth, Novartis, and Medimmune, owns stock in Resources in Physician's Management Services and Mathion Discount Vaccine Alliance, and serves on the Speakers Bureau for Physician's Computer Co. and Sanofi.
Kathryn M. McDonald, MM is a consultant for Peoplechart.
James W. Varni, PhD serves on the Advisory Committee for Amgen and is an industry funded research/investigator for Takeda.

Disclosure of Discussion of Non-FDA Approved Uses for Pharmaceutical and/or Medical Devices:
The University of Virginia School of Medicine, as an ACCME provider, requires that all authors identify and disclose any "off label" uses for pharmaceutical and medical device products. The University of Virginia School of Medicine recommends that each physician fully review all the available data on new products or procedures prior to clinical use.

TO ENROLL

To enroll in the *Pediatric Clinics of North America* Continuing Medical Education program, call customer service at 1-800-654-2452 or visit us online at www.theclinics.com/home/cme. The CME program is available to subscribers for an additional fee of $195.00.

Contributors

GUEST EDITORS

LEONARD G. FELD, MD, PhD, MMM, FAAP
Sara H. and Howard C. Bissell Endowed Chair in Pediatrics and Chief Medical Officer, Levine Children's Hospital at Carolinas Medical Center; and Clinical Professor of Pediatrics, University of North Carolina School of Medicine, Charlotte, North Carolina

SHABNAM JAIN, MD, FAAP
Assistant Professor of Pediatrics and Emergency Medicine, Emory University and Children's Healthcare of Atlanta, Atlanta, Georgia

AUTHORS

RICHARD C. ANTONELLI, MD, MS
Medical Director, Children's Hospital Boston Integrated Care Organization; Interim Associate Medical Director, Quality of Physicians' Organization, Children's Hospital Boston; and Division of General Pediatrics, Children's Hospital/Harvard Medical School, Boston, Massachusetts

MARIA T. BRITTO, MD, MPH
Assistant Vice President and Professor, Divisions of Adolescent Medicine and Health Policy and Clinical Effectiveness, Cincinnati Children's Hospital Medical Center and University of Cincinnati College of Medicine, Cincinnati, Ohio

DAVID G. BUNDY, MD, MPH
Assistant Professor, Department of Pediatrics, Johns Hopkins University School of Medicine, Baltimore, Maryland

CHERYL D. COURTLANDT, MD
Division of General Pediatrics; Co-Director, Center for Advancing Pediatric Excellence; and Director, Asthma Program, Levine Children's Hospital at Carolinas Medical Center, Charlotte, North Carolina

KAREN S. COX, RN, PhD, FAAN
Associate Director, Bi-State Nursing Workforce Innovation Center; and Director, Nursing Workforce and Systems Analysis, University of Missouri Kansas City; Co-Chief Operating Officer, Children's Mercy Hospitals and Clinics, Kansas City, Missouri

MARK DELBECCARO, MD
Professor of Pediatrics, Department of Pediatrics, University of Washington; and Pediatrician-in-Chief, Seattle Children's Hospital, Seattle, Washington

MEGAN ESPORAS, MPH
Director, North Carolina Children's Center for Excellence, North Carolina Children's Hospital; Department of Pediatrics; and Adjunct Associate Professor, Public Health Leadership Program, University of North Carolina at Chapel Hill, Chapel Hill, North Carolina

GERRY FAIRBROTHER, PhD
Professor and Associate Director, Child Policy Research Center, Department of Pediatrics, Cincinnati Children's Hospital Medical Center, Cincinnati, Ohio

LEONARD G. FELD, MD, PhD, MMM, FAAP
Sara H. and Howard C. Bissell Endowed Chair in Pediatrics and Chief Medical Officer, Levine Children's Hospital at Carolinas Medical Center; and Clinical Professor of Pediatrics, Department of Pediatrics, University of North Carolina School of Medicine, Charlotte, North Carolina

DAVID C. GOODMAN, MD, MS
Professor of Pediatrics, The Dartmouth Institute for Health Policy and Clinical Practice; and The Children's Hospital at Dartmouth, Dartmouth-Hitchcock Medical Center, Lebanon; Dartmouth Medical School, Hanover, New Hampshire

PATRICK HAGAN, MHSA
President and Chief Operating Officer, Seattle Children's Hospital, Seattle, Washington

NORMAN (CHIP) HARBAUGH, Jr., MD
Pediatrician at Children's Medical Group; and CEO and Chairman of the Board-Emeritus, Kid's Health First, Atlanta, Georgia; Steering Committee on Quality Improvement and Management, National American Academy of Pediatrics; Section on Administration and Practice Management-Executive Board, National American Academy of Pediatrics; Child Healthcare Financing Committee, National American Academy of Pediatrics; National Conference for Education Committee, National American Academy of Pediatrics; United Healthcare Physician Advisory Committee; Center for Disease Control, Clinical Laboratory Improvement Committee

JAMES HENDRICKS, PhD
President, Seattle Children's Research Institute, Seattle, Washington

CHARLES J. HOMER, MD, MPH
National Initiative for Children's Healthcare Quality, Boston, Massachusetts

DANIEL HYMAN, MD, MMM
Chief Quality Officer, The Children's Hospital of Denver; and Assistant Professor of Pediatrics, University of Colorado School of Medicine, Aurora, Colorado

SHABNAM JAIN, MD, FAAP
Assistant Professor of Pediatrics and Emergency Medicine, Emory University and Children's Healthcare of Atlanta, Atlanta, Georgia

UMA R. KOTAGAL, MBBS, MSc
Professor, Department of Pediatrics and Obstetrics/Gynecology, University of Cincinnati College of Medicine; and Senior Vice President of Quality and Transformation, Division of Health Policy and Clinical Effectiveness, Cincinnati Children's Hospital Medical Center, Cincinnati, Ohio

PAUL KURTIN, MD
Chief Quality and Safety Officer and Director, Sadler Center for Quality, Rady Children's Hospital, San Diego, California

SUSAN R. LACEY, PhD, RN, FAAN
Director, Bi-State Nursing Workforce Innovation Center; and Director, Nursing Workforce and Systems Analysis, University of Missouri Kansas City; Children's Mercy Hospitals and Clinics, Kansas City, Missouri

RICHARD LANDER, MD
Essex Morris Pediatrics Group, Livingston, New Jersey

MARIELLEN LANE, MD
Director of Pediatric Ambulatory Education, Division of General Pediatrics; and Associate Clinical Professor of Pediatrics, Columbia University, Morgan Stanley Children's Hospital of New York-Presbyterian, New York, New York

CHRISTINE A. LIMBERS, MS
Clinical Psychology Doctoral Student, Department of Psychology, College of Liberal Arts, Texas A&M University, College Station, Texas

KEITH E. MANDEL, MD
Associate Professor, Department of Pediatrics, University of Cincinnati College of Medicine; Vice President of Medical Affairs, Physician-Hospital Organization, Division of Health Policy and Clinical Effectiveness, Cincinnati Children's Hospital Medical Center, Cincinnati, Ohio

PETER A. MARGOLIS, MD, PhD
Professor of Pediatrics, Center for Health Care Quality, Division of Health Policy and Effectiveness, Cincinnati Children's Hospital Medical Center and University of Cincinnati College of Medicine, Cincinnati, Ohio

SARA MASSIE, MPH
Communication and Development Specialist, North Carolina Children's Center for Excellence, North Carolina Children's Hospital; Department of Pediatrics; and Manager, Child Health Research Program, North Carolina Translational and Clinical Sciences Institute, University of North Carolina at Chapel Hill, Chapel Hill, North Carolina

KATHRYN M. McDONALD, MM
Senior Research Scholar, Center for Primary Care and Outcomes Research, Stanford University, Stanford, California

STEPHEN E. MEUTHING, MD
Associate Professor, Department of Pediatrics, University of Cincinnati College of Medicine; and Assistant Vice President, Division of General and Community Pediatrics, Cincinnati Children's Hospital Medical Center, Cincinnati, Ohio

PAUL V. MILES, MD
Senior Vice President for Maintenance of Certification and Quality, The American Board of Pediatrics, Chapel Hill; and Adjunct Professor of Pediatrics, Duke University School of Medicine, Durham, North Carolina

DANIEL R. NEUSPIEL, MD, MPH
Director, Ambulatory Pediatrics, Division of General Pediatrics, Department of Pediatrics, Levine Children's Hospital of Carolinas Medical Center; and Adjunct Clinical Professor of Pediatrics, University of North Carolina School of Medicine, Charlotte, North Carolina

LAURA NOONAN, MD
Division of General Pediatrics, Levine Children's Hospital at Carolinas Medical Center, Charlotte, North Carolina; Director, Center for Advancing Pediatric Excellence, Levine Children's Hospital at Carolinas Medical Center, Charlotte, North Carolina; Senior Improvement Officer, Area Hospital Education Center, Charlotte, North Carolina

LLOYD P. PROVOST, MS
Statistician and Improvement Advisor, Associates in Process Improvement, Austin, Texas

GREG RANDOLPH, MD, MPH
Associate Professor, Department of Pediatrics; Co-Director, North Carolina Children's Center for Excellence, North Carolina Children's Hospital; Department of Pediatrics; and Adjunct Associate Professor, Public Health Leadership Program, University of North Carolina at Chapel Hill, Chapel Hill, North Carolina

RAMESH C. SACHDEVA, MD, PhD, JD, FAAP
Executive Vice President and COO, National Outcomes Center; Vice President, Quality Outcomes, Children's Hospital of Wisconsin; Professor of Pediatrics, Medical College of Wisconsin; and Adjunct Professor of Law, Marquette University Law School, Milwaukee, Wisconsin

PAMELA J. SCHOETTKER, MS
Medical Writer, Division of Health Policy and Clinical Effectiveness, Cincinnati Children's Hospital Medical Center, Cincinnati, Ohio

JOSEPH SCHULMAN, MD, MS
Weill Cornell Medical College, Division of Newborn Medicine, Department of Pediatrics; Division of Outcomes & Effectiveness, Department of Public Health; and New York Presbyterian Hospital, New York, NY

LISA A. SIMPSON, MB, BCh, MPH
Professor and Director, Child Policy Research Center, Department of Pediatrics, Cincinnati Children's Hospital Medical Center, Cincinnati, Ohio

F. BRUDER STAPLETON, MD
Professor and Chair, Department of Pediatrics, University of Washington; and Chief Academic Officer, Seattle Children's Hospital, Seattle, Washington

ERIN STUCKY, MD
Pediatric Hospitalist and Medical Director for Quality and Safety, Rady Children's Hospital, San Diego; and Clinical Professor, Department of Pediatrics, University of California San Diego, La Jolla, California

RENEE M. TURCHI, MD, MPH
Clinical Director of Special Programs, St. Christopher's Hospital for Children; and Associate Professor, Department of Pediatrics, Drexel University School of Public Health, Philadelphia, Pennsylvania

KERRY T. VAN VOORHIS, MD
Clinical Associate Professor of Pediatrics, Division of General Pediatrics; and Director of Inpatient Services, Levine Children's Hospital at Carolinas Medical Center, Charlotte, North Carolina

JAMES W. VARNI, PhD
Professor and Vice Chair for Research, Department of Pediatrics, College of Medicine; and Professor, Department of Landscape Architecture and Urban Planning, College of Architecture, Texas A&M University, College Station, Texas

STEVEN E. WEGNER, JD, MD
Medical Director, AccessCare, Morrisville; and Adjunct Clinical Assistant Professor, Department of Pediatrics, University of North Carolina School of Medicine, Chapel Hill, North Carolina

TINA SCHADE WILLIS, MD
Assistant Professor, Division of Pediatric Critical Care Medicine; Medical Director, ECMO and Pediatric Intensive Care Unit; and Co-Director, North Carolina Children's Center for Clinical Excellence, University of North Carolina at Chapel Hill, Chapel Hill, North Carolina

DAVID D. WIRTSCHAFTER, MD
David D. Wirtschafter, MD, Inc., Valley Village, California

ALAN E. ZUCKERMAN, MD
Assistant Professor, Department of Pediatrics; and Assistant Professor, Department of Family Medicine, Georgetown University School of Medicine, Washington, DC

Contents

every practitioner delivering safe, effective, and efficient care. The case study demonstrates how this methodology can be applied in any busy health care setting. Incorporating this approach to quality improvement into daily work will improve clinical outcomes and advance health care delivery and design.

Model for Improvement–Part 2: Measurement and Feedback for Quality Improvement Efforts **779**

Greg Randolph, Megan Esporas, Lloyd Provost, Sara Massie, and David G. Bundy

Measurement and feedback are fundamental to quality improvement. There is a knowledge gap among health care professionals in knowing how to measure the impact of their quality improvement projects and how to use these data to improve care. This article presents a pragmatic approach to measurement and feedback for quality improvement efforts in local health care settings, such as hospitals or clinical practices. The authors include evidence-based strategies from health care and other industries, augmented with practical examples from the authors' collective years of experience designing measurement and feedback strategies.

Modifying the Toyota Production System for Continuous Performance Improvement in an Academic Children's Hospital **799**

F. Bruder Stapleton, James Hendricks, Patrick Hagan, and Mark DelBeccaro

The Toyota Production System (TPS) has become a successful model for improving efficiency and eliminating errors in manufacturing processes. In an effort to provide patients and families with the highest quality clinical care, our academic children's hospital has modified the techniques of the TPS for a program in continuous performance improvement (CPI) and has expanded its application to educational and research programs. Over a period of years, physicians, nurses, residents, administrators, and hospital staff have become actively engaged in a culture of continuous performance improvement. This article provides background into the methods of CPI and describes examples of how we have applied these methods for improvement in clinical care, resident teaching, and research administration.

QI Measures

Approach to Improving Quality: The Role of Quality Measurement and a Case Study of the Agency for Healthcare Research and Quality Pediatric Quality Indicators **815**

Kathryn M. McDonald

Data and well-constructed measures quantify suboptimal quality in health care and play a crucial role in improving quality. Measures are useful for three major purposes: (1) driving improvements in outcomes of care by prioritizing and selecting appropriate interventions, (2) developing comparative quality reports for consumer and payer decision making and health system accountability, and (3) creating incentives that pay for performance. This article describes the current landscape for measurement in

practical help to others seeking to create such networks. The content illustrates concepts with broad applicability for pediatric quality improvement.

Standardize to Excellence: Improving the Quality and Safety of Care with Clinical Pathways **893**

Paul Kurtin and Erin Stucky

Providing practitioners with locally developed, consensus-driven, evidence-based clinical pathways can improve the quality of care by (1) incorporating national guidelines and recommendations into routine care practices, increasing the use of validated practice; (2) reducing unnecessary variation in care by a single physician or group of physicians, improving efficiency and timeliness and reducing disparities; and (3) standardizing care processes, improving safety. Pathways make it easier to identify opportunities for future improvements in care processes while simultaneously making those improvements easier to enact. Pediatric hospitalists have a vital role in creating, implementing, evaluating, and improving clinical pathways. Involving house staff enriches the scholarly components of pathway development while actively engaging them in the science and practice of quality improvement.

Transforming Safety and Effectiveness in Pediatric Hospital Care Locally and Nationally **905**

Keith E. Mandel, Stephen E. Muething, Pamela J. Schoettker, and Uma R. Kotagal

Achieving dramatic, sustainable improvements in the safety and effectiveness of care for children requires a transformational approach to how hospitals individually focus on improvement and learn from each other to achieve national goals. The authors describe a theoretic framework for transformation that includes setting system-level priorities, aligning measures with each priority, identifying breakthrough targets, testing interventions to get results, and spreading successful interventions throughout the organization. Essential key drivers of transformation include leadership, building will, transparency, a business case for quality, patient and family engagement, improvement infrastructure, improvement capability, and reliability and standardization. Improving national system-level measures requires each hospital to pursue its own transformation journey while collaborating with hospitals and other organizations.

Implementing a Pediatric Rapid Response System to Improve Quality and Patient Safety **919**

Kerry T. Van Voorhis and Tina S.Willis

Life-threatening events are common in today's hospitals, where an increasing proportion of patients with urgent admission are cared for by understaffed, often inexperienced personnel. Medical errors play a key role in causing adverse events and failure to rescue deteriorating patients. In-hospital cardiac arrest outcomes are generally poor, but these events are often preceded by a pattern of deterioration with abnormal vital signs and mental status. When hospital staff or family members observe warning signs and trigger timely intervention by a rapid response team, rates of cardiac arrest and mortality can be reduced. Rapid response team involvement can be used to trigger careful review of preceding events to help uncover important systems issues and allow for further improvements in patient safety.

Quality Improvement and Patient Safety in the Pediatric Ambulatory Setting: Current Knowledge and Implications for Residency Training **935**

Daniel R. Neuspiel, Daniel Hyman, and Mariellen Lane

The outpatient environment has been the leading edge of improvement work in pediatrics and it has similarly served as an effective locale for the training of pediatric residents in the science of improvement. This review summarizes what is known about the measurement of quality and patient safety in pediatric ambulatory settings. The current Accreditation Council for Graduate Medical Education (ACGME) requirements for resident training in improvement and their application in these settings are discussed. Some approaches and challenges to meeting these requirements are reviewed. Finally, some future directions that this work may follow are presented; the goal is to strengthen the effectiveness of improvement methods and their linkage to professional education.

The Medical Home—Improving Quality of Primary Care for Children **953**

Steven E. Wegner, Richard C. Antonelli, and Renee M. Turchi

The concept of a medical home appears to be a key driver for enhancing the value of health services as care systems are transitioned to meet the ongoing challenges of improving quality and containing costs. This article provides an overview of the challenges faced in United States health care delivery systems that affect child health, explains how the medical home might address them, describes methods for measuring quality in medical homes, and identifies barriers to implementation of the model.

The Role of Health Information Technology in Quality Improvement in Pediatrics **965**

Alan E. Zuckerman

Health information technology (HIT) will play an important role in most efforts to improve the quality of pediatric medicine, as evident from the range of investigations and projects discussed in this volume. Clement McDonald identified the importance of using information technology as an integral component of quality initiatives early in the development of electronic medical records (EMR). The role of HIT in quality improvement is not limited to tools integrated into EMR, but that remains an important strategy. Today, much attention is focused on interoperability of clinical systems that integrate and share data from multiple sources. There are also additional freestanding quality-improvement tools that can be used without an EMR. This article explores the many roles of HIT in quality improvement from several perspectives.

Nursing: Key to Quality Improvement 975

Susan R. Lacey and Karen S. Cox

Nurses and effective nursing care contribute to quality patient outcomes. This article explains in detail the importance of nursing care in the quality agenda and explores the existing gaps in this field of science. Key stakeholders and groups that advocate and focus on specific quality agendas within the field of pediatrics are briefly described. Pediatric health care uses a multidisciplinary model of delivery; each discipline uses specific domains of knowledge and interventions, making it difficult to separate them when evaluating patient outcomes. Much work needs to be conducted using health services research approaches that link and partition the overall and combined contribution of discipline-specific providers.

THE FUTURE OF QUALITY IN PEDIATRIC PRACTICE

Maintenance of Certification: The Role of the American Board of Pediatrics in Improving Children's Health Care 987

Paul V. Miles

This article describes the evolution of board certification for pediatricians and the current ongoing assessment process called Maintenance of Certification (MOC). To be called a board-certified pediatrician under the MOC framework requires a level of training, competence, and knowledge that can only be achieved by completing a rigorous, defined, closely monitored training program approved by the Accreditation Council for Graduate Medical Education and then demonstrating a level of knowledge comparable to established standards by passing the initial certifying examination. Once this landmark baseline threshold is reached, the emphasis shifts to demonstrating lifelong professional development and the ability to deliver quality care and to continually improving that care through MOC.

A Pediatrician's Opinion 995

Richard Lander

Pediatricians are inundated by phrases such as "pay for performance" and "enhancement of payments tied into quality measurements." Although there is no argument that we must provide high quality care to our patients and must continuously improve ourselves, we need flexibility within the managed care criteria. Medicine is not only a science, but it is also an art with many interpretations.

Pay for Performance: Quality- and Value-Based Reimbursement 997

Norman (Chip) Harbaugh, Jr.

There is urgent need to reform health care reimbursement models, including physician compensation, to address high health care costs, despite numerous quality initiatives. Pay for performance (P4P) is a model that attempts to align financial incentives with better outcomes and value rather than the current system of rewarding volume and intensity of care delivered. P4P has been implemented in other countries besides the United States and is perhaps most advanced in the United Kingdom. Measurement for P4P is evolving, as are the types of incentives; neither is perfect at this time. For P4P to succeed, all health care stakeholders will need to collaborate.

How Health Policy Influences Quality of Care in Pediatrics **1009**

Lisa A. Simpson and Gerry Fairbrother

The primary focus of child health policy for the last twenty years has been on improving health care coverage and access. More recently, the focus has shifted to include not only coverage, but also the quality of the care received. This article describes some "voltage drops" in health care that impede delivery of high quality health care. The growing emphasis on quality is reflected in provisions of the new Child Health Program Reauthorization Act of 2009 (CHIPRA) legislation. In addition to providing funding for health coverage for over four million more children, it also includes the most significant federal investment in pediatric quality to date.

Index **1023**

FORTHCOMING ISSUES

October 2009

Nutritional Deficiencies

Praveen S. Goday, MD, and
Timothy Sentongo, MD, *Guest Editors*

December 2009

Health Issues in Indigenous Children: An Evidence-Based Approach

Anne B. Chang, MBBS, MPHTM, FRACP, PhD, and Rosalyn Singleton, MD, *Guest Editors*

February 2010

Bone Marrow Transplantation

Max Coppes, MD, PhD, MBA,
Terry Fry, MD, and Crystal Mackall, MD, *Guest Editors*

RECENT ISSUES

June 2009

Advances in Neonatology

Lucky Jain, MD, MBA and
David P. Carlton, MD, *Guest Editors*

April 2009

Child Abuse and Neglect: Advancements and Challenges in the 21st Century

Andrew Sirotnak, MD, *Guest Editor*

February 2009

Common Respiratory Symptoms and Illnesses: A Graded Evidence-Based Approach

Anne B. Chang, MBBS, MPHTM, FRACP, PhD, *Guest Editor*

RELATED INTEREST

Pediatric Clinics December 2006 (Vol. 53, Issue 6)

Patient Safety
Anne Matlow and Ronald Laxer, *Guest Editors*
www.pediatric.theclinics.com

Erratum

An error appeared in the article "Molecular and Cellular Basis of Congenital Heart Disease" in the October 2006 issue of *Pediatric Clinics of North America*. In Table 1 on page 997, the incidence of the syndromes listed is incorrect. The incidence should be per 100,000 live births.

Pediatr Clin N Am 56 (2009) xix
doi:10.1016/j.pcl.2009.06.003
pediatric.theclinics.com
0031-3955/09/$ – see front matter

Preface

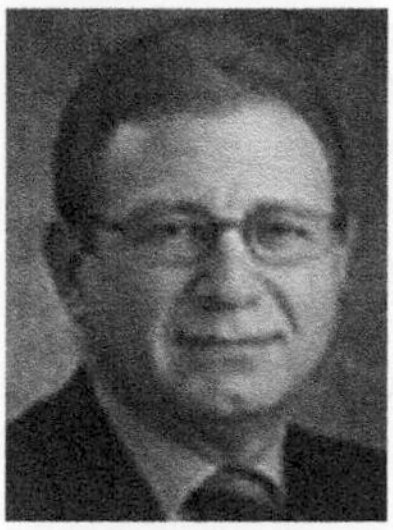

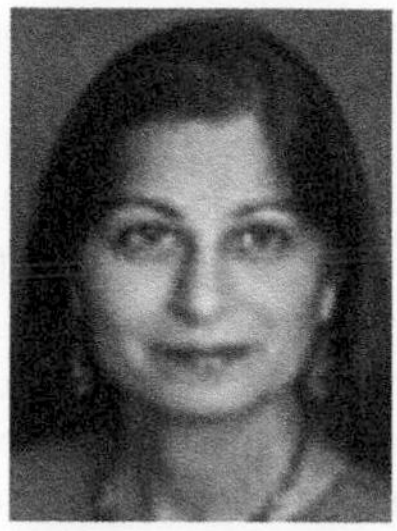

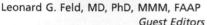

Leonard G. Feld, MD, PhD, MMM, FAAP Shabnam Jain, MD, FAAP
Guest Editors

Few issues are more central to the ongoing debate about health care in the United States than the quality and cost of care. As we start tackling some of these issues, three simple but eloquent statements should be engrained in our minds: (1) Business as usual will not help us achieve the health care system that our children deserve.[1] (2) Every system is perfectly designed to achieve exactly the results it gets.[2] (3) Knowing is not enough; we must apply. Willing is not enough; we must do.[3]

Three years ago, *Pediatric Clinics of North America* published an issue on patient safety. Although safety in health care remains an important goal, improving the quality of the care we deliver entails much more than just ensuring safety. This current issue, devoted to pediatric quality, has a series of articles by leaders in the field on topics addressing multifaceted angles in health care quality improvement (QI).

The issue starts with an introduction by Charles Homer, MD, the "father" of pediatric quality improvement. The quality movement is further along in adults in comparison with pediatrics; however, children have their own unique set of quality needs. Dr. Homer has been a driving force in establishing the agenda for health-care professionals in our journey for "perfect pediatric healthcare."

The first of four sections in this issue of the *Pediatric Clinics of North America* lays a foundation by providing an overview of the urgency to improve the current state of health care quality and costs; some emerging concepts as well as future directions in the quality movement are introduced. Unwarranted variation in health care delivery is prevalent and often goes unrecognized—this important problem is discussed in this section.

Most health professionals today are not formally trained in QI methodology; despite a sincere desire to improve, they often come to the task with a handicap. The second section, QI Methods and Measures, provides a toolkit to help make necessary changes in our clinics and hospitals. This section describes the PDSA/Model for Improvement and the Lean/Six Sigma methodology using a case presentation. This section also

Pediatr Clin N Am 56 (2009) xxi–xxiii
doi:10.1016/j.pcl.2009.05.020 pediatric.theclinics.com

covers how to apply QI models initially used in manufacturing to the inpatient health-care setting.

Deciding which QI method to implement is only half the story; how success is measured is the other half. The section on QI measures discusses the systematic development of a set of pediatric quality indicators by the Agency for Healthcare Research and Quality. Health care quality measurement in relation to existing evidence-based strategies, and the need to establish benchmarks as well as monitoring and feedback strategies to track effectiveness are all discussed in detail in this section.

QI efforts in health care are more established in inpatient hospital settings; the third section of this issue presents a wide array of hospital-based initiatives, using examples of regional and national collaborations to reduce NICU infections, development of pathways and order sets for common pediatric conditions, and rapid response teams to prevent codes in general care units. Pediatric hospitals have a sense of urgency to improve the quality of the care they deliver, yet there are organizational and financial challenges. We learn how a leading children's hospital has aligned its quality agenda to systematically transform pediatric hospital care. The importance of the medical home for the coordination of care, as well as the collaboration with nursing colleagues, particularly in the inpatient setting, is presented in this section.

QI plays a role in both the research and teaching mission of academic institutions; this section discusses how they can be integrated. It is becoming clear that traditional research methodologies need to be supplemented by newer methods of improving systems of care and practice. Well designed studies on quality and safety using a wide range of research methods will help us move from the "era of evidence" to the "era of quality."[4] As a vital part of the teaching agenda, we need to explore how best to train future generations of pediatricians by incorporating QI into trainee curriculums. The section ends with a discussion of the importance of health information technology for improving children's health care quality by bringing all necessary information to the point of care. Recent legislation by the United States government highlights the new horizon of health information technology and importance of its integration into the clinical care delivery system.

Improving healthcare clearly requires involvement of both *p*atients and *p*roviders in health care decisions, but that is not enough. The last section of this issue of the *Pediatric Clinics of North America* notes the importance of the other two "p"s: policy makers and payers. Reform in health care policy and payment systems has begun, but we have far to go to make these efforts endure. Given the rapid pace of health care quality improvement, how do we keep frontline practitioners informed and engaged? We learn about processes implemented by the American Board of Pediatrics related to the maintenance of certification; these will affect all practicing pediatricians in the years to come.

Quality improvement is a hot topic in health care today. We in the United States have certainly embarked on that journey, but we have far to go. Indeed, there is much debate about what works, whether it works in every setting, and how to move it from concept to practice. These questions need urgent attention, and this first ever issue of the *Pediatric Clinics of North America* dedicated entirely to quality attests to that. We are grateful to Carla Holloway at Elsevier for her support, and to all of our colleagues who have contributed to this project.

It is our hope that this compilation of articles by experts in the field will serve as a "handbook" on pediatric quality to help us achieve a pediatric health care environment with the quality of care that all children deserve.

Leonard G. Feld, MD, PhD, MMM, FAAP
Levine Children's Hospital at Carolinas Medical Center
Department of Pediatrics
PO Box 32861
Charlotte, NC 28232, USA

Shabnam Jain, MD, FAAP
Departments of Pediatrics and Emergency Medicine
Emory University
Children's Healthcare of Atlanta
Atlanta, GA, USA

E-mail addresses:
leonard.feld@carolinashealthcare.org (L.G. Feld)
shabnam.jain@oz.ped.emory.edu (S. Jain)

REFERENCES

1. Halfon N, DuPlessis H, Inkelas M. Transforming the US Child Health System. Health Affairs 2007;26:315–3301.
2. Berwick D. Institute of Healthcare Improvement.
3. Phillips DF. "New Look" Reflects Changing Style of Patient Safety Enhancement. JAMA 1999;336(281):217–9.
4. Grol R, Berwick DM, Wensing M. On the trail of quality and safety in health care. BMJ 2008;336(7635):74–6.

Foreword

A Great Start and A Long Way to Go

Charles J. Homer, MD, MPH

Could any of us have imagined how far the field of pediatric quality improvement would come in less than two decades? The number of individuals who were committing their careers to pediatric quality—either through research or management—could likely have fit within a telephone booth, and certainly within a minivan, in the early 1990s. In looking at the contents of this issue of the *Pediatric Clinics of North America*, it is clear how far our field has come—how much greater the breadth and number of individuals involved, how much deeper our understanding of the nature of our quality problem, how much improved our tools are to measure quality and our methods are for taking action to improve performance. We now can point to real beacons of success, actual programs that have made dramatic improvements in removing the excuse that "it cannot be done in health care." At this time of hope, renewal, and opportunity in the United States of America, it is worth reflecting on what has contributed to the successes that these articles describe and the growth in our field, as well as challenges ahead and what we need do to better achieve the goal of our movement—a world in which all children receive the health care they need.

In order to succeed and be sustained through long-term institutional and societal change, all successful movements must build political will, have a solid evidence base, and have a successful social strategy to move forward. The political will in our field comes from an increasing awareness of the gap between what children need and what our health care system provides. For the technicians among us, the evidence of the chasm between what science demonstrated to be effective practice, such as the use of appropriate medications for asthma, and what was the usual practice was sufficient to get this movement started. For others, the continued occurrence of the harm inflicted by the health care system was the motivation for change, particularly when safety science in other disciplines and industries had already proven the capability of complex systems to perform at much higher levels of reliability than did health care. The frustrations of parents and patients, including both those with chronic conditions such as autism and those who have experienced harm from care, with a system that learns too slowly and varies too much, is also driving change. For policy makers and the public, the poor outcomes for the United States health care system, relative to outcomes for children in other developed nations and coupled with the high cost and the limitations in access, have lit a fire for wide scale health system change. The emergence of new public health concerns, such as obesity, for which the delivery system is ill prepared, that threaten to swamp the health care system in the future is also motivating professionals, the public, and policymakers to focus on improving the performance of our health care system. And while children's health care concerns traditionally are marginalized in conversations about larger health system reform, the dedication of professionals such as those writing these articles, the power of the family voice, the critical role of visionary philanthropic foundations at critical points, the

Pediatr Clin N Am 56 (2009) xxv–xxvii
doi:10.1016/j.pcl.2009.05.019

importance of children's health issues to the public, and even the prolonged political struggle over reauthorization of the Child Health Insurance Program has kept these issues on the table and moving forward.

The scientific basis on which to make improvements in care is amply documented throughout this issue and constitutes its major contribution. The articles highlight the key role of measurement—and the availability of more and more proven measures—in identifying gaps and variation in care, in tracking success, and in communicating to the public and each other how well (or how poorly) we are doing. They indicate the importance of a systematic approach to changing processes, approaches such as the model for improvement, lean and six sigma, as well as the value of reliability science in reducing harm. Several contributors elaborate on the value of standardization as one key mechanism for enhancing quality and safety, reflected in mechanisms such as order sets and guidelines. Others note how collaboration amongst many organizations working together—using measurement, benchmarking, and the systematic approaches to process change—often accelerates the change and improvement process. An underlying theme in several of the articles is the critical role of families in driving the change process as well as being the most important voice in the care process. The critical role of a well-prepared workforce is amplified in separate articles that detail the role of nursing and training resident physicians.

Despite these tremendous advances, we also know, or at least strongly suspect, that the overall performance of the health care system for children as a whole has not yet made dramatic strides forward. We cannot yet confidently assure a parent that, regardless of which practice they bring their child to, that their child will receive appropriate developmental surveillance and that the family will receive the most effective counseling on health behaviors to position their child for a healthy life; that if diagnosed with a condition, their child will consistently receive evidence-based treatments and do so in a way that is consistent with family preferences and cultural values. We cannot yet promise families that when their child is admitted to a hospital, he or she will not be exposed to unnecessary harm from medication errors or nosocomial infections, or that all of the important aspects of their care will be communicated across institutional boundaries (such as home, hospital, and school) either accurately or on a timely basis. This despite the vast good intentions of the child health community, the increased but still imperfect technical knowledge of how to provide safer, more effective care, and the good work of demonstration programs and collaborative ventures.

What will it take to get us from here to there? In my opinion, there are two critical steps that are needed. The first is greater specificity to the design of an ideal health care system for children and families, one that contributes to a larger system that better promotes and maintains health. I have articulated the need for a comprehensive child and family health home, a multidisciplinary, team-oriented health program that incorporates the current framing of the medical home and not only extends and reframes its disciplinary base and explicitly incorporates mental health services, but also links it to broader community health monitoring and programming and explicitly includes families and the broader community in setting priorities and driving improvement. Another team of thought leaders convened by Nemours[1] has published an even broader model that places strong emphasis on prevention and calls for integrated planning and financing of health, education, social support, and other child services and shared accountability across these systems. Demonstrations of these and other transformational approaches are needed to inform policymakers of the potential of such new designs to provide better care and better systems that will reap a return on investment through societal gains.

The other necessary step is a set of the social strategies to move this transformational agenda forward. Maintenance of certification, a professionally oriented strategy, should broaden the motivation for pediatricians to engage in improvement and learn some of the core methods. Other strategies are needed to engage other disciplines, promote team-based approaches to care, and promote more transformational changes in health and health care systems. Payment reform is a necessary part of system reform. The current payment systems reward transactions between physicians and patients, rather than either relationships or outcomes; moreover, they value certain types of transactions (those with procedures or using high technology) far greater than transactions involving cognitive and social approaches. Providing incremental incentives for preferred practices within the current fee for service environment may well promote the targeted specific processes in either ambulatory or hospital settings; major system change, however, will require more dramatic restructuring of payment systems. Moving this forward will require a broader coalition involving not only physicians, but consumers and state and federal leaders.

This type of coalition has been fruitful in building a stronger emphasis on quality measurement and improvement into the Child Health Insurance Program Reauthorization Act noted above, now signed into law by President Barack Obama. Leaders in child health policy that represent not only provider groups (hospitals and pediatricians) but also consumers and quality experts took advantage of the need to renew this program by working with Congress to include federal support—for the first time—for the development and use of consistent pediatric quality measures by Medicaid and State Child Health Insurance Program (SCHIP) programs. These measures, linked to demonstration programs focused on care coordination and medical home and significant investment in pediatric health information technology, provide an important foundation in the strategy for more widespread improvement. Other near-term policy actions that could promote this would be the creation of national and state technical assistance centers for children's quality, creation of a national child health improvement corps modeled on the Centers for Disease Control's Epidemiology Intelligence Service to strengthen state capacity for supporting improvement, federal support for the creation of national disease registries for chronic conditions, and funding comparative effectiveness research for children's health care. But the key element is to build a broad coalition that can advocate for such system changes.

Our field has made tremendous advances over the past two decades. We have reduced harm and improved quality in numerous settings. While we continue to refine both measurement and quality improvement technical approaches, we must also define the system changes that will lead to dramatically better outcomes, identify the policies that will promote the adoption of this system, and build the coalitions and seize the opportunities to move these policies into practice.

Charles J. Homer, MD, MPH
Chief Executive Officer
National Initiative for Children's Healthcare Quality
30 Winter Street, 6th Floor
Boston, MA 02108, USA

E-mail address:
chomer@nichq.org

REFERENCE

1. Nemours Health and Prevention Services. Helping parents raise healthy, happy, productive children. In: Lesley B, editor. Big ideas for children: investing in our nation's future. Washington DC: First Focus; 2008. p. 146–58.

Making the Case to Improve Quality and Reduce Costs in Pediatric Health Care

Ramesh C. Sachdeva, MD, PhD, JD, FAAP[a,b,c], Shabnam Jain, MD[d,*]

KEYWORDS

- Quality improvement • Health care costs • Pediatrics
- Value in health care • Legal implications of quality movement

The United States health care system is in the midst of a crisis in terms of both quality and costs. The need to implement quality improvement strategies is critical for several reasons. First, there are unwarranted variations in health care delivery with patients receiving different amounts of health care for the same clinical situation without measurable differences in outcomes.[1] Not only is there variation in health care delivery, but only about half of the time do adults and children receive recommended care.[2,3] This unwarranted variation and underuse of effective care can in large part be improved by physicians, and underscores the professional obligation of physicians and pediatric institutions to ensure that quality improvement strategies are in place. Second, there is a growing amount of concern about patient safety. A recent study found that among 1000 children in 12 independent children's hospitals, 1 in 15 children was exposed to wrong medications, side effects, or drug interactions.[4] Patient safety an integral component of quality, is included as one of the six dimensions of quality proposed by the Institute of Medicine (IOM).[5] Third, the cost of health care in the United States is high and is continuing to escalate. Despite this, there are major gaps in the quality of health care. These gaps are also present in pediatric health care delivery. Finally, there is growing dissatisfaction in health care among patients, providers, and payers. Improving health care quality is the right thing to do for children. It is timely, and pediatricians must take an affirmative role in getting engaged and leading the quality movement.

[a] National Outcomes Center and Children's Hospital of Wisconsin, 9000 W. Wisconsin Avenue, MS-950, Milwaukee, WI 53226, USA
[b] Department of Pediatrics, Medical College of Wisconsin, 8701 Watertown Park Road, Milwaukee, WI 53226, USA
[c] Marquette University Law School, 1103 West Wisconsin Avenue, Milwaukee, WI 53233, USA
[d] Emory University and Children's Healthcare of Atlanta, 1645 Tullie Circle, Atlanta, GA 30322, USA
* Corresponding author.
E-mail address: sjain@emory.edu (S. Jain).

doi:10.1016/j.pcl.2009.05.013
pediatric.theclinics.com

WHAT IS QUALITY?

The IOM has defined quality in health care as "the degree to which health care services for individuals and populations increase the likelihood of desired health outcomes and are consistent with current professional knowledge."[6] Further, the IOM has proposed six dimensions of quality in health care.[5] **Fig. 1** illustrates these six dimensions and how they can be put into operation. While outcomes and patient safety are traditional elements of quality, "nonclinical" attributes, such as efficiency and access, are also elements of quality.

Another important concept in quality is the "structure-process-outcome" model proposed by Donabedian.[7,8] Structure in health care relates to the various organizational aspects for health care delivery in the outpatient and inpatient settings.[8] Electronic health records and registries are examples of the structure aspect of this model.[8] Process relates to physician-patient interaction.[8] An asthma management plan provided to the family is an example of the process aspect.[8] Outcome relates to the final outcome after health care is delivered.[8] Outcome measures can be objective or subjective.[9] In the acute care setting, an objective outcome measure may be survival (eg, infant mortality rate or risk-adjusted survival in intensive care units) or, increasingly, functional status.[9] Subjective outcome measures may include health-related quality-of-life measures and patient-satisfaction indicators.[9]

THE CHANGING APPROACH TO QUALITY

Historically, efforts for improving quality focused on "quality *assurance*" (**Fig. 2**). The goal was to minimize "defects" as measured by audits. Although quality assurance still has a role and can be used to address quality issues, there has been a paradigm shift toward "quality *improvement*." Quality improvement focuses on moving the entire performance curve forward toward a greater level of performance by adopting best practices, instead of simply focusing on low performers.[10] "Quality science," along with electronic health records, can help spread and sustain improvements.

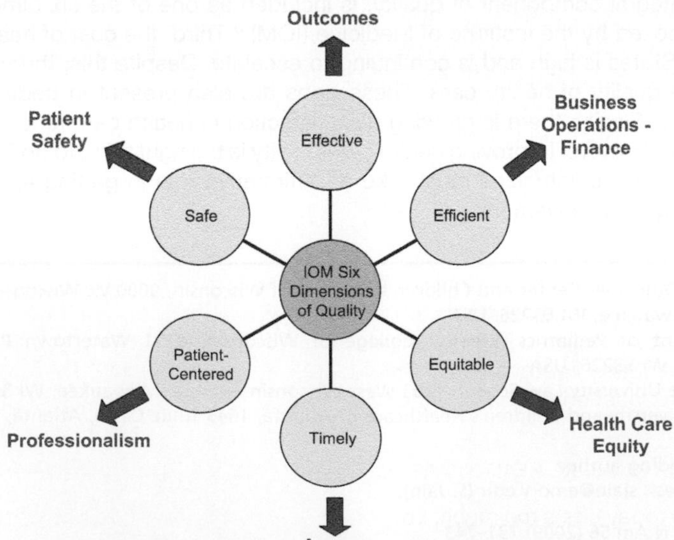

Fig. 1. Putting the six dimensions of quality into operation.

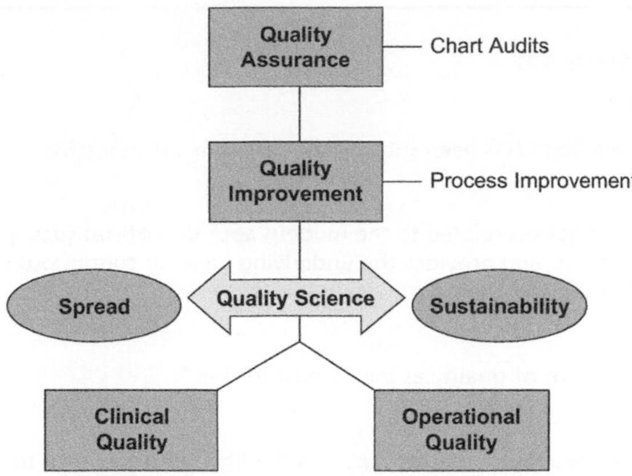

Fig. 2. The changing paradigm of quality.

Finally, quality improvement efforts can have a clinical and operational perspective. Most physicians view improvements in quality as improvements in their clinical practice. Another aspect of quality is "operational quality," which focuses on systems improvement and can result in significant enhancements in efficiencies of health care delivery systems. The concept of operational quality is aligned with IOM's quality dimension of efficiency, and can reduce waste. Methodologies, such as the Toyota Production System, Lean, and Six Sigma, which are frequently used in non–health care settings, have significant potential for improving operational quality in office-based practices and in inpatient hospital settings.[11]

Another aspect of enhancing operational quality relates to the use of management science, which provides a quantitative and scientifically robust approach for planning. Management science, which stems from the field of operations research, has been successfully used in non–health care settings, such as airlines, banking, and the defense sector.[12] Examples of its use in health care include planning for hospital expansion to ensure optimal capacity, planning ambulance services to improve efficiencies, and managing capacity and patient flow in emergency departments and in ambulatory clinic settings.[13–16] Management science has been successfully used in many European health care settings, including those in the United Kingdom, and is gaining popularity in the United States.[17] Improvement methodologies, such as Six Sigma and Lean, focus primarily on improving operational quality of existing systems and tend to be more "reactive" in nature. Management science provides a unique perspective to build better systems and is more "proactive" in nature. It has the potential to minimize processes that lead to creation of waste in health care systems. Ultimately, a multifaceted approach that combines both proactive and reactive methodologies (eg, management science, the Model for Improvement, Six Sigma, and Lean) needs to be tailored for the particular clinical setting to optimize quality improvement. These quality improvement methodologies for application in health care build on the strong foundation of quality principles developed in other industries (**Box 1**).

THE CASE FOR REDUCING HEALTH CARE COSTS

Health care today costs too much, covers too few, and isn't as good as we like to think it is. In recent years, there has been a lot of emphasis on improving health care quality, but little or no success in addressing health care costs. Part of this disconnect stems

Box 1
Quality principles from industry

Deming

Deming's Fourteen Steps has been successfully used in many industries.

Shewhart

Development of principles related to the modern approach of statistical process control, focusing on variations, and provides the underlying basis for continuous quality improvement and the Shewhart Cycle: Plan, Do, Study, Act.

Juran

Focuses on the concept of quality as the "fitness for use."

Crosby

Focuses on the philosophy of the concept that quality is free and aims to achieve "zero defects."

Data from Vonderheide-Liem DN, Pate B. Total quality management. In: Applying quality methodologies to improve healthcare. Marblehead (MA): HCPro, Inc; 2004.

from the unsatisfactory experience with cost containment efforts of managed care in the 1990s. However, the rapid and unrelenting rise in health care costs, whether measured in absolute dollars, as a proportion of the gross domestic product (GDP), or as it relates to wages and inflation, makes it imperative that health care costs be urgently addressed.

Annual health care expenditure for the United States was $2.2 trillion in 2007, with per-capita health care expense at $7421, more than twice that of other industrialized nations. This constituted 16.2% of GDP.[18] The Centers for Medicare and Medicaid Services estimate that health expenditure was $2.4 trillion in 2008. Predictions are that health care spending will reach $4.4 trillion annually by 2018 and constitute a whopping 20% of GDP. Medicare threatens to become insolvent by 2019, and only by decreasing health care costs can this albatross be shaken off. Economists warn that unless we eliminate excess spending in health care and put those dollars to better use, rising health care costs will continue to threaten our long-term fiscal security.

One could justify some or all of the United States spending on health care if the quality of the resulting health care compared favorably to that in other countries. Health indicators show that this is not the case. Despite spending more per capita on health care than any other nation, numerous measures indicate that the country lags in overall health outcomes: It ranks 29th in infant mortality, 48th in life expectancy, and 19th out of 19 industrialized nations in preventable deaths.[19] Even as health care expenditures rise, the number of uninsured (46 million in 2007) and underinsured continues to grow. It is not hard to see that the United States health care system is in crisis and needs urgent fixing. We cannot afford to continue on our present course.

DRIVERS OF HEALTH CARE COSTS

Box 2 summarizes major factors contributing to high health care costs. Advances in medical technology are the number-one factor driving health care costs, chief amongst which are new imaging technologies. Technology accounts for between one and two thirds of the growth in health spending.[20,21] Industry stakeholders agree

Box 2
Factors contributing to high health care costs

- New technologies, especially those related to diagnostic imaging
- Specialty drugs
- Population health status (including increasing rates of obesity)
- Misaligned payment systems
- Emphasis on subspecialty care
- Lack of care coordination
- Insurance administrative costs
- Defensive medical practice (redundant, inappropriate, or unnecessary tests and procedures)

that improved evaluation methods are needed to accurately weigh the risks and benefits of new technologies and procedures to avoid misallocation of health care dollars.[22]

Not lagging far behind, specialty drugs account for $54 billion in drug spending with the annual cost per treated patient ranging from $10,000 to more than a $1 million.[23] By 2010, the United States specialty prescription spending is expected to reach $99 billion, as new specialty products continues to pour into the market. Aside from imaging, specialty drugs are the largest growth sector in health care and it is believed that this trend will continue to increase. New technology and specialty drugs need to be evaluated from an effectiveness standpoint to determine if the investments result in improved quality.

Finally, and most importantly, current incentives in the United States health care system focus health care services on acutely ill patients requiring episodic care, rather than on programs for preventing illness. Across all age groups, the proportion of the population with preventable conditions, such as obesity and chronic illnesses, is increasing. Obesity accounts for about 12% of the growth in health spending,[24,25] while a handful of preventable, chronic illnesses, such as heart disease and diabetes, account for 75% of health care costs. Pediatrics as a specialty emphasizes health maintenance and disease prevention. However, fewer than half of children receive recommended preventive care.[2] Many factors with significant direct impacts on long-term health care costs are under the control of individuals and families, and are determined by their day-to-day choices about diet, exercise, stress management, and tobacco use. There is a growing consensus that successful efforts to stem rising health care costs will necessitate a focus on consumers and their health behaviors as well as emphasis on primary, as opposed to subspecialty, care. This will entail a shift to preventing and managing chronic diseases, so patients will not need as much health care in the future. This calls for a method of macroefficiency or demand management.

MUDA: THE ROLE OF WASTE IN HEALTH CARE

Muda is a Japanese term for waste. The IOM describes waste as activities, or resources, that do not benefit patients. Waste can also be defined as costs that could have been avoided without diminishing quality. Health economists agree that at least one third of the country's spending on health care is unnecessary (see **Box 2**).[26] Some examples of *muda* include the cost of recovering from preventable events; simple inefficiency; and unnecessary diagnostics, therapeutics, and interventions with minimal added value (eg, aggressively marketed blockbuster drugs that are often no more effective or safer than existing treatments, but are certainly more expensive).

Factors that contribute to this waste and overuse include misaligned provider reimbursement systems and liability issues. Contrary to popular belief, while defensive practice does lead to some amount of unnecessary testing and treatments, medical malpractice is not a major driver of spending trends (see **Box 2**).[27] Research on the effect of defensive medicine on spending is challenging because liability risk pushes physicians in the same direction as fee-for-service payment incentives (ie, toward providing more services). Liability coverage premiums contribute to health spending, but they are not a large factor, nor are they a significant factor in the overall growth of health care spending.[28]

A major reason for the prevailing climate of waste and overuse is the current fee-for-service payment system, which encourages volume-driven, rather than value-driven, health care. Under current payment systems, physicians, hospitals, and other health care providers have strong financial incentives to deliver more services to more people with notable absence of incentives for providing better services and improving health. There is also an imbalance in payment systems such that the provision of specialty care is rewarded more than primary and preventive care (see **Box 2**). Reducing unwarranted resource use and thereby reducing costs requires changing the way we pay for care, so as to reward hospitals and physicians for providing high-quality, high-value care and for prudent stewardship of resources.

THE LINK BETWEEN QUALITY AND COST

Contrary to traditional thinking that "quality" means "sparing no expense," pursuit of high quality can lead to substantially reduced costs. This is just as true for health care as it is for other industries. Recent research has demarcated two major areas—quality waste and inefficiency—in which high health care quality can lead to substantially lower costs.[29] Estimates suggest that health care quality waste and inefficiency waste (recovering from preventable events, unnecessary diagnostics and therapeutics, and simple inefficiency) may account for more than 50% of all American health care expenditures.[30]

A recent study by the Commonwealth Fund on health system performance ranked the 50 states in the United States by potentially avoidable hospital admissions (as the quality metric) and Medicare reimbursements (as the cost metric).[31] The study found that as quality goes up, cost goes down (**Fig. 3**).[31] Poor quality care is a major contributor to runaway health care costs. The pursuit of high quality in health care can lead to substantially lower health care costs; improving quality is a key part of making health care affordable. Efforts to rein in health care costs cannot be made in isolation; rather, they have to be made in the context of solving the broader problems of the health care system, including improving quality and access.

NATIONAL DRIVERS FOR QUALITY IMPROVEMENT

Three major national drivers are serving as catalysts for the quality movement. These will significantly affect pediatricians and their practices. The first is the Maintenance of Certification (MOC) requirements being adopted by the American Board of Pediatrics for implementation in 2010.[10,32] This is part of a larger process adopted by the American Board of Medical Specialty Boards.[33] Under these new requirements, all pediatricians and pediatric subspecialists with time-based certificates must demonstrate an understanding of quality improvement principles and how to apply such principles.[10,32] The second major driver is the changing reimbursement landscape favoring pay-for-performance (P4P), which significantly affects physician and hospital revenues. P4P relates to the concept of linking certain amounts of reimbursement for

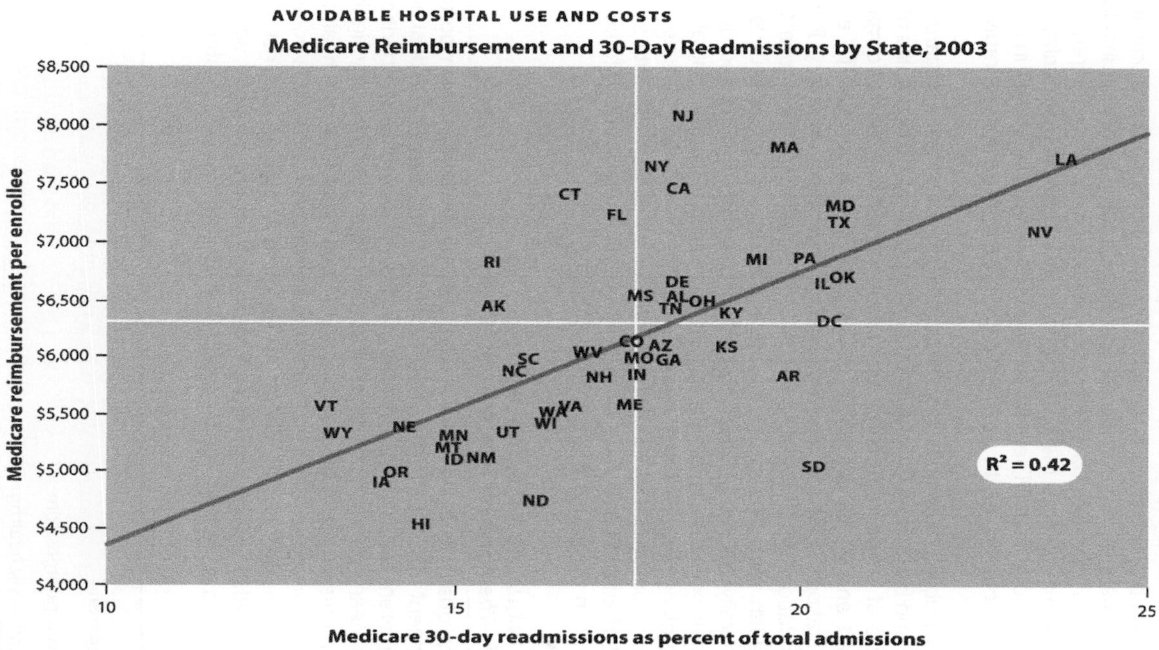

DATA: Medicare reimbursement – 2003 Dartmouth Atlas of Health Care; Medicare readmissions – 2003 Medicare SAF 5% Inpatient Data

Fig. 3. Correlation between quality and cost based on 2003 Medicare data. Quality is shown as Medicare 30-day readmissions as percent of total admissions (avoidable hospital use). Cost is shown as Medicare reimbursement per enrollee. (*From* Commonwealth Fund State Scorecard on Health System Performance, 2007; with permission.)

physicians and hospitals to quality metrics.[34] P4P has already been implemented in Medicare in the adult clinical setting and is gradually permeating the pediatric arena. Although the long-term impact of P4P strategies remains controversial, its spread to Medicaid and other private insurers will affect reimbursement for pediatricians and pediatric health care facilities. The new policy adopted in 2008 by the Centers for Medicare and Medicaid Services (CMS) for nonpayment of "Never Events" further underscores the impact of P4P-related strategies.[35] Hospitals cannot seek reimbursement from CMS for patient care that is delivered related to any condition included in the list of Never Events (eg, serious preventable events, hospital-acquired injuries and infections). The third driver is the movement for transparency of quality, which will likely affect consumer choice. The transparency movement will result in patients, families, and payers choosing health care options that promise demonstrably better quality.[36]

Currently, several publicly available Web sites provide information regarding the quality of physician and hospital services. **Box 3** summarizes some examples of these Web sites. The value of online information sources is limited because information is not always validated and is not presented in a standardized manner. To address this concern, the National Quality Forum created a Technical Advisory Panel to develop recommendations for the public reporting of quality.[37] The move toward transparency in health care has governmental support: A 2006 executive order requires that all federally insured programs have transparency in price and quality.[38] This national direction poses some unique challenges in the pediatric clinical setting by, for example, making apparent the need to develop valid and reliable quality measures that can be easily tracked in general pediatric and subspecialty settings. The push toward P4P and transparency further underscores the urgency to establish meaningful measures in pediatrics to achieve quality goals.

FUTURE DIRECTIONS IN QUALITY IMPROVEMENT

Comparing Quality—The Need for Risk Adjustment

When evaluating the quality of health care by comparing outcomes, it is important to understand the concept of risk adjustment. Risk adjustment allows statistical adjustment of patient differences, such as severity of illness, to make comparisons of outcomes clinically meaningful.[39] This enables the translation of statistically significant tests into clinically meaningful results. Risk adjustment methods for health care outcomes are better developed in the inpatient and acute care settings as compared with the outpatient ambulatory care setting. An example of an inpatient risk adjustment system is the PRISM (Pediatric Risk of Mortality) scoring system, which has been successfully used to adjust for differences in outcomes in pediatric critical

Box 3
Examples of public reporting

- RateMD: http://www.ratemds.com
- Healthgrades: http://www.healthgrades.com/consumer
- DrScore: http://www.drscore.com
- The Joint Commission Quality Check: http://www.qualitycheck.org
- CMS hospital compare: http://www.hospitalcompare.hhs.gov
- WebMD quality services: http://www.selectqualitycare.com

care units.[40,41] Although an initial evaluation of the outcomes from these units showed that the survival from large tertiary care units was worse than that for smaller non-tertiary care units, after performing severity risk adjustment, these differences disappeared and allowed more accurate and meaningful comparisons of outcomes.[41] The science of severity risk adjustment is undergoing rapid growth with the development of new methods for risk adjustment. Although not as robust as the physiologic risk adjustment methods, such as that of the PRISM system, APR-DRGs (All Patient Refined Diagnosis Related Groups) have also been frequently used for purposes of risk stratification when comparing outcomes within patient groups in many settings.[42] Recently, Sachdeva and colleagues[43] proposed the need for the next generation of diagnosis-based physiologic risk adjustment approaches to compare outcomes. As newer risk methods are refined, it will become increasingly possible to risk adjust and compare the quality and outcomes of health care in many settings.

The Value Proposition

Many people feel that a big problem in health care is the disconnect between "what we pay for" and "what we get." A helpful concept to understand this is *value*, which is measured as quality per unit of cost (**Fig. 4**). Value can be defined as the quality (sum of outcomes, safety, and service) achieved for the resources committed and costs incurred. High-value clinical care results from the most efficient expenditure of resources to achieve an established high level of clinical quality.

In health care, improving quality is essential but not enough; cost has to be addressed simultaneously. According to the Agency for Healthcare Research and Quality 2007 National Healthcare Quality and Disparity Report, health care quality is improving modestly, but health care spending is rising much faster, underscoring the urgency to improve the value Americans are getting for their health care dollars. In other words, the quality agenda has to put the cost of health care in the same equation to get the most benefit. A value-based national health care movement is taking shape and gaining momentum, and may be one of the cornerstones of reimbursement in the future.[44] This approach will also be relevant to the evolving concept of comparative effectiveness research, which is aimed at achieving the highest quality and greatest value from health care spending.

Whose Responsibility is Quality?

As the United States attempts to revamp health care quality, a fundamental question that arises is: Who should hold that responsibility? As discussed by Wharam and Sulmasy,[45] quality is the responsibility of several stakeholders. Historically, quality has been defined from the perspective of administrators and, more recently, clinicians. It becomes important to further expand the definition of quality to incorporate the perspective of families. Sachdeva and colleagues[46] have shown that families can successfully define quality measures using the six dimensions proposed by the IOM

$$Value = \frac{Quality}{Cost}$$

$$\text{Quality} = \text{Outcomes} + \text{Safety} + \text{Service}$$

$$\text{Service} = \text{Satisfaction} + \text{Access}$$

Fig. 4. Value equation in health care.

in both ambulatory pediatrics and inpatient subspecialty settings. As future quality measures are developed, it may be prudent to involve families to provide a unique insight and enrich the scope of the measures.

Expanding Quality Measurement from a Systems Level to the Level of Individual Physicians

Most quality strategies focus on systems improvement. More recently, new policies being implemented by The Joint Commission require that quality be measured at the level of individual practitioners through such tools as the Ongoing Professional Practice Evaluation (OPPE) and Focused Professional Practice Evaluation (FPPE).[47] These policies will affect all physicians who have medical staff privileges in hospitals. The implementation of OPPE and FPPE, currently underway, provides an opportunity for physicians in leadership roles to ensure that this process is developed in a meaningful and effective manner.

The Unintended Legal Implications of the Quality Movement

The movement toward transparency of health care quality may have significant legal implications. No one yet fully knows how data easily gleaned from electronic health records, such provider performance and quality measures, will affect issues related to medical malpractice. The impact will likely vary among states because of differences in state laws.[48] However, quality and related outcomes information cannot be hidden. This is illustrated in the prominent case of Bristol Children's Hospital in the United Kingdom.[49] The class action litigation that emerged from the failure to share outcomes information regarding cardiac surgery has served as the catalyst for a significant movement toward transparency of cardiac outcomes in the United Kingdom. Furthermore, the case illustrates that outcomes information cannot and should not be hidden, and that transparency is the right policy to improve the care for children.

Availability of quality and outcomes information may even create a duty for physicians to include such information when obtaining informed consent. In the case of *Johnson v Kokemoor* decided by the Supreme Court of Wisconsin,[50] a surgeon was held liable for failure to obtain informed consent after neglecting to share with the patient available comparative outcomes information related to the surgical procedure. This highlights the importance of transparency and the potential legal liability that may be created by not sharing quality data with patients. There is a unique interaction between health care and law. It will be important to follow how the law evolves with the changing direction in health care quality, and also how the health care quality national agenda influences new laws.

Shared Savings Model

As quality improves, costs go down for patients, purchasers, and payers. How would providers fare in this new era of reduced health care expenditures? While P4P initiatives reward improvements in quality, current reimbursement systems do not necessarily reward behavior that reduces the cost of health care services. The shared savings model is a novel concept based on sharing the savings generated from efforts aimed at improving quality and reducing costs. Some places, such as California, are beginning to experiment with this approach. However, its application at a broad level will require major payment system reform to better align financial incentives.

SUMMARY

Our current mix of suboptimal quality, escalating costs, and eroding coverage reflects a health care system in chaos and underscores the urgent need for quality improvement efforts. Quality can be defined and encompasses the concept of operational quality, which is more than the traditional concept of clinical quality. Unsustainable increases in health care costs make it imperative that we understand the drivers of cost, including a significant component of waste. Quality and cost are linked, and it is important to include both in the equation to maximize the value obtained from health care expenditures.

The field of quality improvement, which continues to experience a paradigm shift, needs to be led and executed by physicians. Changing national drivers, including maintenance of certification requirements, P4P policies, and the transparency movement, will accelerate the adoption of quality improvement initiatives. Quality improvement and measurement is not perfect, and may have unintended consequences, including legal implications. However, embracing quality improvement and reducing health care costs is the right thing to do, so that we can make a real difference in our care of children.

ACKNOWLEDGMENTS

The authors would like to thank Lisa Ciesielczyk for her assistance in the preparation of this manuscript.

REFERENCES

1. Wennberg JE. Understanding geographic variations in health care delivery. N Engl J Med 1999;340(1):52–3.
2. Mangione-Smith R, DeCristofaro AH, Setodji CM, et al. The quality of ambulatory care delivered to children in the United States. N Engl J Med 2007;357(15):1515–23.
3. McGlynn EA, Asch SM, Adams J, et al. The quality of health care delivered to adults in the United States. N Engl J Med 2003;348(26):2635–45.
4. Takata GS, Mason W, Taketomo C, et al. Development, testing, and findings of a pediatric-focused trigger tool to identify medication-related harm in US children's hospitals. Pediatrics 2008;121:e927–35.
5. Institute of Medicine, Committee on Quality Health Care in America. Crossing the quality chasm: a new health system for the 21st century. Washington, DC: National Academies Press; 2001.
6. Institute of Medicine, Committee to Design a Strategy for Quality Review and Assurance in Medicare. In: Lohr KN, editor, Medicare: a strategy for quality assurance, Volume 1. Washington, DC: National Academies Press; 1990.
7. Donabedian A. Evaluating the quality of medical care. Milbank Mem Fund Q 1966;44(Suppl 3):166–206.
8. Steering Committee on Quality Improvement and Management and Committee on Practice and Ambulatory Medicine. Principles for the development and use of quality measures. Pediatrics 2008;121(2):411–6.
9. Sachdeva RC. Functional outcomes in pediatric models. Curr Opin Crit Care 1997;3(3):179–82.
10. Miles P. Health information systems and physician quality: role of the American Board of Pediatrics maintenance of certification in improving children's health care. Pediatrics 2009;123:S108–10.
11. Spear SJ. Fixing health care from the inside, today. Harv Bus Rev 2005;83:78–91.

12. Sachdeva RC. Mixing operational research methodologies to achieve organizational change: a study of the pediatric intensive care unit. Thesis for Doctorate in Business Administration (DBA), University of Strathclyde, UK, 2005.
13. Ashton R, Hague L, Brandreth M, et al. A simulation-based study of a NHS walk-in center. J Oper Res Soc 2005;56:153–61.
14. Boldy DP, O'Kane PC. Health operational research—a selective overview. Eur J Oper Res 1982;10:1–9.
15. Lehaney B, Paul RJ. The use of soft systems methodology in the development of a simulation of out-patient services at Watford General Hospital. J Oper Res Soc 1996;47(7):864–70.
16. Van der Meer RB, Rymaszewski LA, Findlay H, et al. Using OR to support the development of an integrated musculo-skeletal service. J Oper Res Soc 2005;56:162–72.
17. Sachdeva R, Williams T, Quigley J. Mixing methodologies to enhance the implementation of healthcare operational research. J Oper Res Soc 2007;58:159–67.
18. Hartman M, Martin A, McDonnell P, et al. National Health Expenditure Accounts Team. National health spending in 2007: slower drug spending contributes to lowest rate of overall growth since 1998. Health Aff (Millwood) 2009;28(1):246–61.
19. World health statistics, 2003. Geneva, Switzerland: World Health Organization; 2005.
20. Peden EA, Freeland MS. A historical analysis of medical spending growth, 1960–1993. Health Aff 1995;14(2):235–47.
21. Cutler DM. Technology, health costs, and the NIH. Paper prepared for the National Institute of Health Economics Roundtable on Biomedical Research. September 1995.
22. Redberg RF. Evidence, appropriateness, and technology assessment in cardiology: a case study of computed tomography. Health Aff (Millwood) 2007; 26(1):86–95.
23. Express scripts 2006 drug trends report. Available at: http://www.expressscripts.com/industryresearch/industryreports/drugtrendreport/2006/forecast.pdf. Accessed February 11, 2009.
24. Thorpe KE, Florence CS, Howard DH, et al. Trends: the impact of obesity on rising medical spending. Web Exclusive, October 20. Health Aff 2004.
25. Congressional Budget Office. Technological change and the growth of health care spending (No. 2764). Washington, DC: Congressional Budget Office; 2008.
26. The PricewaterhouseCooper Health Research Institute 2008: The price of excess—identifying waste in healthcare spending. Available at: https://www.pwc.com/nz/healthcare/HC_PriceOfExcess_May09.pdf. Accessed July 16, 2009.
27. Ginsburg P. High and rising health care costs: demystifying U.S. health care spending. Princeton, NJ: Robert Wood Johnson Foundation Research Synthesis Report; 2008.
28. Sloan FA, Chepke LM. Medical malpractice. Cambridge (MA): Massachusetts Institute of Technology; 2008.
29. James BC, Quality management for health care delivery. 2005 HRET Trust Award; 2005.
30. James B, Bayley KB. Cost of poor quality or waste in integrated delivery system settings. Rockville, MD: Agency for Healthcare Research and Quality; 2006.
31. Cantor JC, Schoen C, Belloff D, et al. Aiming higher: results from a state scorecard on health system performance. The Commonwealth Fund Commission on a High Performance Health System 2007. Available at: http://www.commonwealthfund.org/Content/Publications/Fund-Reports/2007/Jun/Aiming-Higher–Results-from-a-State-Scorecard-on-Health-System-Performance.aspx. Accessed July 16, 2009.

32. Available at: www.abp.org. (Last Accessed February 10, 2009).
33. Horowitz SD, Miller SH, Miles PV. Board certification and physician quality. Med Educ 2004;38(1):10–1.
34. Pay for performance improving health care quality and changing provider behavior; but challenges persist. Available at: http://www.rwjf.org/newsroom/newsreleasesdetail.jsp?productid=21847. (Last Accessed February 10, 2009).
35. Centers for Medicare and Medicaid Services. Press Release: Eliminating serious, preventable, and costly medical errors—Never Events. Available at: http://www.cms.hhs.gov/apps/media/press/release.asp?Counter=1863; May 18, 2006. (Last Accessed February 10, 2009).
36. Patients' hospital ratings hit the Web: Federal agency's ads aim for more users. Milwaukee Journal Sentinel, May 21, 2008.
37. Guidelines for consumer-focused public reporting. Available at: http://www.qualityindicators.ahrq.gov/downloads/usermeeting2008/Cronin_Consumer%20focused%20public%20reporting.ppt. September 2008. (Last Accessed February 10, 2009).
38. Kent C. White House orders health information standards as states move ahead. National Conference of State Legislatures. Available at: http://www.ncsl.org/programs/health/shn/2006/news474a.htm. (Last Accessed February 10, 2009).
39. Sachdeva RC, Jefferson LS, Coss-Bu J, et al. Effects of availability of patient-related charges on practice patterns and cost containment in the pediatric intensive care unit. Crit Care Med 1996;24(3):501–6.
40. Pollack MM, Ruttimann UE, Getson PR. Pediatric risk of mortality (PRISM) score. Crit Care Med 1988;16:1110–6.
41. Pollack MM, Alexander SR, Clarke N, et al. Improved outcomes from tertiary center, pediatric intensive care: a statewide comparison of tertiary and non-tertiary care facilities. Crit Care Med 1991;19:150–9.
42. Sachdeva R, Pedretti J. Enabling informed choice through quality and outcomes communications. NACHRI Annual Meeting, October 2007, San Antonio, TX.
43. Sachdeva RC, Kuhn EM, Gall CM, et al. A need for development of diagnosis-specific severity of illness tools for risk adjustment. Crit Care Med 2008;36(12): A83 (Suppl).
44. Value-driven health care. Available at: http://www.hhs.gov/valuedriven/index.html. (Last Accessed February 11, 2009).
45. Wharam JF, Sulmasy D. Improving the quality of health care: Who is responsible for what? JAMA 2009;301(2):215–7.
46. Sachdeva RC, Lenzner SM, Christensen CS, et al. Has including families in quality really made a difference? NACHRI Annual Meeting, October 2008, Salt Lake City, UT.
47. Medical staff update from the president of the medical staff at Stanford Hospital and Clinics. Available at: http://med.stanford.edu/shs/update/archives/FEB2007/president.htm. (Last Accessed February 10, 2009).
48. Sachdeva RC. Electronic healthcare data collection and pay-for-performance: translating theory into practice. Ann Health Law 2007;16(2):291–311.
49. The Bristol Royal Infirmary Inquiry. Learning from Bristol: the report of the public inquiry into children's heart surgery at the Bristol Royal Infirmary 1984–1995. Bristol Royal Infirmary Inquiry; july 2001. (CM 5207.) Available at: www.bristol-inquiry.org.uk. (Last Accessed February 10, 2009)
50. Johnson v. Kokemoor, 199 Wis. 2d 615 1996. Discussing the application of sharing outcomes data as a requirement for obtaining informed consent in health care.

Unwarranted Variation in Pediatric Medical Care

David C. Goodman, MD, MS[a,b,c,*]

KEYWORDS

- Small area analysis • Physician practice patterns • Quality
- Workforce • Child • Infant

The findings from studies of unwarranted variation in medical care rival the decoding of the human genome in the potential for improving patients' health and well-being. Small area analysis has revealed myriad ills in our health care system and at the same time has led the way in improvement efforts and reform. Although child health researchers in the United States were relatively slow in initiating analysis of medical care variation, there has been notable progress in the past 15 years, and some research has surpassed that of adult health care. In other areas, the study of pediatric variation substantially lags, suffering from an absence of conceptual frameworks and from incomplete data about pediatric health care resources and delivery. This deficiency has impeded the child health care community from fully engaging in the current national debates about health care system reform.

This article provides a survey on the concepts, methods, and applications of the study of unwarranted variation in health care with particular attention to children's medical services. Unwarranted variation is the variation in medical care due to differences in health system performance. Originally, analyses examining unwarranted variation were termed *small area analysis* in reference to their examination of variation of health care resources (eg, hospital beds, physicians) and utilization across empirically defined health care service areas. With improvements in data quality, recent efforts have been directed toward the measurement of variation across providers such as hospitals and clinicians. Regardless of the units that define the population or patient

This article was supported, in part, by the Robert Wood Johnson Foundation and the National Institute on Aging (P01 AG019783).

[a] The Dartmouth Institute for Health Policy and Clinical Practice, 35 Centerra Parkway, Suite 202, Lebanon, NH 03766, USA

[b] The Children's Hospital at Dartmouth, Dartmouth-Hitchcock Medical Center, Lebanon, NH 03756, USA

[c] Dartmouth Medical School, Hanover, NH, USA

* The Dartmouth Institute for Health Policy and Clinical Practice, 35 Centerra Parkway, Suite 202, Lebanon, NH 03766.

E-mail address: david.goodman@dartmouth.edu

Pediatr Clin N Am 56 (2009) 745–755
doi:10.1016/j.pcl.2009.05.007 pediatric.theclinics.com

denominators, the study of health care variation faces similar challenges in methods and interpretation.

ORIGINS OF SMALL AREA ANALYSIS

Tonsillectomies in England and Wales from 1908 to 1938

Although the connection of place with health is an ancient concept, the idea that medical practice might also vary across locales, haphazardly and without apparent reason, was initially recognized in England in the first half of the twentieth century. In response to growing concerns about the "physical deterioration" of the public, Parliament included a clause in the 1907 Education Bill which provided for the universal medical inspection of children at entry to schools and periodically thereafter. Parliament initially deferred funding treatment, a policy reflecting worries about the costs, but included the vague language, "... the power to make such arrangements as may be sanctioned by the Board of Education for attending to the health and physical condition of children educated in Public Elementary Schools."[1] For advocates of publicly funded treatment, this was a clever compromise. As the full picture of the ill health of school-aged children developed, the provision of pediatric medical services inevitably followed.

In the 1920 annual report of Chief Medical Officer of the Board of Education, the most common "defects" identified were dental disease, nose and throat disease, defective vision, uncleanliness, and malnutrition. About 4% of children were diagnosed with "adenoids and enlarged tonsils," a figure that rose to 6% by 1931.[2,3] Treatment did indeed follow diagnosis. In 1923, the majority of local education authorities provided adenoid/tonsillectomies either through their own clinics or at local hospitals. The surge in diagnosis and surgical treatment was a surprise to the Chief Medical Officer and led to the establishment of the Committee on Enlarged Tonsils and Adenoids in 1924.[4] The Committee issued cautions against the indiscriminate use of tonsillectomies and worked to improve surgical safety; however, no consensus could be reached on the function of the tonsils, the definition of tonsillar disease, or the indications for the procedure. In the absence of professional consensus within the Board of Education or the larger medical community, the total number of procedures grew to 84,000 by 1931, representing three quarters of the total procedures in English and Welsh school-aged children.[3]

Although no one knew what to do with the information, the Board of Education medical staff conducted exquisite epidemiologic analyses of the tonsillectomy epidemic that reached their full maturation in 1938 with the publication of "The Incidence of Tonsillectomy in School Children" in the *Proceedings of the Royal Society of Medicine* by J.A. Glover.[5] This article was the first extant academic report using the study design we now call small area analysis and was nearly the only publication for 35 years.

Dr. Glover's article is essential reading for all students interested in unwarranted variation of pediatric medical care. He documents the remarkable rise of the use of operative treatment for enlarged tonsils in epidemiologic terms, calling it an "epidemic," and notes the over tenfold variation in rates across local educational authorities. He also identified an intriguing difference in procedure rates between two communities with prominent medical schools, noting that the 1936 annual incidence in children aged 5 to 14 years was 0.3% in Cambridge and 3.1% in Oxford. In a prescience and forthright discussion, he argued that "A study of the geographic distribution in elementary school children discloses no correlation between...any other factor, such as overcrowding, poverty, bad housing, or climate. In fact it defies any explanation, save that of variation of medical opinion on the indications for operation."[5]

The convergence of circumstances and ideas that led to these novel and provocative studies of pediatric tonsillectomies reveals a great deal about the methods and usefulness of small area analysis. First, the identification of unwarranted variation requires good population-based data. Education funding in England, including for the School Medical Service, was highly centralized, with money flowing from and data flowing to London. In an era when the tools of data tabulation were ledger books and pencils, the School Medical Service kept meticulous records that were hand tabulated into tables and figures that rival any of today. These records about the numbers of children, "defects," and treatments could have been doomed to obscurity except for the second important condition—the close alignment of the Department of Health with its epidemiologists and the School Medical Service. Indeed, for many years they were both directed by Dr. George Newman, a renowned leader in British public health. The application of epidemiologic methods led to precise denominator and event definitions, stratification by student characteristics, and, ultimately, to calculation of incidence rates by place. For the first time, the methods used to measure and characterize diphtheria and rheumatic fever were applied to the study of medical care.

By using local educational authorities as units of analysis, Drs. Newman and Glover attributed tonsillectomy rates to the medical staff responsible for the delivery of tonsillectomies. The use of other political boundaries might have been easier but would have smoothed the variation and obscured the connection between procedure rates and the local medical staff.

John Wennberg and Medical Care in Vermont, Circa 1970

After Glover's 1938 article, few publications described regional variation in medical care,[6,7] and none were about children until John Wennberg and Alan Gittelsohn published their seminal report "Small Area Variation in Health Care Delivery" in the journal *Science* in 1973.[8] Using population-based hospitalization data, Wennberg assigned Vermont towns to hospital service areas based on the patterns of travel for inpatient care. The geography of Vermont was particularly favorable to small area analysis, with scattered population centers that were principally reliant on a single hospital and its associated medical staff. The population of each hospital service area was linked to an identifiable supply of hospital beds and physicians. Despite the relatively homogenous population, the per capita number of hospital beds, hospital personnel, and physicians varied over 50% across hospital service areas. Hospital discharge rates for medical and surgical conditions varied more than twofold, and tonsillectomy rates varied more than tenfold. Wennberg could find little relation between greater utilization rates and need, such as would be indicated by higher mortality rates. Costs were higher in the areas with higher capacity (beds, physicians) and utilization.

Given today's recognition of the irrationalities in health care delivery, it may be difficult to appreciate that in the 1970s these findings were initially ignored, later attacked[9] before being replicated,[10,11] and then widely embraced by clinicians, health system administrators, and policy makers. The most common criticism of small area analysis was that the variation in capacity and utilization was expected and reflected needed treatment for sicker populations.[12–14] Some attributed the variation to chance and imprecision in the rates, leading to the publication of several reports on statistical inference in measuring variation.[15,16] Other cited causes were patient preferences for more care or differences in malpractice environments.[17]

A notable testament to the seminal character of Wennberg's article in *Science* is its citation by over 750 other academic reports.[18] Subsequent studies by Dr. Wennberg and his Dartmouth colleagues examined a large number of different types of medical care and populations. In addition to studies across regions, access to Medicare claims permitted examination of variation in the care of the elderly across specific hospitals. Cohort study designs were used in addition to cross-sectional designs, and ecologic studies were supplanted by increasingly sophisticated hierarchical models with the patient as the unit of analysis.[19] With funding from the Robert Wood Johnson Foundation, Wennberg, Fisher, and colleagues[20] developed the *Dartmouth Atlas of Health Care* series as a dissemination tool directed toward nonacademic audiences such as health care administrators, health policy makers, and congressional staffers. In the past 35 years these and other studies of unwarranted variation have had an unparalleled influence on the practice of medicine, the organization of delivery systems, the financing of medical care, and federal health care policy.[21]

PIONEER STUDIES IN UNWARRANTED VARIATION IN PEDIATRIC MEDICAL CARE

Studies of variation in children's health care took root as a distinct field of study in the 1980s. Although Wennberg studied pediatric hospitalizations in Vermont and Maine,[22,23] these analyses were primarily an outgrowth of adult medical care research. In 1982, Connell and colleagues[24] conducted a specific study of hospitalization rates in Medicaid children across small areas in Washington State and noted 18-fold differences in gastroenteritis and 15-fold differences in lower respiratory infections. Wissow and colleagues[25] also observed tenfold differences in asthma hospitalizations across small areas in Maryland. In 1989, Perrin and colleagues reported that Boston children were more than twice as likely (relative risk, 2.65; 95% CI, 2.53–2.78) to be hospitalized for medical conditions when compared with children residing in Rochester, New York. The relative risk for children in New Haven, Connecticut was 1.80 (95% CI, 1.68–1.93). This pattern persisted in specific diagnosis-related groups, including bronchitis and asthma, fractures and sprains, and gastroenteritis. For conditions in which the diagnosis was certain and hospitalization requisite, little variation was observed. The relative risk between Boston and Rochester for femur fractures was 1.0 (95% CI, 0.7–1.4), for appendectomy 1.1 (95% CI, 0.9–1.4), and for bacterial meningitis 1.3 (95% CI, 0.8–1.9). A lower degree of variation was noted for surgical hospitalizations. These three studies stimulated several studies of pediatric medical care using similar methods.

METHODOLOGICAL CONSIDERATIONS

Because analyses of variation are now associated with a diverse set of research questions including racial and socioeconomic disparities, it is helpful to discuss the methods needed to measure health system performance. Studies of unwarranted variation require methods that link either locations or providers of care with populations through data with a high degree of locational specificity. For studying common causes of hospitalization and physician care, the minimal location information are data with the zip codes of populations and providers. As important as counties and states might be for examining public policy driven variation, these geopolitical units are usually too large or are geographically discordant with health markets.[26] Zip code referenced utilization data permit classic small area analysis in which the records are used to define geographic representations of health care markets, such as hospital service areas[27,28] or primary care service areas.[29] These areas are then used in calculating population-based utilization rates. Counties can be appropriate for developing health markets for care that is highly regionalized, such as in defining neonatal intensive care regions.[30]

Unfortunately, this research has been slowed by a scarcity of population-based utilization data. For example, the bare minimum data elements necessary for small area analysis of hospitalization rates are patient zip code, provider zip code, patient characteristics (eg, age, sex, race/ethnicity), diagnoses, and procedures. To date, no national data set with these fields is available to pediatric researchers. The Health Care Cost and Utilization Project (HCUP) Kids' Inpatient Database is a national sample of hospitalizations and does not provide the geographic information necessary to conduct small area analysis.[31] Some states offer discharge records through HCUP with the necessary zip code information,[31] although prohibitions against directly or indirectly identifying providers limit the analyses to analyzing overall variation phenomena, removing one of the most basic reasons for studying unwarranted variation, that is, to provide public accountability through open description of specific health system performance.

Medicare data, in comparison, provide (for non-HMO–enrolled beneficiaries) information about 100% of beneficiary hospitalizations and, for a 20% sample of beneficiaries, all physician and other provider claims. These claims are linkable to other utilization of a patient irrespective of Medicare data file or year and to a denominator file with beneficiary characteristics including date of death. Institutional providers' (eg, hospitals, ambulatory surgical centers) names and associated data are releasable to the public. The Centers for Medicare and Medicaid require that tabulations with less than 11 events for a patient or a clinician are suppressed, and neither patients nor clinicians can be publicly identified. The Medicare data sets allow for national analyses using cross-sectional and cohort study designs and hospital-specific analyses with public release of hospital rates.[20,32]

Because pediatric studies have been shaped by data availability, most of the early research used hospitalization data to study variation in discharge rates, with more recent efforts reliant on registry data of participating practices or care units. Although the quality of the research conducted has generally been excellent, the research questions are severely limited in scope when compared with studies in adults and are usually reported without identification of pediatric facility names.

INTERPRETING VARIATION IN PEDIATRIC MEDICAL CARE

An expanded definition of unwarranted variation is that it is the variation in medical resources, utilization, and outcome that is due to differences in health system performance. Not all variation is unwarranted. Dozens of alternative reasons might explain why medical care utilization rates are different across places or providers. Even if the underlying probabilities of a health care event are the same, rates may have large standard errors, suggesting the variation is a chance phenomenon. More importantly, population characteristics differ, such as in median age. Differences may also occur in underlying health risk as reflected in obesity or infant mortality rates. Areas with children having higher health risks as measured directly or through surrogate metrics such as zip code median household income are expected to have higher physician and hospital utilization and to have more physicians and hospital beds to provide that care.

Child clinicians and researchers are particularly attuned to the socioeconomic determinants of children's health and health care. Although health status contributes to differences in pediatric hospitalization rates, it is not the sole or even the primary cause.[27,33–37] In fact, in the evaluation of health system performance, these population differences are not of primary interest and are considered cofounders. "Unwarranted" refers to the portion of the variation that is explained not by population difference but by the quality, appropriateness, and efficiency of health care. In small area analysis, health status is controlled through study design or statistical models.

Over the past two decades, the most unifying classification of medical care variation has been developed by Wennberg and colleagues. Variation of utilization is parsed into three parts—effective, preference-sensitive, and supply-sensitive care. Variation in health care capacity, such as hospital beds and physicians, is a fourth nonutilization category.

Variation in Effective Care

Variation in effective care reflects differences in technical quality. Usually, the "right" rate is known for a given population. Immunization rates are the obvious pediatric example. Deviation from near 100% reflects less than ideal health system performance. Pediatrics has been actively involved in developing effectiveness data and is a leader in promoting system change and improvement to achieve the right rate.

Although the absence of population-based data that are comparable to Medicare claims has limited some variation research, pediatric health service researchers have excelled in developing patient registries through practice networks. For example, the Vermont-Oxford Network collects primary data on infants with birth weights ranging from 401 to 1500 g cared for in 750 member neonatal intensive care units, representing about two thirds of all very low birth weight infants in the United States.[38] Data on processes of care and outcomes are tabulated and reported back to individual units for use in quality improvement efforts.[39] There are some disadvantages to this approach. The rates are not population based in the epidemiologic or small area analysis sense of reporting the experience of an entire population, and they cannot be used to study predictors of admission to a neonatal intensive care unit. Similar to most other practice-based registries, the unit data are not publicly available, and each unit's data are also blinded to other units. The advantage of this strategy is that units do not have to worry about the consequences of public reporting. Perhaps as a result, the Vermont-Oxford Network has a high level of unit participation and high quality data.

The Cystic Fibrosis Foundation's Patient Registry was developed along similar lines, but all cystic fibrosis centers in the foundation are required to participate. Although the registry also reports data about care processes and outcomes to each center, the Cystic Fibrosis Foundation has recently made seven center-specific measures publicly available.[40]

Variation in Preference-based Care

Variation in preference-based care refers to differences in rates for diagnostic and therapeutic procedures where there is uncertainty in the outcome or when there is a complex balance of possible benefits and harm. In this type of variation, there is no single right rate. The right rate reflects the decisions of fully informed patients and families. It is expected that the care choice will differ across families and, in turn, across regions.

The original analyses that led to this concept were studies of benign prostatic hypertrophy in adult men,[41] decidedly a nonpediatric problem. In the early 1980s, there was high regional variation in the use of transurethral prostatectomies, with the decisions driven by the local theories of benefit and harm held by urologists. The literature on outcomes was not complete, but to the extent that it existed, it appeared to be ignored by urologists. Today there is a full effectiveness literature on the ever widening available treatment choices, and formal decision aids[42] are used to assist men in making a choice that is consistent with their own utilities (ie, values). Often, but not always, the introduction of decision aids reduces utilization rates. A list of available decision aids and their sources can be found at the Ottawa Health Research Web site (http://decisionaid.ohri.ca/index.html). These aids greatly differ in quality; only a relatively few are available for pediatric illness.

Preference-based care remains a fruitful area of pediatric research. Some of the pediatric diseases that would seem to lend themselves to preference-based care include management of middle ear disease, chronic sinusitis, allergies, acne, and enuresis. Practice guidelines are an unsatisfactory solution to the complexity of decision making, often mixing physician opinion with evidence. Naturally, the recommendations will differ depending on the membership of the committee authoring the guideline. Variation in use rates reflects local practice styles and, in some instances, the relative dominance of the pediatrician or pediatric surgeon in the child's care. Even if all of the outcomes and associated probabilities are known, an individual child's outcomes are likely to be maximized when the child or family can participate fully in evaluating the treatment choices and making the medical care decision.

Variation in Supply-sensitive Care

Supply-sensitive care refers to medical services for which use rates are sensitive to the local availability of health care resources such as beds and physicians. Although in some instances effective care may be constrained by the lack of resources, this category is principally concerned with the many types of medical care for which there is weak or no evidence of effectiveness, and for which the complexity of the decision making and the rich number of alternatives make efficacy and effectiveness studies difficult. These services are also termed *discretionary*. Generally, the right rate is the lowest rate with comparable outcomes.

Medical admissions are often considered supply-sensitive care.[43,44] Medical discharge rates vary 200% to 300% across hospital services areas and are strongly influenced by area bed supply.[27,45] Asthma hospitalizations are a useful pediatric example. A clinician caring for a child with an asthma exacerbation has the option of longer treatment and monitoring in the office or emergency department or hospitalization, and will decide after considering physiologic parameters, past medical history, social support available to the family, and parental preferences. Although this seems to be a rational judgment, clinical opinions will differ frequently, and the guidelines available for management of an acute ill asthmatic patient do not provide clear guidance.[46] Invisible to the clinician is the supply of beds and its subtle influence on local practice patterns. There is no evidence that hospital beds are explicitly rationed in lower supply areas or that patients are harmed by fewer hospital days.

In the 1990s, McConnochie and colleagues[47] studied the variation in pediatric discharge rates in New York State using counties and small areas in Monroe County as units of analysis. Discharge rates for lower respiratory illness varied over threefold and were inversely correlated with area socioeconomic indicators. These analyses were extended to a wider set of conditions with similar findings.[34,48] Capacity measures, such as bed supply, were not explicitly examined. Although these and other studies[49] confirm the known relationship between wealth and health, the studies suffer from possible ecologic biases and provide little insight into relative health system performance. Indeed, Gorton's study of pneumonia discharges in Pennsylvania children suggests differences in illness levels may be relatively unimportant.[37]

Other studies of pediatric hospitalization variation have focused on the appropriateness of admissions[50] or the quality of ambulatory care.[51] Differences in the quality of ambulatory care are thought to be an important cause of varying hospitalization rates, although the empiric evidence remains weak. When studies have examined the association of capacity and pediatric use, a strong association has been observed.[27,45]

Perhaps both the quality of ambulatory care and capacity will turn out to be important explanations of unwarranted variation in pediatric hospitalization rates.

Other types of adult care that have been shown to be supply sensitive include ICU days, imaging studies, and physician visits.[52,53] Unfortunately, the lack of population-based pediatric data linked to provider and patient location has severely limited comparable studies.[45]

Variation in Health Care Capacity

Measuring the variation in the number of child health physicians has proven to be easier than counting pediatric beds. Although the literature has been relatively silent on the former, several studies have shown marked variation in the per capita (eg, child or newborn) number of general pediatricians and pediatric subspecialists. Chang and Halfon[54] showed a lack of association between general pediatrician supply across states and indicators of child health needs. Mayer[55] observed a high degree of variation across *Dartmouth Atlas* regions for different pediatric subspecialists, and Goodman and colleagues[56] found little relation between the supply of neonatologists and regional differences in perinatal risk. None of these studies linked capacity to the utilization of pediatric services.

FUTURE DIRECTIONS

Since Glover's 1938 report, studies of unwarranted variation in pediatric medical care have taken root but have only flourished in studies of technical quality (ie, evidence-based care). The causes of differences in utilization rates and costs have been largely attributed to differences in patient need, although these conclusions are based upon a small set of studies with limited data. This view places the child health delivery system in a disadvantageous position as the debate about health system performance and reform is driven by considerations of the efficiency (ie, cost controlled by quality) of providers. Further research in unwarranted variation in pediatric care will require the use of commercial payer claims data sets that include the location or provider variables necessary to conduct small area analysis of hospital and physician care over large and diverse child populations.

ACKNOWLEDGMENTS

Andrew Goodman, MPH student, provided indispensable assistance in the literature search for this article.

REFERENCES

1. Harris B. The health of the schoolchild: a history of the school medical service in England and Wales. Buckingham (UK): Open University Press; 1995.
2. Board of Education. Health of the schoolchild 1920. Annual Report of the Chief Medical Officer of the Board of Education for 1920. London: Board of Education; 1920.
3. Board of Education. Health of the schoolchild 1931. Annual Report of the Chief Medical Officer of the Board of Education for 1931. London; 1931.
4. Board of Education. Health of the schoolchild 1924. Annual Report of the Chief Medical Officer of the Board of Education for 1924. London; 1924.
5. Glover JA. The incidence of tonsillectomy in school children. Proc R Soc Med 1938;31:95–112.

6. Lembcke PA. Measuring the quality of medical care through vital statistics based on hospital service areas. 1. Comparative study of appendectomy rates. Am J Public Health 1952;42:276–86.
7. Lewis CE. Variations in the incidence of surgery. N Engl J Med 1969;281(16): 880–4.
8. Wennberg J, Gittelsohn A. Small area variations in health care delivery. Science 1973;182:1102–8.
9. Moore FD. Small area variations in health care delivery. J Maine Med Assoc 1977; 68:49–57.
10. Wennberg J, Gittelsohn A. Variations in medical care among small areas. Sci Am 1982;246:120–34.
11. Shaheen P, Clark J, Williams D. Small area analysis: a review and analysis of the North American literature. J Health Polit Policy Law 1987;12(4):741–809.
12. Blumberg MS. Inter-area variations in age-adjusted health status. Med Care 1987;25(4):340–53.
13. Wennberg JE. Population illness rates do not explain population hospitalization rates: a comment on Mark Blumberg's thesis that morbidity adjusters are needed to interpret small area variations. Med Care 1987;25(4):354–9.
14. Wennberg JE, Fowler FJ. A test of consumer contribution to small area variations in health care delivery. J Maine Med Assoc 1977;68(8):275–9.
15. Diehr P, Cain K, Connell F, et al. What is too much variation? The null hypothesis in small area analysis. Health Serv Res 1990;24(6):741–71.
16. Wennberg J. Small area analysis and the medical care outcome problem. In: Sechrest L, Perrin E, Bunker J, editors. Research methodology: strengthening causal interpretations of nonexperimental data. Washington,DC: Agency for Health Care Policy and Research; 1990. p. 177–206.
17. Baicker K, Fisher ES, Chandra A. Malpractice liability costs and the practice of medicine in the Medicare program. Health Aff (Millwood) 2007;26(3):841–52.
18. ISI web of knowledge 2009; Accessed January 22, 2009.
19. Goodman D, Fisher E, Little G, et al. The relation between the availability of neonatal intensive care and neonatal mortality. N Engl J Med 2002;346(20): 1538–44.
20. Wennberg J, Fisher E, Goodman D, et al. Tracking the care of patients with chronic illness: the Dartmouth Atlas of Health Care 2008. Hanover (NH): The Dartmouth Institute for Health Policy and Clinical Practice; 2008.
21. Institute of Medicine. John E. Wennberg receives 2008 Lienhard Award. Available at: http://www.iom.edu/CMS/28312/5010/59060.aspx. Accessed January 29, 2009.
22. Wennberg J, Kimm SYS. Common uses of hospitals: a look at Vermont. In: Sechrest L, Perrin E, Bunker J, editors. Developing a better health care system for children. Cambridge (MA): Ballinger; 1977. p. 353–82.
23. Wennberg J, McPherson K, Caper P. Will payment based on diagnosis-related groups control hospital costs? N Engl J Med 1984;311:295–300.
24. Connell FA, Day RW, LoGerfo JP. Hospitalization of Medicaid children: analysis of small area variations in admission rates. Am J Public Health 1981;71(6):606–13.
25. Wissow LS, Gittelsohn AM, Szklo M, et al. Poverty, race, and hospitalization for childhood asthma. Am J Public Health 1988;78(7):777–82.
26. Guagliardo MF, Ronzio CR. Is region of country a useful variable for child health studies? Pediatrics 2005;116(6):1542–5.
27. Goodman DC, Fisher ES, Gittelsohn A, et al. Why are children hospitalized? The role of nonclinical factors in pediatric hospitalizations. Pediatrics 1994;93(6 Pt 1): 896–902.

28. Guagliardo MF, Jablonski KA, Joseph JG, et al. Do pediatric hospitalizations have a unique geography? BMC Health Serv Res 2004;4(1):1–9.
29. Goodman DC, Mick SS, Bott D, et al. Primary care service areas: a new tool for the evaluation of primary care services. Health Serv Res 2003;38(1 Pt 1):287–309.
30. Goodman DC, Fisher ES, Little GA, et al. The uneven landscape of newborn intensive care services: variation in the neonatology workforce. Eff Clin Pract 2001;4(4):143–9.
31. Healthcare Cost and Utilization Project. Introduction to the HCUP Kids' inpatient database (KID) 2006. Rockville (MD): Agency for Healthcare Research and Quality; 2008.
32. Goodman DC, Stukel TA, Chang CH, et al. End-of-life care at academic medical centers: implications for future workforce requirements. Health Aff (Millwood) 2006;25(2):521–31.
33. Wise PH, Eisenberg L. What do regional variations in the rates of hospitalization of children really mean? N Engl J Med 1989;320(18):1209–11.
34. McConnochie KM, Roghmann KJ, Liptak GS. Socioeconomic variation in discretionary and mandatory hospitalization of infants: an ecologic analysis. Pediatrics 1997;99(6):774–84.
35. Perrin J. Variations in pediatric hospitalization rates: why do they occur? Pediatr Ann 1994;23(12):676–83.
36. Bergman DA, Mayer ML, Pantell RH, et al. Does clinical presentation explain practice variability in the treatment of febrile infants? Pediatrics 2006;117(3): 787–95.
37. Gorton CP, Jones JL. Wide geographic variation between Pennsylvania counties in the population rates of hospital admissions for pneumonia among children with and without comorbid chronic conditions. Pediatrics 2006;117(2):176–80.
38. Vermont Oxford Network. About us: database. Available at: http://www.vtoxford.org/home.aspx?p=about/network_db.htm. Accessed February 5, 2009.
39. Horbar J, Badger G, Lewit E, et al. Hospital and patient characteristics associated with variation in 28-day mortality rates for very low birth weight infants. Pediatrics 1997;99(2):149–56.
40. Cystic Fibrosis Foundation. Care Center Network. Available at: http://www.cff.org/LivingWithCF/CareCenterNetwork/. Accessed February 5, 2009.
41. Wennberg J, Mulley A Jr, Hanley D, et al. An assessment of prostatectomy for benign urinary tract obstruction: geographic variations and the evaluation of medical care outcomes. JAMA 1988;259(20):3027–30.
42. Barry M, Fowler F Jr, Mulley A Jr, et al. Patient reactions to a program designed to facilitate patient participation in treatment decisions for benign prostatic hyperplasia. Med Care 1995;33(8):771–82.
43. Wennberg JE, Freeman JL, Culp WJ. Are hospital services rationed in New Haven or overutilised in Boston? Lancet 1987;1(8543):1185–9.
44. Roemer MI. Bed supply and hospital utilization: a natural experiment. Hospitals 1961;35:36–42.
45. Wennberg J, Wennberg D. Dartmouth Atlas of Health Care in Michigan. Detroit (MI): Blue Cross Blue Shield of Michigan; 2000.
46. National Asthma Education and Prevention Program. Expert panel report 3: guidelines for the diagnosis and management of asthma. Bethesda (MD): National Heart, Lung, and Blood Institute; 2007.
47. McConnochie K, Roghmann K, Liptak G. Hospitalization for lower respiratory tract illness in infants: variation in rates among counties in New York State and areas within Monroe County. J Pediatr 1995;126(2):220–9.

48. McConnochie K, Russo M, McBride J, et al. Socioeconomic variation in asthma hospitalization: excess utilization or greater need? Pediatrics 1999;103(6):1–8.
49. Garg A, Probst JC, Sease T, et al. Potentially preventable care: ambulatory care–sensitive pediatric hospitalizations in South Carolina in 1998. Southampt Med J 2003;96(9):850–8.
50. Payne SM, Donahue C, Rappo P, et al. Variations in pediatric pneumonia and bronchitis/asthma admission rates. Is appropriateness a factor? Arch Pediatr Adolesc Med 1995;149(2):162–9.
51. Homer C, Szilagyi P, Rodewald L, et al. Does quality of care affect rates of hospitalization for childhood asthma? Pediatrics 1996;98(1):18–23.
52. Fisher ES, Wennberg DE, Stukel TA, et al. The implications of regional variations in Medicare spending. Part 1. The content, quality, and accessibility of care. Ann Intern Med 2003;138(4):273–87.
53. Fisher ES, Wennberg DE, Stukel TA, et al. The implications of regional variations in Medicare spending. Part 2. Health outcomes and satisfaction with care. Ann Intern Med 2003;138(4):288–98.
54. Chang RK, Halfon N. Geographic distribution of pediatricians in the United States: an analysis of the fifty states and Washington, DC. Pediatrics 1997; 100(2 Pt 1):172–9.
55. Mayer M. Are we there yet? Distance to care and relative supply among pediatric medical subspecialties. Pediatrics 2006;118(6):2313–21.
56. Goodman D, Fisher E, Little G, et al. Are neonatal intensive care resources located where need is greatest? Regional variation in neonatologists, beds, and low birth weight newborns. Pediatrics 2001;108:426–31.

Model for Improvement - Part 1: A Framework for Health Care Quality

Cheryl D. Courtlandt, MD, FAAP[a,b,c,*], Laura Noonan, MD, FAAP[a,b,d],
Leonard G. Feld, MD, PhD, MMM, FAAP[b,e]

KEYWORDS

- Quality Improvement • PDSA cycle • Model for improvement
- Healthcare improvement • Pediatric quality

Health care expenditures represent a staggering portion of the United States government spending.[1] Competitive pressures and scarce resources are forcing health care organizations to reduce costs, eliminate waste, increase productivity, and ensure patient safety.[2] Continuous quality improvement is an imperative mandate for the success of health care organizations.[3] The use of formal improvement strategies is new to health care but has a long history in industry especially manufacturing. Industrial improvement initiatives were oriented toward decreasing waste, increasing efficiency, eliminating duplication and creating opportunities for expansion in industry or increasing market share.

The earliest industrial quality improvement efforts were pioneered by Joseph Juran, W. Edward Deming, and Philip Crosby.[4–6] Juran's theory[4–6] postulated the concept of fitness for use. This approach built interdisciplinary teams using various diagnostic tools to understand why certain manufacturing processes produced products that are unusable. His theories focused on determining the causes of inferior production and using that information or set of circumstances to decrease production of substandard product. A theory proposed by Philip Crosby,[6] defined quality in terms of

[a] Division of General Pediatrics, Department of Pediatrics, Levine Children's Hospital at Carolinas Medical Center, P.O. Box 32861, Charlotte, NC 28232-2861, USA
[b] Center for Advancing Pediatric Excellence, Department of Pediatrics, Levine Children's Hospital at Carolinas Medical Center, P.O. Box 32861, Charlotte, NC 28232-2861, USA
[c] Asthma Program, Levine Children's Hospital at Carolinas Medical Center, P.O. Box 32861, Charlotte, NC 28232-2861, USA
[d] Area Health Education Center, P.O. Box 32861, Charlotte, NC 28232-2861, USA
[e] Department of Pediatrics, Levine Children's Hospital at Carolinas Medical Center, P.O. Box 32861, Charlotte, NC 28232, USA
* Corresponding author. Division of General Pediatrics, Levine Children's Hospital at Carolinas Medical Center, P.O. Box 32861, Charlotte, NC 28232-2861.
E-mail address: cheryl.courtlandt@carolinashealthcare.org (C.D. Courtlandt).

Pediatr Clin N Am 56 (2009) 757–778
doi:10.1016/j.pcl.2009.06.002
pediatric.theclinics.com

performance, a quality performance produces zero defects. If defects are produced, these defects increase the cost of production or delivery of service and impacted on profit margin or consumer safety.

Deming[5,7] made key contributions by outlining a framework of knowledge necessary for the application of the science of improvement. Deming's theory focused on four components: an appreciation of a "system," understanding variation, acquisition of knowledge, and the knowledge of psychology. These factors and their interaction represent the cornerstone of improvement science. All improvement theories include the following concepts: commitment of the organization to quality; focus on the customer or consumer; modification of systems, not people; ability to foster teamwork; and encouraging group problem solving. Using improvement science, decisions are made based on objective not subjective information.

The effectiveness of these improvement methods in manufacturing was acknowledged by health care management. Twenty years ago, the Institute for Healthcare Improvement (IHI) launched its first project called "The National Demonstration Project on Quality Improvement in Healthcare" which explored the application of modern quality improvement methods to health care.[8] In 1990, the landmark book *Curing Healthcare*,[8] introduced the concept of creating a culture of continuous quality improvement in health care. *Crossing the Quality Chasm*, published in 2001 by the Institute of Medicine, defined six aims of health care quality. These quality indicators recommended that patient care should be timely, effective, efficient, patient centered, safe, and equitable.[2] Even though the health care industry has made strides in improving quality of health care, major gaps persist in performance of health care systems and these gaps represent significant risk to patient safety.[9]

Currently, the focal point of quality improvement in health care has shifted from institutions to include individual providers. The question is often asked, "What is quality?" "How is it measured?" Health care providers are expected to assess and improve their patients' outcomes but lack training in quality improvement and limits their ability to fully implement quality initiatives.[10,11] Future trends in health care delivery will require practitioners to participate in continuous quality improvement as part of their daily practice. Acquisition of this skill set will become as important as the underlying medical knowledge used to diagnose and treat disease.[12] The process of quality improvement requires careful planning, thorough documentation, consistent analysis, and openmindedness to results. Fortunately, there are methods and tools to assist the practitioner in the development of quality improvement skills.[13]

THE MODEL FOR IMPROVEMENT

All methodology of quality improvement is based on the same underlying theories of improvement science.[4–6,13] Associates in Process Improvement (API) developed the Model for Improvement in 1996[13] to illustrate how to facilitate change. The Model for Improvement is an effective and easily understood method that can be implemented by either large health care systems or a small office practice. This model uses methodology that produces specific, measurable results. The IHI and other leading health care quality improvement organizations utilize the Model for Improvement to advance health care quality projects (**Fig. 1**).

In any complex system, change can be difficult to accomplish; incorporation of several key elements is necessary to produce system change.[13]

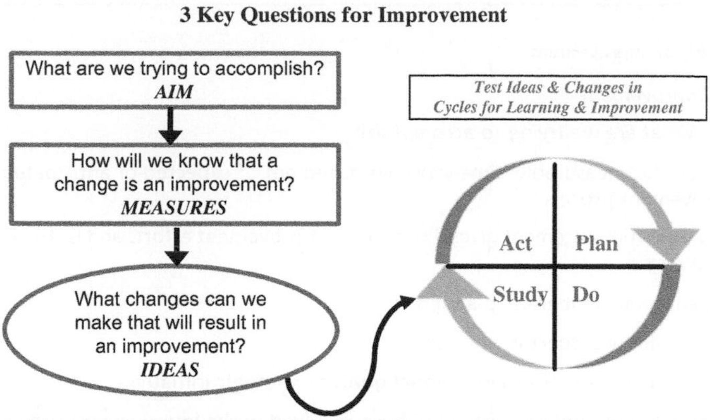

Fig. 1. Model for improvement. (*Data from* Langley G, Nolan K, Nolan T, et al. The improvement guide: a practical approach to enhancing organizational performance. San Francisco (CA): Jossey-Bass Pub; 1996.)

Key elements to system change

1) The *will* to do whatever it takes to make a change to a system
2) The *ideas* on which to base the design of the new system
3) The *execution* of the changes to the system.

The Model Asks Three Fundamental Questions

What are we trying to accomplish?

The Aim statement is a written statement of the *expected* or *anticipated* accomplishments from an improvement effort (**Box 1**). The key components include: a general description of the Aim, a clear description of what is trying to be accomplished, the rationale and importance of the effort, some guidance for executing the work, specifying the target population, establishing a time period for the project, and setting measurable goals.

An Aim statement captures early decisions, aligns the team, communicates with others and acts as a touchstone throughout an improvement project. This document is key to successful projects, many projects fail due to flaws in the Aim statement. The goals included in the Aim statement should be measurable, numeric and preferable absolute rather than relative. Attaining the goals should be a stretch, achievable not impossible, not business as usual.[13,14]

How will we know if a change is an improvement?

"*All improvement is change but not all change is an improvement*" (**Box 1**).[13] "How will we know that a change is an improvement?" is a question often asked during the improvement process. To adequately assess change, three types of measures are used in improvement science: outcome, process, and balancing measures.[13] *Outcome* measures are global measures, directed related to the Aim statement. In the ideal scenario, they reflect the desired outcome of the improvement effort. Process or intermediate measures are related to key changes to be implemented during the improvement effort. A process measure evaluates the interval change or steps to attain the outcome of the improvement effort. These measures are usually proximal to the overall outcome. Balancing measures are used to evaluate if a change is

Box 1
Key questions for improvement

Model for Improvement

Question 1: What are we trying to accomplish?

Aim: A specific, measurable, time-sensitive statement of expected or anticipated results of an improvement process.

A strong clear Aim statement gives direction to improvement efforts and is characterized by the following:

- Intentional, deliberate, planned
- Unambiguous, specific, concrete
- Aligned with other organizational goals or strategic initiatives
- Agreed upon and supported by those involved in the improvement project and leadership

Include:

- A general description of the Aim - should answer, "What are we trying to accomplish?"
- Rationale/importance
- Specify target population and time period
- Measurable goals

Question 2: How will we know that a change is an improvement?

Measures: measures are indicators of change.

These measures can also be used to monitor a system's performance over time. Project measures should:

- Be directly linked to Aims and goals
- Seek usefulness over perfection.
- Be integrated into daily work whenever possible.
- Be graphically and visibly displayed, usually as run charts.
- Include outcome, process, and balancing measures.

Note these system or project measures are not the same as the "study" measures for PDSA cycles described below.

Question 3: What changes can we make that will result in an improvement?

Ideas: Ideas for change or *change concepts* to be tested in a P-D-S-A cycles can be adapted from:

- Evidence - results of research/science
- Critical thinking or observation of the current system
- Creative thinking and extrapolations from other situations

When selecting ideas to test, consider the following:

- Direct link to the Aim
- Likely impact of the change (avoid low-impact changes.)
- Potential for learning and adding to knowledge base

- Feasibility
- Logical sequencing
- Series of tests that will build on one another
- Scale of the test (cycle of one)
- Shortness of the cycle (1 day or week NOT 1 month)

causing unexpected effects. Change can improve one part of a system but undermine another. The most skeptical person of a group is a source for balancing measures, often they outline credible reasons why a particular project will fail or why certain goals are impossible.[14]

The optimal measure set includes four to eight measures; at least one should be a balancing measure. All of the measures must be aligned with the Aim statement. The most successful improvement projects have measures that are easily collected and improvement can be shown quickly.[14,15] Methods for data collection should be simple and easily integrated into daily work. The results of any improvement efforts should be displayed graphically over time through the use of simple run charts. A run chart shows a pattern or trend over time. These charts should be annotated to show implementation of a change, explain a result or note an unusual circumstance[16,17] (**Fig. 2**). Additional information on measurement for quality improvement can be found in the article by Randolph and colleagues found elsewhere in this issue.

What changes can we make that will result in an improvement?

The Model for Improvement permits testing of ideas or changes or implementing change concepts that have worked in other settings (**Box 1**). Change concepts are general approaches to change, the rationale is to generate specific ideas to test.[13] These concepts may be feasible and effective in one setting but may need adaptation to a new setting. Change concepts need to be altered to fit the existing culture, resources, or institutional goals. Ideally, a change concept initially is a vague or innovative strategic idea that is further whittled down to a specific actionable idea or change that can be tested.[13]

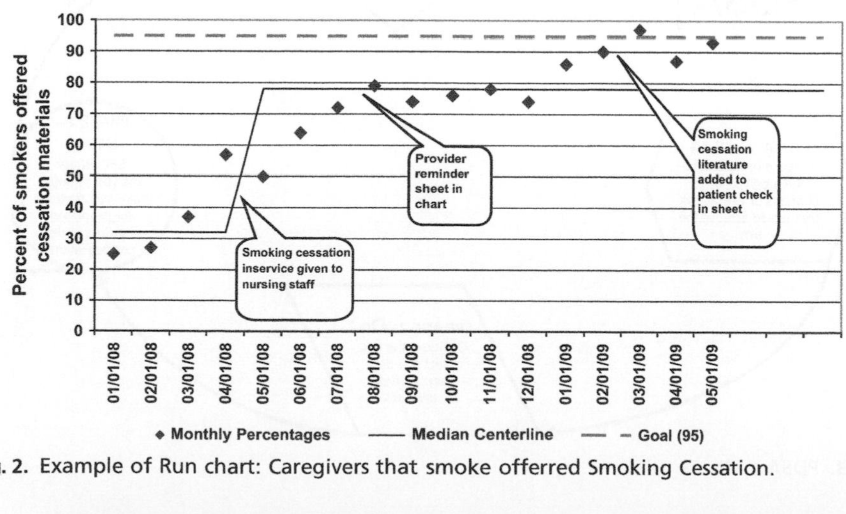

Fig. 2. Example of Run chart: Caregivers that smoke offerred Smoking Cessation.

Another method to support change is a *change package*. A change package is a group or set of changes that through evidence-based study can affect a particular outcome. For example, the of use asthma action plans, the use of inhaled corticosteroids in moderate asthma, and having an identified primary care provider/pediatric medical home are elements of an asthma care change package. These items used as a group, have been shown to produce improvement of asthma care in some health care settings.

Using Plan-Do-Study-Act Cycles to Test an Idea or Change

Walter Shewart, in 1924, penned a one-page memo outlining his idea of quality processes.[18] From his work came the PDCA cycle, later referred to as the PDSA cycle. The plan-do-study-act cycle (PDSA cycle) is a short rapid cycle used to test an idea or a change (**Fig. 3**).

The P phase

The objective for the learning should be stated with clear assumptions. All details of the plan serve as documentation for the implementation of subsequent phases.

The D phase

The data collection phase indicates the collection process, any barriers to the process or unexpected occurrences that may affect the interpretation of the data.

The S phase

During this phase, data are studied and interpreted. The analysis is then compared with the initial predictions or assumptions. Data should be displayed in a run chart or Pareto chart. (A Pareto chart is a bar graph reflecting the frequency of occurrence, illustrating the predominance of a specific cause.) PDSA cycles may use either qualitative or qualitative data. This phase should review the data collection instrument, its use, and ease of collection. The data are specific to the cycle and end with the cycle.

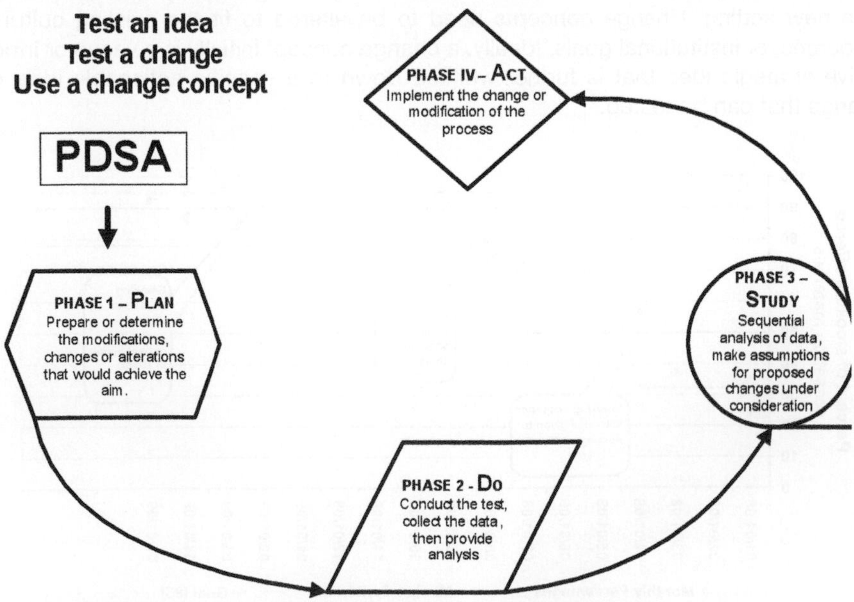

Fig. 3. PDSA cycle.

The A phase

The last step in the cycle, analyzing the data collected to attain new learning or knowledge, addresses required changes in the testing process and poses additional questions to be answered before implementing a change.

PDSA cycles assist improvement teams in adapting good ideas to their specific situation. When used appropriately, PDSA cycles force small-scale thinking. The PDSA cycle promotes detailed stepwise thinking, allows for making predictions, forces thoughtful deliberation on the increased knowledge, and subsequently facilitates change. Use of small-scale change can cause rapid adaptation and implementation of change in various health care settings (**Fig. 3**).[13,14,18]

CASE STUDY

Super Smart Pediatrics is a suburban practice, with a diverse patient base, that includes numerous insurance plans. The practice has 7 full-time doctors, 3 part-time doctors, several midlevel providers, 10 nurses, and 15 front office and medical record staff. The practice has grown significantly over the past 15 years and currently serves 15,000 patients.

The practice manger of Super Smart Pediatrics noted that recently there were more complaints from office staff, practice providers, and patients. During a casual discussion with the practice manager, one of the partners revealed her frustration with working harder and harder, and feeling overwhelmed especially by patients with chronic diseases. She felt there was never enough time to address all the necessary patient issues. Her partners treated illnesses in different fashions leading to confusion among patients. In addition, the number of new patients enrolling in the practice had decreased over the past 2 years and two neighboring practices were growing and adding additional staff.

After several discussions with other staff members, Super Smart Pediatrics' employees and partners realized many of them were concerned with the direction of the practice. Two of the partners and the office manager visited several other practices and had some frank discussions with their colleagues. They observed different approaches that were successful in other offices but were unsure where to begin.

Fortunately, the practice manger had kept a log of all the complaints from the previous year, he was able to divide the complaints into three categories: Office Efficiency, Staff Efficiency, and Provider Efficiency. The Pareto chart in **Fig. 4** illustrates the data.

The office manager used a Pareto chart (www.lchcape.org) and displayed the complaint data for discussion at the staff meeting. The providers and staff of the Super Smart Pediatrics were surprised by the data and requested an examination of potential causes for the relatively large proportion of complaints regarding provider efficiency. The practice manager conducted a simple three-question survey to assess of the causes of provider inefficiency. The survey was given to providers, staff, and patients over 5 days at three different times. The results are displayed in the Pareto chart in **Fig. 5**.

Identifying the Problem

Super Smart Pediatrics identified a problem through frustration and job dissatisfaction of a partner and office manager. Identification of a concern, problem, or deficiency may come from various sources. Sources may include the work environment, recurring problems or a special interest of the staff. Strategic thinking will identify projects that are sensible and feasible for a particular group, practice, or organization. A focus may be suggested by a compelling issue on at the national, state, regional, or local level. New evidence-based practice guidelines not implemented in a particular setting are another source of quality improvement projects. Every attempt should be made to

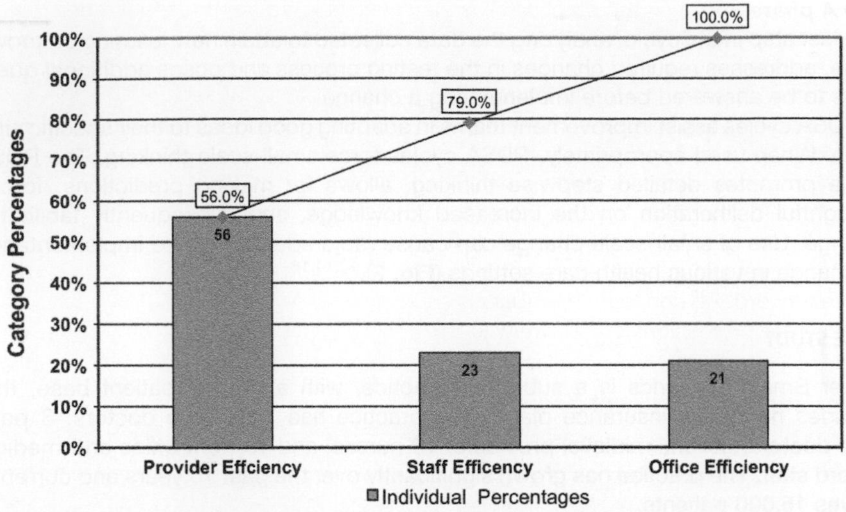

Fig. 4. Pareto Chart: complaints collected by Super Smart Pediatrics.

develop a passion factor in any improvement project, because change is difficult. Topics should attract attention or generate the necessary interest to move the project forward. Finally, external pressures on providers may be the driving force of improvement projects. For example, recently established requirements for Part IV of Maintenance of Certification are "sparking" the interest of many providers to participate in office-based quality improvement projects.[11,13–15]

Development of a Team

Case study (continued)

After several staff meetings, Super Smart Pediatrics decided to focus on provider variability. The practice decided to focus on asthma since it was the most common

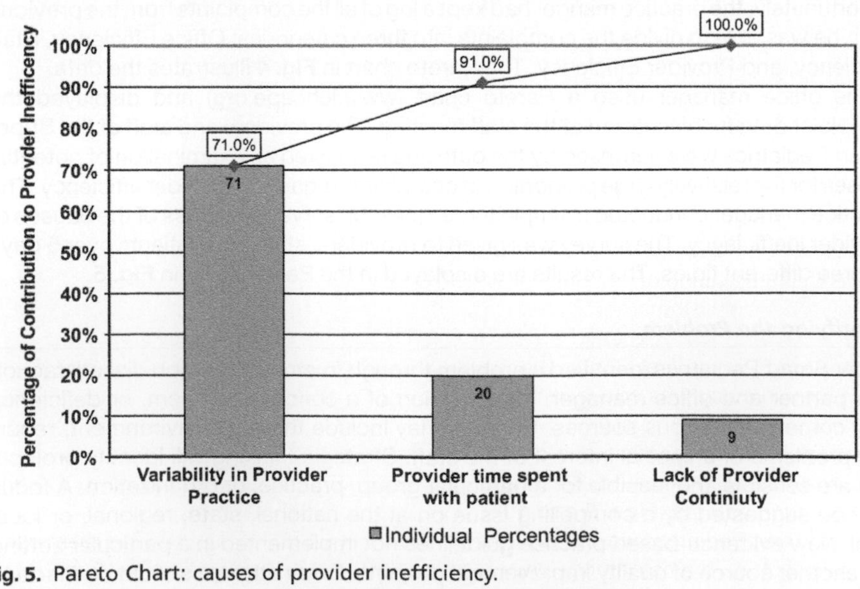

Fig. 5. Pareto Chart: causes of provider inefficiency.

chronic illness seen in the practice. The new National Asthma Education and Prevention Program (NAEPP) guidelines were not being implemented uniformly in the practice and subsequently this lead to confusion by both staff and patients. An improvement team was assembled from front office, billing, nurses, midlevel providers, and physicians. A future goal was to add an interested parent or patient.

Once a project has been identified, it is important to assemble a team because quality improvement is not a solo endeavor but a "team sport." Successful projects recruit team members from all disciplines. Several team options exist ranging from a small core group to larger groups that include all the stakeholders. The ideal size is 4 to 8 team members, as larger groups may limit ability to make decisions and move forward. Ad hoc team members may include specific content experts and allied health care professionals[19–21] (www.lchcape.org for team chart).

Using Quality Improvement Tools to Start a Project

As the project progresses, there are several useful QI tools to smooth the progress of the project. Several tools are described or illustrated in the case study and additional tools are on the Web site, www.lchcape.org. Using these tools requires practice, but once mastered accelerates the improvement effort.[22,23]

Case study (continued)

The Super Smart Pediatrics Asthma Team met twice weekly during lunch time for 30 minutes using the 7-step meeting agenda (www.lchcape.org), with a weekly report to the entire practice incorporated into the existing staff meeting.

Meetings should be incorporated into an existing scheduled meeting. Meeting frequency may limit the involvement of some group members so meetings should be focused and brief to continue momentum and interest.[19] The Aim statement developed by Super Smart Pediatrics outlines their Aim, the goals, the measures, and some ideas for initial PSDA cycles (www.lchcape.org) (**Box 2**).

Sharing the Aim statement with others not directly involved in the project often provides a new perspective on the problem. The objectives should be clear even to those not involved with the project. Feedback should be sought about goals and their measurement. It is critical that the Aim statement is reviewed by supervisors and senior leadership or practice management. Is project compelling? Is it aligned with strategic objectives of the organization or practice? A project without leadership support will be difficult to implement and impossible to sustain.[24–26]

Case study (continued)

Super Smart Pediatrics Asthma Team developed their Aim statement using existing change concepts. The Super Smart Pediatrics Asthma Team realized that identification of asthma patients in the practice was necessary for all future steps. The first PDSA cycle (PDSA Planner 1) illustrated that the providers had different criteria for the diagnosis of asthma and coded/billed differently. The team used a simple check sheet to gather data and used a Pareto chart to display the results (**Figs. 6** and **7**).

As a result of the first PDSA, the practice realized that the first step in decreasing provider variability was education and reaching a consensus.

The second PDSA cycle (PDSA Planner 2) was focused on decreasing provider variability around diagnosis and coding of asthma (**Fig. 8**).

The third PSDA cycle (PDSA Planner 3) examined ways for the office to identify patients with asthma (**Figs. 9** and **10**).

Smart Start Pediatrics was slowly identifying the patients with asthma. The team used the concept of brainstorming (www.lchcape.org) to cultivate ideas to speed the

Box 2
Super Smart Pediatrics Aim statement

Aim statement:

A specific, measurable time-sensitive statement of expected results of an improvement project

Super Smart Pediatrics will improve the care of their patients with asthma by implementing evidence-based changes to improve care. They will accomplish this by involving the entire health care team to ensure patient staff and provider satisfaction. We will accomplish this by January 2009

Goals

>90% of asthma patients will have an asthma action plan

>90% of asthma patients will receive flu vaccine

>90% of asthma patients will have an asthma flow sheet

>90% of asthma patients will have planned visits for asthma care.

Measures

Clear indicators of change, related to Aim statement.

Most useful when integrated into daily work

% of asthma patients with an asthma action plan

% of asthma patients who receive the flu vaccine

% of asthma patients with an asthma flow sheet

% of asthma patients with asthma who have planned visits

% of no-shows for planned asthma visits

Plan for data collection: Survey 20 charts every week for flu shots, action plans, flow sheets, and planned visits. Report these results in run charts

Ideas

These changes or change concepts will be the basis for PDSA cycles

Changes are based on current research or evidence

Critical observation of current system

Feasibility

Identification of patients with asthma to Implement current guidelines

Establish practice guidelines for diagnosis

Implement planned asthma visits

Implement asthma flow sheet

process. During discussions, they realized that another system problem may be part of the solution. The practice experienced a tremendous demand for flu shots that they were unable to meet during the winter and realized better planning was needed. The practice decided on a mass mailing survey to gauge patient interest in a flu shot clinic. The team added one question to the survey: "Does your child have asthma?" Using an informal survey to assess flu shot interest, the practice identified 658 additional patients with asthma. The total number of identified patients with asthma in the practice was similar to the 5% of the practice previously expected. The Super Smart Pediatric Asthma Team decided to trial a flow sheet for patient's charts to decrease the variation

PDSA Planner
PDSA 1
PLAN
Can Super Smart Pediatrics identify patients with asthma using billing data and the office computer?
1. Using all the billing codes can the computer identify all children, age 2 to 18 in the practice with asthma.
2. What are the various diagnosis codes used by the providers for asthma?
3. When compared to billing data will all patients with asthma be identified?

Predictions/Hypotheses
The computer will be able to identify all patients with asthma in the practice.
There are approximately 5% of the practice patients have asthma

Plan for data collection: The office manger will run a test report to identify all children age 2-18 using all of the billing codes of asthma
Pull 20 charts to verify the diagnosis of asthma
Pull 20 charts of patients that providers identify as having the diagnosis of asthma

---

DO
Only 170 patients identified by office computer
16/20 charts pulled matched billing with diagnosis code
14/20 provider identified charts had a diagnosis of asthma
Wheezing, reactive airway disease and cough were alternative diagnoses.

STUDY
80% of patients were identified correctly using chart verification using diagnosis codes and billing data
A smaller than expected numbers of patients were identified using asthma billing codes
Alternative Diagnoses have been used for patients with asthma

---

ACT
Patient Identification for asthma may be limited due to numerous codes used by providers.
The diagnosis of asthma varies with provider
Need to survey providers and reach a consensus on diagnosis and codes to be used
Next PDSA cycles will include surveying providers about how they make the diagnosis of asthma

Fig. 6. Super Smart Pediatrics Asthma Team PDSA Planner 1.

of asthma care received by each patient. Several of the measures from the Aim statement were readily assessable from the flow sheet (**Fig. 11**).

Initial cycles should be done on a small scale. A cycle of one can yield valuable information (**Fig. 12**).

Several cycles should be run to increase knowledge before instituting major change. Failed cycles are good learning opportunities when small (**Fig. 13**).

Super Smart Pediatrics expected to easily identify all the patients with asthma. Several PDSAs were needed to identify those patients targeted in their quality improvement project. To increase learning during a failed test, the following questions should be asked: Was the test conducted well? Does the change tested need

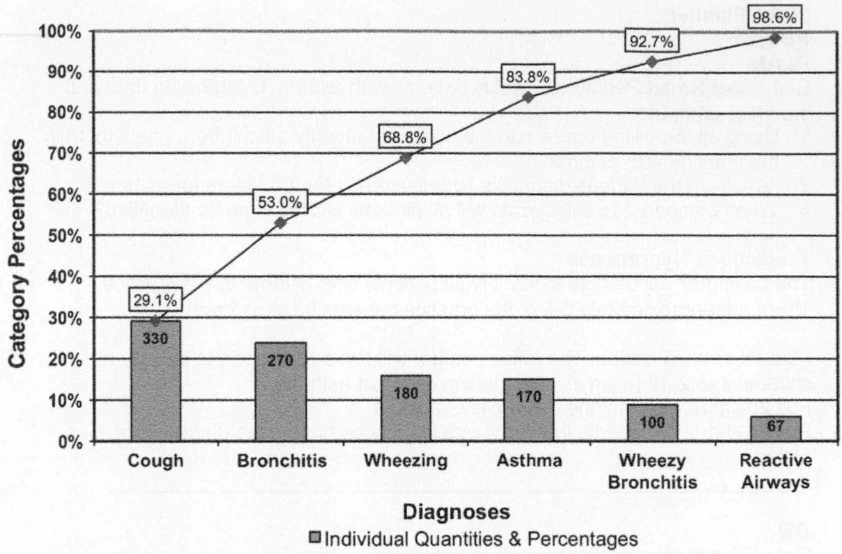

Fig. 7. Pareto Chart: diagnosis codes.

modification in our setting? Could the measures detect improvement or were they insufficient? Was the prediction or theory wrong?[13,14]

With successful tests, knowledge and learning will increase. As implementation of the change nears, testing should occur under as many conditions as possible. Prior thinking to special situations, busy times, vacations, or other factors are essential for successful change. Effective changes are made by conducting many test cycles to increase learning before implementing the changes to the entire practice or setting. After making a change a team should ask "What did we expect to happen? What did happen? Where there unintended consequences? What was the best thing about this change, the worst? What might we do next?" Reflection on the cycle is as important as the performance of the cycle. The learning and knowledge from a failed test is as important as a successful test.

After testing a change on a small scale, learning and refining from each PDSA allows for implementation on a broader scale. Implementation is the permanent change to the way work is done.[13] This step involves building the change into the system or workflow. Hardwiring change effects documentation, written policies, hiring, training, and possibly compensation. For example, testing a change may include a small number of providers using the asthma flow sheet as portrayed in PDSA 4 and 5 (**Fig. 14**). Implementation is the extension to the entire group of practitioners.

By using the Model for Improvement, health care providers can successfully identify areas that require change or improvement, set goals and determine measures, test changes and ideas using the PDSA cycle and then implementing those changes also using the PDSA cycle.

SUSTAINING CHANGE

"There will come a time when you think you are finished. That will be the beginning."

Louis L'Amour

PDSA Planner

PDSA 2

PLAN

Decrease Provider variability in the diagnosis of asthma and coding so patients can be identified and the guidelines can be better implemented

Predictions/Hypotheses

After reaching consensus, using the same diagnosis criteria and billing codes all patients the asthma in the practice will be identified.

Plan for change or test: All Providers at Super Smart Pediatrics will be reviewing the current guidelines for the diagnosis of asthma.

A local pulmonologist will consult with the practice to develop a working definition for asthma. The practice will establish specific codes to be used for billing asthma visits.

DO

Over a two week period, the providers met and established criteria for the diagnosis of asthma for the practice and some common billing codes.

Two weeks after the meeting the practice manger pulled 20 charts of patients recently seen using the new criteria and billing codes

---

STUDY

Practice manager realized that several patients identified as having asthma previously were seen in the practice for other reasons and were not coded for asthma as well

19/20 patients matched diagnosis and billing codes

1/20 patients with the diagnosis of asthma did not have an appropriate code

4 patients with asthma were seen for other reasons but were not coded for asthma

---

ACT

Using the established criteria >90% of patients with asthma were identified correctly

The practice manger will each month pull 20 charts to check the consistency of diagnosis and billing codes

Future questions identified for PDSA cycles

1) How will the patients not recently seen be identified as having asthma?
2) Should charts have an external method of identification so can be coded if seen for another reason?

Fig. 8. Super Smart Pediatrics Asthma Team PDSA Planner 2.

Change is difficult but sustaining change is even more complex. Once change has been implemented, there is a tendency to revert to the old system. To overcome this tendency, several sustainability strategies must be introduced. These strategies include assigning ownership, hardwiring the change into the system, periodic measurement and feedback, and involvement of senior leadership.[25]

Hardwiring sustainability into a new system is imperative. "The old way" has to be more difficult or inconvenient to perform. Organizations that are successful in sustaining improvement involve all staff and build the improvement-related expectations into job descriptions, evaluations, and merits. These organizations are not just focused on "the project" but incorporate improvement into the fabric of daily work. Concrete plans for turnover and absences, staff orientation, and training are all methods to sustain an improvement effort. Accountability is a core principle of sustaining improvement. Finally, educating patients about the improvement effort encourages staff to remain consistent and extends accountability.[14,25]

PDSA Planner

PDSA 3

PLAN

Attempt to identify patients with asthma not recently seen or seen for other reasons and mark charts.

Predictions/Hypotheses

There are too many patients in the practice for every chart to be examined if the child has asthma by the new consensus criteria therefore the practice has decided to place a blue stripe on charts when they come for well visits or sick visits for other reasons.

Plan for change or test: Upon registration of all patients the staff will ask "Does your child have asthma "if yes a blue stripe will be applied. If no, the chart will be reviewed by the nurse to see if the patients meet the practice asthma criteria. If yes, Blue stripe applied and provider notified. If provider makes a new diagnosis of asthma, a request to have chart marked with a blue stripe is made.

DO

Over a one week period, a blue stripe will be placed on every encounter form and on every chart of patients with asthma, regardless of the reason they are seen in the practice.

STUDY

Summarize data:

36 additional patients were identified with asthma using the new criteria and billing codes patients matched diagnosis and billing codes

ACT

Additional patients were identified but small numbers. The practice manger will each month pull 20 charts to check the consistency of diagnosis and billing codes and correctly identified with blue stripes. Need to identify more patients more quickly.

Future questions identified

1) If the practice sent out letters to all patients about a flu shot clinic and listed asthma as one of the target chronic illness , how many more patients would be identified
2) Will sending out the letter to entire practice overwhelm the practice with requests for flu shots and cause dissatisfaction in other patients

Fig. 9. Super Smart Pediatrics Asthma Team PDSA Planner 3.

Ongoing measurement is vital to sustaining any improvements.[16,17] The measurement process is shifted into audit mode. Data collection should occur with a frequency to detect if the process is losing gains; depending on the project this may be monthly or weekly. Data should be openly displayed and discussed. Successes, no matter how small, should be celebrated. By showcasing the staff and their successes, a culture that is data driven will slowly emerge. These victories can be used for marketing or further accreditation. A more in-depth discussion of data during the sustainability phase of improvement is available in the article by Randolph and colleagues found elsewhere in this issue.

The final strategy for sustaining improvement is the involvement of senior leadership.[27,28] Senior leadership involvement enables a shift from a project view to a strategic vision. The creation of a shared vision is essential to sustaining improvement. "The one-year project view," must be eliminated by senior management to guarantee success of any improvement project. The effort required to sustain improvement is often more than is needed to spread improvement. Sustaining and spreading of

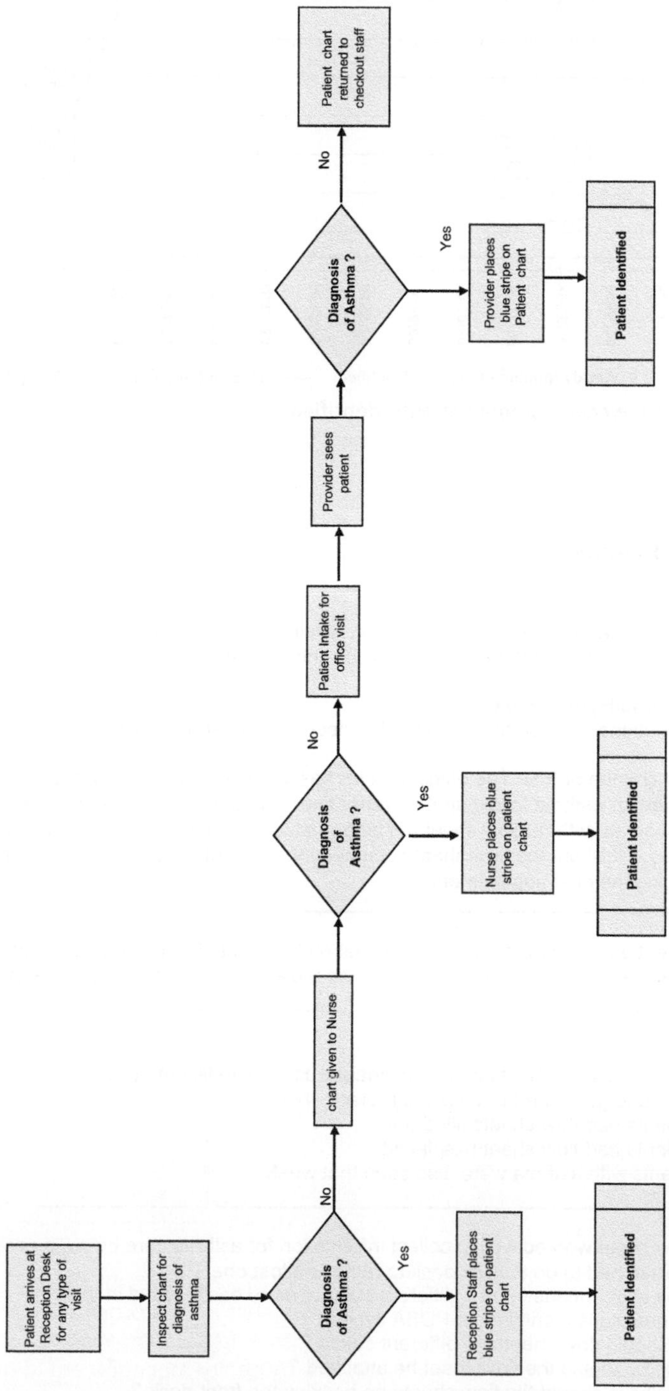

Fig. 10. Asthma Patient Identification Process flow chart.

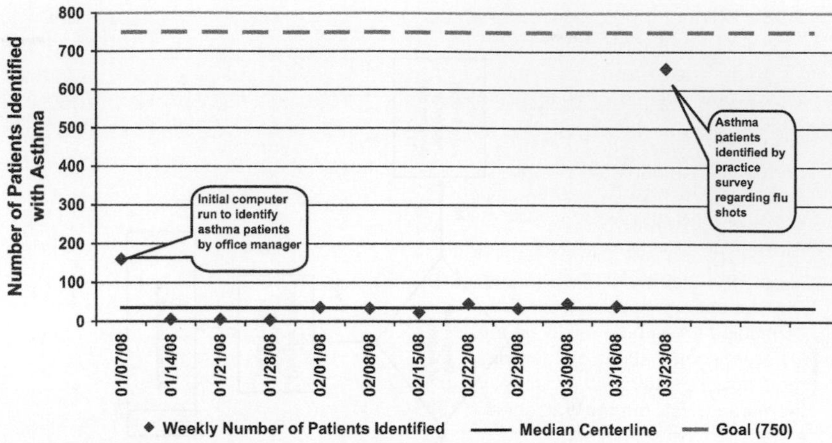

Fig. 11. Run Chart: weekly asthma patients identified.

PDSA Planner

PDSA 4

PLAN

Dr. Exceptional will use a flow sheet while seeing 3 patients for asthma follow up this week. The flow sheet is one that is currently utilized by a similar practice in the area.

Predictions/Hypotheses

Dr. Exceptional will use the flow sheet to decrease variation of asthma care

Plan for change or test: The office manger has identified 3 patients that are scheduled for asthma follow up this week. Their charts have been flagged. At registration an asthma flow sheet will be added to the chart. Dr. Exceptional and the nurse will fill out the flow sheet documenting the continued asthma care and scheduling the next appointment.

DO

Dr. Exceptional and nurse used flow sheet on 3 patients for asthma follow up. The flow sheet was lost once and had to be replaced prior to the end of the visit.

STUDY

Summarize data:
3 patients had flow sheets done, the sheet was easy to fill out but got lost once. Nurse had to go to the front desk to replace sheet.
3/3 patients had flow sheets filled out
1/3 patients had flow sheet misplaced
34 patients with asthma were also seen that week

ACT

The flow sheet worked well to collect information for asthma care but was easily lost . Nurse had to go to front desk to retrieve a lost one.
The flow sheet needs to be a different color or more easily found in the chart
Future questions identified for PDSA cycles

1) Should flow sheets be different colors ?
2) How should the flow sheet be attached ?
3) Where should the flow sheets be besides the front desk ?.

Fig. 12. Super Smart Pediatrics Asthma Team PDSA Planner 4.

PDSA Planner
PDSA 5
PLAN
Dr. Exceptional and 2 mid level providers will use the flow sheet while seeing 9 patients each for asthma follow up this week. The flow sheet will be colored white or blue or yellow. The flow sheet will be attached with a paper clip or permanently mounted or fastened to the chart. The flow sheet will located in provider and nurse work space as well as the front desk.

Predictions/Hypotheses
Dr. Exceptional and the mid level providers will use the 3 different colored flow sheet and 3 different attachments to find out the best combination
Plan for change or test: The office manger has identified 27 patients that are scheduled for asthma follow up this week. Their charts have been flagged. Different combinations of flow sheet and attachment have been assigned. At registration an asthma flow sheet will be added to the chart. Dr. Exceptional and the nurse will fill out the flow sheet documenting the continued asthma care and scheduling the next appointment.

DO
Dr. Exceptional and providers decided to eliminate the blue form immediately because writing could not be seen well on it. The trial continued with the 2 color combinations and 3 attachments. No flow sheets were misplaced. Nurse pulled permanently mounted sheet out to fill out his portion

STUDY
26 patients had flow sheets done 1 patient rescheduled
3/3 providers preferred the yellow flow sheet
3/3 providers preferred the flow sheet fastened
3 additional patients with asthma were also seen that week
Less than 2 minutes was added in filling out flow sheet, decreased time searching for information

ACT
The flow sheet worked well to collect information for asthma care and fastening it was the best option. The yellow sheet was preferred over the white.
The flow sheet will be trialed by the rest of the practice using the yellow flow sheet fastened to the chart, the flow sheet needs to be a different color or more easily found in the chart
Future questions identified for PDSA cycles
1) How well will the flow sheet copied?
2) Will the flow sheet work as well when used by entire practice?

Fig. 13. Super Smart Pediatric Asthma Team PDSA Planner 5.

improvement often overlap, spreading an improvement project, particularly in large organizations, is often started before improvement gains are sustained.

Case Study (Continued)

Super Smart Pediatrics had many successes to celebrate and reached their goal one month before the date expected (**Figs. 14–16**).

After 3 months of continued improvement, the team decided to develop a sustainability plan.

Super Smart Pediatrics sustainability plan

The practice manager was assigned ownership of the improvement project; written specific quality improvement tasks and expectations into all staff job descriptions. Evaluations and merits were linked to participation in the asthma care system.

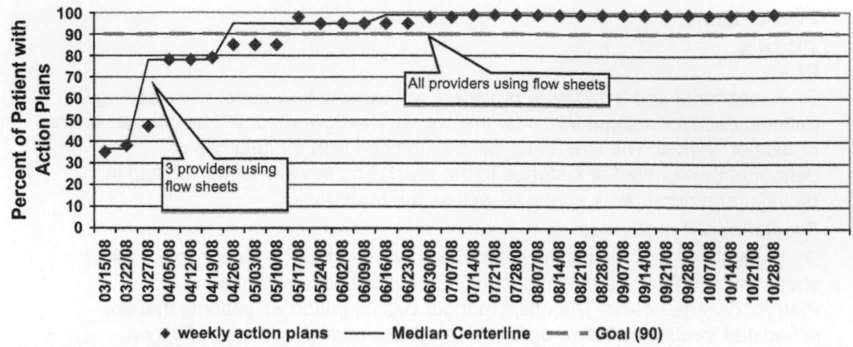

Fig. 14. Run Chart: asthma action plans.

SPREADING CHANGE

The basis for spread comes from Everett Rogers, *Diffusion of Innovations*. "Diffusion or spread, is the process by which and innovation is communicated through certain channels over time, among members of a social system."[29]

This work has become the landmark writing on spreading improvement. Spread of improvements in health care is different from spread of other innovations.[30] When making an assessment of improvements gained, several factors that impact spread must be considered.[29]

- Relative advantage over current practice
  - Compatibility with current practice
  - Simplicity of change
  - Trialability—test change with little investment (risk/cost/time)
  - Observability of change, results need to be seen by those adopting the change

The improvement must be communicated effectively, this may occur person to person, or through much broader channels.[14,29] Time is required for the spread of the improvement to occur. Spread does not occur all at once in a population, rather it is linear across people depending on their receptivity to change and the kind of evidence they need.

Spread may be more difficult in a group of independent practices versus an integrated health care system. Spread can occur at different levels: from one physician

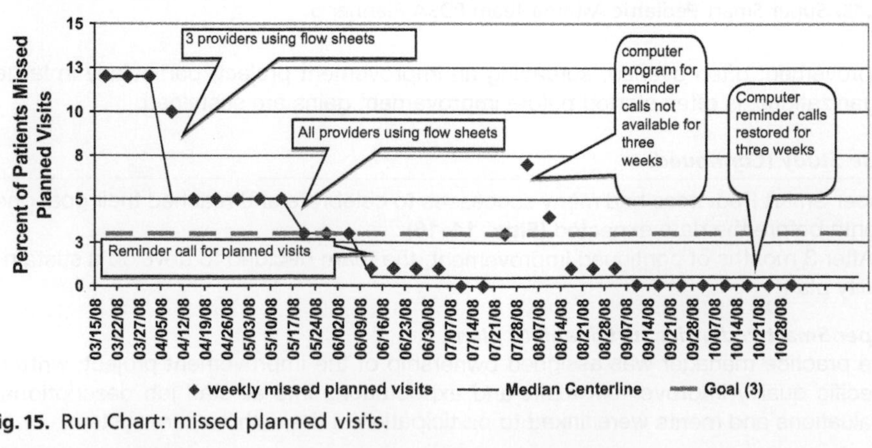

Fig. 15. Run Chart: missed planned visits.

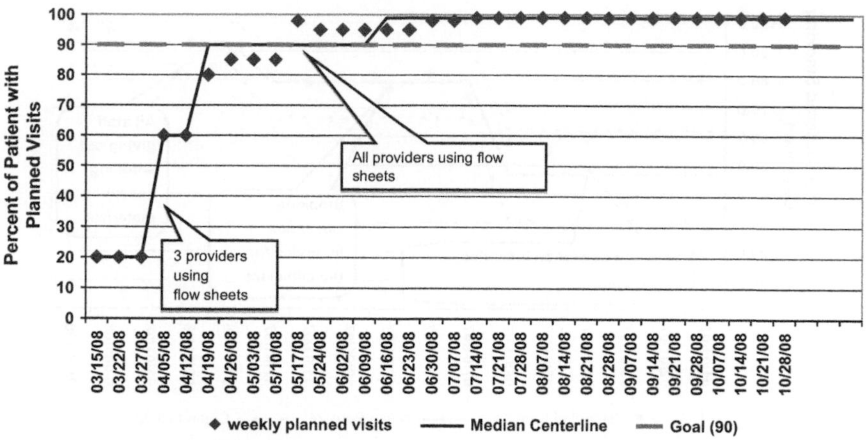

Fig. 16. Run Chart: planned visits.

in a practice to the entire practice; from one practice site to all the sites of that practice; or between organizations or hospitals. Each level will require different motivators and incentives. In health care, spreading improvements does depend on key individuals, the messenger, and the "stickiness" of the message. "*This change will save money for the health care system versus. this change will help get you home earlier.*"[30]

One critical success factor for spread is the role of leadership.[24,27,28]

There are islands of improvement in many organizations or practices, but without commitment from leadership most improvements fail to spread. For further information on spread, refer to the white paper "A Framework for Spread" is available on the IHI Web site, www.ihi.org, and can be used at all levels of spread.[31] Leaders must inspire and communicate a shared vision; model the way; challenge the current process, no longer accepting the status quo; enable others with resources, training, and time; and encourage the heart by celebrating the successes.[27]

In our case study, Super Smart Pediatrics' level of spread was from one physician to the entire practice. The leadership of the founding partner was a key element in the success. The changes made by the pilot physician and the team demonstrated improved asthma care. Measurement and feedback became a routine part of their monthly provider meetings.

Advanced Improvement Methods

Using the model of improvement, any quality initiative can be successful. Once an improvement project is under way, run charts can be converted to control charts and the process of improvement can be analyzed. Statistical control charts are frequently used in industry to monitor quality in production. This method can be readily extended to health care. These control charts illustrate if a process is in "control," or within limits of acceptable variation. Data points are plotted around a mean and confidence intervals are established. Monitoring the control chart of process can detect problems with a process or special causes that are outliers to a controlled process. There are numerous types of control charts, applicable to many health care indices. For example, charts can be used to monitor the proportion of patients with a particular disease and their outcome or rare events such a central line infections that are monitored by days between infections (**Fig. 17**).

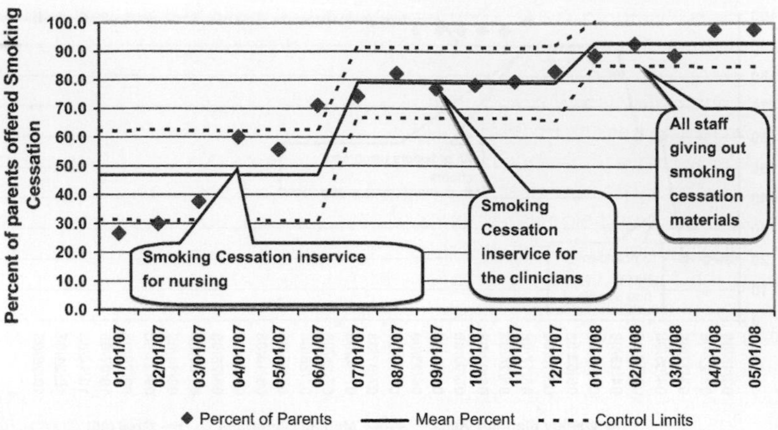

Fig. 17. Control Chart: parents offered Smoking Cessation.

Another advanced improvement methodology is planned experimentation. This method conducts a series of tests under varying conditions. This methodology is different from most familiar scientific experimentation. Under traditional experiments, factors under study are tightly controlled. Planned experimentation uses series of tests that are performed by changing levels of factors and background variables and observing the effects. In planned experimentation, factors are not controlled but are used in combination to see what effect is achieved. This type of experimentation is more oriented toward real world occurrences, because rarely can the health care system operate in perfectly controlled situations.

Case study (continued)

Super Smart Pediatrics has worked diligently on asthma care for their patients and has made impressive gains. They realized their patients with asthma were improved but continue to have exacerbations. They postulated that smoking by parents was having some impact on their patients' asthma and they wanted to encourage smoking cessation. After implementing several office changes they reached their goal for offering smoking cessation materials to most of their parents that smoked (**Fig. 17**). After several weeks and improvements, their process of delivery of smoking cessation

Response Variables:
- Smoking Cessation
- Asthma Exacerbation

		Quit Line Referral		No Quit Line Referral	
		Patch	Gum	Patch	Gum
Quit Smoking Contract	Follow up calls				
	No follow up calls				
No Quit smoking contract	Follow up calls				
	No follow up calls				

Fig. 18. Factorial design to improve asthma care by Smoking Cessation.

materials was noted to be in control. The practice noticed they were all offering different advice on smoking cessation and were unsure what method to endorse. They decided to do a small planned experiment using a factorial design in the practice offering many options and combinations for smoking cessation to determine which methods seem to have success in their practice (**Fig. 18**).

Using planned experimentation, several short test cycles can be performed in order to identify factors that may effect a particular outcome. Using factorial design, many factors can be studied simultaneously using only a few patients. As more knowledge is accumulated, more assumptions regarding the effect of the factors and their interaction can be made. Initial factorial results for Super Smart Pediatrics showed the combination of the quit line, patch and follow up calls were the most strongly associated with smoking cessation and lack of asthma exacerbation. As a factor, a smoking contract seemed not to have any impact. As more knowledge is obtained, the number of factors can be revised and their interaction studied further. For further information on Planned Experimentation and Factorial design, see the book *Quality Improvement through Planned Experimentation*.[32]

SUMMARY

The Model for Improvement is a rigorous and reasonable method for busy health care practitioners to use to improve patient outcomes. Use of this model requires practice for clinicians to be comfortable, however it is critical to develop the necessary skills to participate in quality improvement initiatives. The future of health care in the United States depends on every practitioner delivering safe, effective, and efficient care. The case study demonstrates how this methodology can be applied in any busy health care setting. Incorporating this approach to quality improvement into daily work will improve clinical outcomes, advance health care delivery and design. The techniques of planned experimentation can further an improvement project, refine interventions, gain further improvement, and standardize processes to ensure reliability. Further information, training, and resources can be found in the many organizations now dedicated to improving the quality of health care.

REFERENCES

1. Department of Health and Human Services Centers for Medicare and Medicaid Services national health expenditure data. Available at: www.cms.hhs.gove/nationahealthexpenddata. Accessed December, 2008.
2. Institute of Medicine. Crossing the quality chasm: a new health system for the 21st century. Washington, DC: National Academy Press; 2001.
3. Shortall SM, Bennett CL, Byck GR. Assessing the impact of continuous quality improvement on clinical practice: what it will take to accelerate progress. Milbank Q 1998;76(4):593–624.
4. Juran JM. Juran's quality handbook. 5th edition. New York: McGraw-Hill; 1999.
5. Deming WE. The new economics for industry, government, education. Cambridge (MA): Massachusetts Institute of Technology, Center for Advanced Engineering Study; 1993.
6. Crosby P. Completeness: quality for the 21st century. New York: Dutton; 1992.
7. Deming WE. Out of the crisis. Cambridge (MA): Massachusetts Institute of Technology; 1986.
8. Berwick DM, Godfrey AB, Roessner J. Curing health care: new strategies for quality improvement. 2nd edition. San Francisco (CA): Jossey-Bass; 2002.

9. Mangione-Smith R, Decristofaro AH, Setodji CM, et al. The quality of ambulatory care delivered to children in the United States. N Engl J Med 2007;357:1515–23, Number 15.
10. Accreditation Council for Graduate Medical Education: competencies of practice-based learning and improvement and systems-based practice, 2008. www.acgme.org/acwebsite/home.asp. Accessed Feb 10th 2009.
11. American Board of Medical Specialties; Maintenance of Certification. www.abms.org/MOC. Accessed on Feb 10th 2009.
12. Accreditation Council for continuing medical education: essential areas and elements for CME, 2007. www.accme.org. Accessed Feb 10th 2009.
13. Langley G, Nolan K, Nolan T, et al. The improvement guide: a practical approach to enhancing organizational performance. San Francisco (CA): Jossey-Bass Pub; 1996.
14. Stuart J, Randolph G, Taylor J, et al. QI 101: a toolbox for quality improvement, North Carolina Area Health Education Center, North Carolina Hospital Association Course delivered on February 2005.
15. Fraser SW. Rolling out your project: thirty five tools for healthcare improvers. UK: Kingsham Press; 2002.
16. Tufte ER. The visual display of quantitative information. 2nd edition. Cheshire (CT): Graphics Press; 2001.
17. Carey RG, Lloyd RC. Measuring quality improvement in healthcare: a guide to statistical process control applications. New York: American Society for Quality; 2001.
18. Shewhart WA. The economic control of quality of manufactured product (1931). Reprinted by. Milwaukee (WI): ASQC; 1980.
19. Sholtes PR, Joiner BL, Streibel BJ. The team handbook. 3rd edition. Madison (WI): Oriel Incorporated; 2003.
20. Leading Teams. Expert solutions to everyday challenges. Boston: Harvard Business School Press; 2006.
21. Lencioni PM. The five dysfunctions of a team. San Francisco (CA): Jossey-Bass; 2002.
22. Tague N. The quality toolbox. 2nd edition. Milwaukee (WI): ASG Quality Press; 2005.
23. Ransom SB, Joshi MS, Nash DB. The healthcare quality book; vision, strategy, and tools. Chicago (IL): Health Administration Press; 2005.
24. Juran JM. Juran on leadership and quality, an executive handbook. New York: The Free Press; 1989.
25. Smith D, Bell GD, Kilgo J, et al. The Carolina way: leadership lessons from a life in coaching. New York: Penguin Press; 2004.
26. Rockart JF. Chief executives define their own data needs. Harv Bus Rev 1979; 57(2):81–93. Year is correct.
27. Kotter JP. Leading change. Boston (MA): Harvard Business School Press; 1996.
28. Kouzes JM, Posner BZ. The leadership challenge. 3rd edition. San Francisco (CA): Jossey-Bass; 2003.
29. Rogers EM. Diffusion of innovations. 5th edition. New York: The Free Press; 2003.
30. Bodenheimer T. The science of spread: how innovations in care become the norm. Oakland CA: California Healthcare Foundation; Sept 2007.
31. Massoud MR, Nielsen GA, Nolan K, et al. A framework for spread: from local improvements to system-wide change. IHI Innovation Series white paper. Cambridge (MA): IHI; 2006.
32. Moen Ronald D, Nolan Thomas W, Provost Lloyd P. Quality improvement through planned experimentation. New York: McGraw Hill Books; Jan 1998.

Model for Improvement - Part Two: Measurement and Feedback for Quality Improvement Efforts

Greg Randolph, MD, MPH[a,b,c,*], Megan Esporas, MPH[a,b,c], Lloyd Provost, MS[d], Sara Massie, MPH[a,e], David G. Bundy, MD, MPH[f]

KEYWORDS

- Quality improvement • Measurement • Feedback
- Health care quality • Organizational performance

WHY THIS TOPIC AND WHY NOW?

The public, government, payors, and health care professionals increasingly agree that the quality of health care in the United States is in urgent need of improvement.[1] Measurement and feedback are fundamental aspects of quality improvement (QI); thus, national and local health care organizations are paying more attention to the selection and use of quality measures. To date, most of the attention and effort has been directed at developing measures at the national level to compare the performance of physicians and health care organizations, ie, what is referred to as national performance measures or standards. Little attention has been directed at measurement and feedback to guide QI projects, which represents the frontline of QI work.

[a] Department of Pediatrics, North Carolina Children's Center for Clinical Excellence, North Carolina Children's Hospital, CB# 7230, Chapel Hill, NC 27599-7230, USA
[b] Department of Pediatrics, University of North Carolina at Chapel Hill, CB# 7230, Chapel Hill, NC 27599-7230, USA
[c] Public Health Leadership Program, University of North Carolina at Chapel Hill, CB# 7230, Chapel Hill, NC 27599-7230, USA
[d] API –Austin, 115 East Fifth Street, Suite 300, Austin, TX 78701, USA
[e] Child Health Research Program, N.C. Translational and Clinical Sciences Institute, University of North Carolina at Chapel Hill, CB# 7230, Chapel Hill, NC 27599-7230, USA
[f] Department of Pediatrics, Johns Hopkins University School of Medicine, CMSC 2-121, 600 N Wolfe Street, Baltimore, MD, USA
* Corresponding author. Department of Pediatrics, University of North Carolina at Chapel Hill, CB# 7230, Chapel Hill, NC 27599 7230.
E-mail address: randolph@unc.edu (G. Randolph).

Pediatr Clin N Am 56 (2009) 779–798
doi:10.1016/j.pcl.2009.05.012

A substantial knowledge gap exists among health care professionals about how to select and use measures to guide QI projects.

In this article, the authors attempt to address this gap by providing evidence-based strategies from health care and other industries, augmented with practical examples from the authors' collective years of experience designing measurement and feedback strategies for frontline health care improvement teams. The article's focus is on the design and development of measurement and feedback strategies for QI projects in local settings, such as health care systems, hospitals, and clinical practices. The article also briefly discusses organizational measures, such as those included in dashboards or scorecards, which guide decision-making and priority setting for system-wide improvements.

The authors use a broad definition of quality measures, including not only clinical, but also satisfaction and financial measures, which are critical to health care organizations.[2] This focus aligns with the Institute of Medicine's definition of quality: "The degree to which health services for individuals and populations increase the likelihood of desired health outcomes and are consistent with current professional knowledge."[1]

This article does not address measurement for QI research, which is typically too slow, too expensive, too much of a data collection burden, and too complex for clinicians and staff engaged in QI efforts in local settings.[3] In addition, the authors do not address national performance standards used for quality assurance and accreditation, such as those established by the Joint Commission and the Center for Medicare & Medicaid Services (CMS). These types of data are regularly collected and reported by hospitals, but they are infrequently used, and rarely sufficient, to guide improvement projects. For example, accountability measures are insufficient for QI teams because they are designed for external groups (eg, payors and regulators for comparison or public reassurance) and typically focus on only outcomes, not processes, making it impossible to link any process changes to changes in outcomes.[3]

BACKGROUND AND HISTORY

The current use of measurement and feedback in health care QI originates from both medicine and industrial/business QI. In the mid-1800s, two pioneers, Florence Nightingale and John Snow, introduced the use of data in health care. Nightingale used measures of mortality to document the low quality of care injured British soldiers received during the Crimean War in Turkey. These data provided a compelling argument for reform by demonstrating that better sanitation in the field hospital could prevent deaths. Subsequent field hospital reforms reduced the death rate from greater than 40% to less than 5%. Nightingale also developed graphical methods to present data, clearly demonstrating that measures provide an organized way of approaching improvements in medical and surgical practice. Nightingale's achievements led to the adoption of formal record keeping in British hospitals.

Also in the mid-1800s, John Snow tracked the incidence and geographic location of cholera in London. By mapping the clusters of cholera cases, Snow provided convincing evidence that homes supplied by the Broad Street water pump had a much higher incidence of cholera than homes supplied with water from other sources. Despite the lack of a clear causal explanation (Snow postulated a "cholera poison"), the data demonstrating the pattern of disease outbreak was convincing enough to persuade authorities to remove the handle from the Broad Street pump, which greatly reduced the incidence of cholera.

The first American to publish on performance measurement in health care was Ernest Codman, a surgeon at Massachusetts General Hospital. Codman advocated for hospital reform and systematic health care performance assessment, and in 1910, proposed the "end result system of hospital standardization,"[4] whereby a hospital would track every patient it treated long enough to determine whether treatment was effective. By tracking patient outcomes, adverse events could be identified and changes could be made to improve the care of future patients.

Modern QI science originated in the 1920s and is often attributed to the work of Walter Shewhart of Bell Telephone Laboratories.[5] Shewhart's work made measurement fundamental to QI activities. He published principles and techniques basic to the use of measurement, including concepts of statistical control, operational definitions, and visual display of data. He postulated two rules for presentation of data:

1) Data has no meaning apart from its context.
2) Data contains both signal and noise; to be able to learn, one must separate the signal from the noise.

One of Shewhart's colleagues, W. Edwards Deming, an American statistician and physicist, popularized his ideas in the industrial production and management sector beginning in the 1940s.[6] Deming applied Shewhart's concepts in government and industry, described the Plan-Do-Study-Act (PDSA) Cycle as an approach to QI, and taught these concepts and methods to thousands of people, primarily in industries other than health care.

In the 1970s, physician Avedis Donabedian proposed a model for assessing health care quality, describing seven pillars of quality: efficacy, efficiency, optimality, acceptability, legitimacy, equity, and cost. He posited, "*Structure* is the environment in which health care is provided, *process* is the method by which health care is provided, and *outcome* as the result of the care provided."[7] Focusing on structure, process, and outcome, he emphasized the importance of measurement and evaluation of health care quality, assuring completeness and accuracy of medical records, observer bias, patient satisfaction, and cultural preferences for health care.

The 1980s saw an emphasis on outcome measurement in the health care literature as a result of variability in medical practice, evidence-based medicine, and regulatory agency requirements. During this time, physicians Paul Batalden and Don Berwick were among many health professionals who began to study and apply Deming's ideas to health care. In 1991, Batalden and Berwick helped form the Institute for Healthcare Improvement (IHI), which has led the application of QI science to health care in the United States and internationally.[8] The IHI has been influential in promoting the adoption of measurement and feedback to improve the quality of health care.

THE FUNDAMENTALS OF QUALITY IMPROVEMENT PROJECTS

A cornerstone of QI science is the concept of a system.[9–12] Systems are complex and dynamic, and a system's nature has a profound effect on the measurement and feedback of QI projects undertaken within it. A system is "an interdependent group of items, people, or processes working together toward a common purpose". A system's identification of its common purpose aligns its parts. Those parts are interdependent, meaning that all parts of the system, and all relations between and among those parts, can influence system performance. Thus, QI projects require multiple measures, at multiple levels, to understand the effects of change on the different components of the system, and on the system as a whole.

The aim of a QI project must guide the selection of project measures. Project measures must be specific to the processes and outcomes being targeted for improvement and specific to the local target audience (within a health care system, hospital, or clinical practice). Stakeholders, those who can affect or be affected by changes in a system, especially frontline clinicians and staff, should receive feedback on the QI effort to understand how the work is helping to achieve the improvement aim. This type of measurement and feedback answers the fundamental question, "Are the changes we are making (via QI projects) leading to improvement?"

In the following sections, the authors describe the process of developing, testing, and implementing measurement and feedback strategies in a typical QI project. **Fig. 1** presents a summary of this process, and a glossary of QI terms used in our discussion is available at the end of the article.

PURPOSES OF MEASUREMENT AND FEEDBACK

In QI, measurement and feedback are used to: (1) identify problems and establish baseline performance; (2) inform and guide QI projects; (3) select and test changes for improvement; and (4) assess progress toward organizational goals.

One strategy for evaluating performance and identifying potential areas for improvement is careful review of patient feedback from complaint systems, feedback forms, written and telephone surveys, and focus groups. Analysis of these data can help define gaps and create the case for conducting QI projects to address those gaps. Another mechanism for evaluating current performance is through continuous monitoring of system-level measures. For example, if performance gaps are detected in the hospital-wide infection rate, the leadership team can initiate a portfolio of improvement projects with the objective of improving this overall measure.

The second purpose of measurement in QI, which is the primary focus of this article, is to inform and guide QI projects. At the beginning of a QI project, a balanced set of measures, including outcome, process, and balancing measures, is established to support the team's aim statement (ie, the project goals).[13] These measures are then reported graphically (typically monthly) on run charts (see previous article on the model for improvement for an example of a run chart). Statistical process control charts[14] can also help monitor the progress of the project in accomplishing the improvement team's aim.

The third purpose of measurement and feedback is to develop, test, and implement changes. One common approach is to use PDSA cycles,[13] where each cycle is designed to answer specific questions about changes that the improvement team is testing. The "plan" step of the PDSA cycle involves specifying these questions and developing measures and a data collection plan to that will answer them. The previous article about the model for improvement shows several examples of PDSA cycles. Usually the measures used in these small tests of change are specific process measures related to the change(s) being evaluated in the cycle; sometimes, they are the project outcome measures stratified for the clinicians or patients who were part of the cycle. Often, the most important part of feedback in a PDSA cycle comes from qualitative data, particularly from comments staff or patients make about the changes being tested.

The fourth purpose of measurement is to assess progress toward organizational goals. The authors briefly discuss the use of organizational scorecards and dashboard in a later section of this article.

OPTIMAL ATTRIBUTES OF QUALITY IMPROVEMENT MEASURES

Selecting measures for QI projects can be challenging. Fortunately, there is increasing knowledge and experience to help improvement teams select useful measures. In this section, the authors describe the most important attributes of QI measures based on

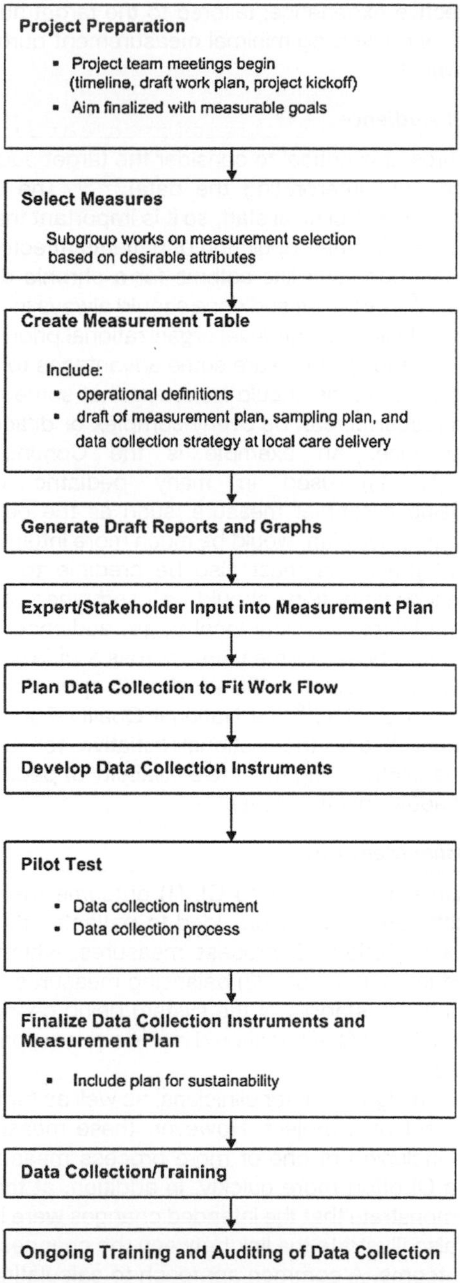

Fig. 1. Flow chart demonstrating the stages of development, testing, and implementation of a measurement and feedback plan during a typical QI project.

the literature and collective experience: tailored to the target audience, comprehensive, carefully defined, and involving minimal measurement burden. These attributes are summarized in **Table 1**.

Tailoring to the Target Audience

When selecting measures, it is critical to consider the target audience (ie, those who will be viewing, using, and interpreting the data).[15–17] The target audience will invariably include clinicians and clinical staff, so it is important that measures address high-impact clinical targets for the population of patients affected by the project (eg, using a common chronic condition like asthma for a chronic disease management improvement project).[15,16] The target audience should always include system leaders; therefore, measures should link to high-level organizational priorities such as strategic and financial goals.[16,17] Although there are some advantages to borrowing measures used by peer organizations, teams should be aware that some measures, especially those originating from research, can be overly complex or difficult to understand for the local target audience. An example is the Continuity of Care index ($coc = (\Sigma_{j=1}^{8} n_j^2 - N)/N(N-1)$) used in many pediatric continuity of care research studies.[18] Using a simpler measure, such as the percentage of patients seen by their primary care physician, would be much more intuitive for most clinicians.

Quality improvement measures must also be credible to the target audience. Measures from national organizations should be used when applicable, as long as they align well with the interests of the local target audience. Good resources for publicly available, evidence-based QI measures across a wide variety of clinical topics include the National Quality Measures Clearinghouse sponsored by the Agency for Healthcare Research and Quality,[16] the National Quality Forum,[19] the Institute for Healthcare Improvement,[20] and the National Initiative for Children's Healthcare Quality.[21] However, it is worth noting that the availability of pediatric-specific national measures lags that of adult-specific measures.

Including Comprehensive Measures

Three types of measures are essential to QI: (1) outcome measures, or those that address how the health care services provided to patients affect their health, functional status, and/or satisfaction; (2) process measures, which address the health care services provided to patients; and (3) balancing measures, which evaluate unintended consequences or the stability of the system being changed in the project. A balanced set of measures for a QI effort should include at least one outcome, process, and balancing measure.[16,17,22]

Outcome measures are significant for clinicians, as well as for leaders, who want to know the ultimate impact of a project. However, these measures can be slow to change over time, so inclusion of one or more process measures allows the team to see the effects of a QI effort more quickly. In addition, at the end of the project, process measures demonstrate that the intended changes were indeed implemented.

Process measures also illustrate the link between the changes made to the system and changes in the outcome. A common approach to calculating improvement is by an item-by-item measurement, such as the proportion of patients who receive each individual component of a health care service. Another approach, all-or-none measurement, is potentially advantageous in some situations. In this approach, the numerator is the number of patients who receive all of the measured components and the denominator is the total number of patients. All-or-none measures are ideal for a process that includes a series of critical steps, all of which must be completed to produce desirable outcomes, such as the process of inserting a central line.[23] If all-or-none measurement is not appropriate, other types of composite measurement can be used.[24]

Any improvement project, which by definition involves making changes to one or more processes, can have unintended consequences. Balancing measures assess these potential unintended consequences and assure teams that they have indeed improved their overall system, rather than optimizing one part of the system at the expense of another.[17] Balancing measures can also be important in helping address the concerns of those who are resistant to the proposed changes. For example, in a project to improve immunization delivery in a private pediatric practice, a balancing measure might be the effect of changes to this high-volume process on office visit wait times.

Carefully Defining Measures

It is important to define measures in such a way that the baseline levels (ie, the level of performance before the QI project starts) are neither too high (difficult to detect improvement) nor too low (may be deflating or seem implausible to the target audience). Measures must also be responsive (show improvement in a timely fashion) to the planned changes in the system, and minimize the impact of variation unrelated to process changes, thereby improving the "signal-to-noise ratio" for detecting improvements to the system.[23,25] For example, a difference in wait times on Mondays versus Wednesdays related to differences in patient volumes on those days would be "noise" in an initiative attempting to lower overall wait times.

During a QI project, a measure's responsiveness to detecting change is affected by the time between piloting a change on a small scale and having the change fully implemented, as well as the time to have the change affect a patient's care and the time to sampling the affected patients. The last issue is particularly important in pediatrics because researchers often sample by age group (eg, sampling 24-month to 30-month olds for immunization status for vaccines given between 0 to 15 months). Thus, months may elapse between the introduction of changes and the measurement of their effects. Optimizing how a measure is defined and sampled can often minimize these delays. For example, changing a measure's denominator to "all children seen in the past month with asthma" rather than "all children seen in the past quarter with asthma" would allow for more rapid detection of the results of a change to asthma care processes.

Minimizing Measurement Burden

Finally, and most importantly, teams should minimize the burden of measurement for their QI project.[17,25,26] Effort spent creating, collecting, displaying, analyzing, and interpreting data, although absolutely critical to improvement, is nonetheless time taken away from making changes to the system. The measurement burden is much like the burden of carrying water on a hike up a mountain: hikers must carry water on the way to the top, but carrying too much water will slow them down unnecessarily, or worse, tire them to the point of not being able to reach the top at all. A small, balanced set of five to eight measures will usually suffice for most improvement projects. **Table 1** lists several strategies to minimize the burden of measurement, such as using data that already exist in your organization.

Putting it All Together: A Balancing Act

Measurement selection involves making tradeoffs among these desirable measure attributes. For example, a measure that is more responsive to changes in a system, such as measuring immunizations by 18 months rather than by 24 months, may

Table 1
Key attributes of measures to support QI projects

Measure Attributes	Considerations
Tailored to the target audience	
Meaningful, important and relevant to target audience	Address areas with substantial effect on the health of population High burden of illness, high volume, problem-prone process, poor quality and/or high variation Relevance to financial and strategic issues
Understandable to target audience	Avoid unnecessary complexity
Credible for target audience	Use nationally recognized practice guidelines when possible If using nationally recognized practice guidelines, measures should account for patient preferences and clinician judgment
Comprehensive (ie, includes outcome, process, and balancing measures)	
Outcome measures	Outcome measures address how the health care services provided to patients affect their health, functional status, and/or satisfaction
Process measures	Process measures address the health care services provided to patients Consider all or none measures
Balancing measures	Balancing measures address potential unintended consequences of changes to processes
Carefully defined	
Definition assures baseline levels are neither too high nor too low	If too high, difficult to show improvement If too low, may be discouraging or cause disbelief
Definition assures measures are responsive to changes in the system	Minimize delay between improvements and measuring the effects of improvements

Definition minimizes the impact of variation	Reduce known causes of variation through stratification (eg, time of day, location/unit, staff or clinicians) to allow for more sensitivity in detecting improvement Seasonal variation - avoid measures with this when possible or handle with rolling averages or year over year comparisons
Measurement burden minimized	
A small, balanced set of measures	Strive for a set of measures that describes a system as much as possible with as few measures as possible Use or adapt existing measures when possible
Data collection built into the flow of work	Understand work flow (eg, through process mapping) and find best place to collect data in work flow and best person(s) to collect Use existing data where possible
Small sample sizes	20–40 observations when collected frequently are often adequate (eg, medical record abstraction on 25 patients collected monthly)
Simple data collection instruments and methods	Use simple and quick instruments like check sheets, checklists Leverage technology (eg, email surveys, scannable forms)

Data from Refs. [2,16,17,22,23].

have a very low baseline level in a particular practice. Improvement teams are well served if they are aware of these attributes and can weigh these tradeoffs as they strive to create useful, though never perfect, measures for their project. **Table 2** presents an example of one project team's measure set to illustrate a product of this balancing act.

THE MEASUREMENT DEVELOPMENT PROCESS

After identifying robust candidate measures with the attributes described above, it is time to commence the measurement development process. The process of measurement development involves establishing operational definitions, collecting data, pilot testing, establishing baselines, and setting goals. During this process, it is also important to plan for sustainability after the project is complete. The next section describes the measurement development process in detail.

Establishing Operational Definitions

The first step of the measurement development is establishing operational definitions. Well-intentioned measures often fail to yield actionable information because of a lack of clear operational definitions.[6] For example, a QI team aiming to improve the emergency department (ED) care of children with pneumonia might select the measure: "Percentage of children with pneumonia who receive their first dose of antibiotics within four hours of arrival to the ED." Operational definitions for this measure would need to include, at a minimum, how target children are defined (eg, age restrictions, chronic disease exclusions); how the presence of pneumonia is defined (eg, clinical versus radiologic versus administrative [eg, billing] diagnosis); and how children are accounted for if they received antibiotics before their arrival in the ED or left the ED in less than four hours.

Table 2
Example of project measurement set used by the UNC Division of Pediatric Gastroenterology for improving care for children with inflammatory bowel diseases

Measure	Project Goal
Process measures	
% patients seen this month with disease activity recorded	95%
% patients seen this month with active disease that have a documented plan to escalate therapy	95%
% patients seen this month with classified steroid status	95%
% chronic steroid users (per clinician) seen this month with documented plan for tapering (± maintenance medication)	95%
% patients seen this month with growth and nutritional status classified at visit	95%
% patients seen this month classified as "at risk" or "failure" for nutrition with documented intervention	95%
Outcome measures	
% of patients with active disease (mild, moderate, severe) measured by physician global assessment this month	< 20%
% patients classified as satisfactory growth status	95%
Balancing measure	
Waiting time	N/A

When defining measures, many QI teams have found it helpful to create a table that summarizes the relevant features of each measure. Measure name, numerator, denominator, source, frequency of collection, and inclusion and exclusion criteria are a minimal set of features, but more detailed specification is often necessary. In addition to defining individual measures, it is important to consider whether to track measures independently (eg, whether each of five steps in a ventilator care bundle were performed daily) or in an all-or-none fashion (eg, whether all five steps in the ventilator care bundle were performed daily), as stated earlier.[10]

Collecting Data

A critical step in developing a data collection strategy is careful consideration of the utility and accessibility of existing data sources. In many health care settings, the electronic medical record (EMR) serves as a valuable source of data. For example, an immunization improvement effort might involve querying the EMR monthly to assess the immunization status for all children of a certain age. These electronic systems are often a robust source of data, but they can be difficult to access. Using an EMR can be a challenge unless improvement team members have both administrative access to the data and the technological expertise required to extract and analyze the data.

Another strategy involves analyzing data collected in an existing patient registry. For example, patient registries of children with chronic health conditions can be used to monitor performance on outcome, process, and even balancing measures. One advantage of registry data is that they typically provide information on the entire population of interest (eg, all children with sickle cell disease seen in a hematology clinic). A disadvantage of registry data is that data specifications are typically already in place before the initiation of an improvement project, limiting the scope of what can be tracked to what already exists in the registry.

Regardless of the means of data collection, it is essential to develop a collection strategy that yields a maximal quality of actionable data with a minimal amount of extra effort. Data collected for other purposes (eg, clinic billing) can often be used in improvement efforts, and may involve substantially less time and effort to collect than data collected specifically for a QI project. Nonetheless, it is often worth comparing a small sample of billing data with more robust data sources (eg, EMR) to ensure that billing data accurately reflect the results they are intended to measure. For example, a review of 20 visits for which the billing data indicate a principal diagnosis code of bronchiolitis could be compared with EMR notes from each of the 20 visits to confirm the accuracy of the billing data as a means of identifying bronchiolitis visits.

Pilot Testing

Measures that appear conceptually strong often fail in the implementation process. For example, using a validated questionnaire is a logical approach to measuring and tracking patient satisfaction; however, if patient flow in the setting of interest is such that patients rarely have time to complete the survey, data collection will be problematic. By pilot testing measures and the data collection process on a small scale, improvement teams can determine whether the measurement system functions as planned. Shortening the survey, administering it at a different point in the visit, conducting it as an interview instead of a survey, or mailing it to patients might all be reasonable alternatives. These strategies would also need to be pilot tested to directly observe potential barriers to their effectiveness. Often, correctable errors (eg, "which provider did you see today?" inadvertently omitted from the patient satisfaction survey) can be identified after pilot testing the survey with a few patients.

Establishing Baselines and Setting Goals

Establishing baseline performance and setting performance goals are essential steps in developing the measurement strategy. In simple terms, measuring baseline performance answers the question, "where are we now?" and setting a goal establishes "where do we want to go and how soon do we want to get there?" The period of baseline measurement should be long enough to provide convincing data to recipients but short enough to avoid impeding initiation of QI efforts.

In the authors' experience, QI efforts are frequently derailed by attempts to collect "perfect" baseline data when more concise (or approximate) data would suffice. Depending on the frequency of the events being measured, prospective versus retrospective baseline data collection may be considered. For example, in a project aimed at reducing catheter-associated bloodstream infections in a pediatric intensive care unit (ICU), historical (ie, retrospective) data from the preceding year may be the best approach for establishing an accurate baseline, given the rarity of the event. In contrast, a 1-week, prospective hand-washing observation period may provide sufficient baseline data for a hand-hygiene QI project.

Goal setting is typically focused on process and outcome measures and can be conceptualized in several ways. First, QI teams can set absolute goals (eg, "90% receiving a preventive service"), which may be consistent with external standards (such as Healthy People 2010). Absolute goals may help team members see linkages between their local efforts and larger regional and national efforts to improve care, as well as compare their performance directly against a standardized benchmark. Some teams choose to set across-the-board, though arbitrary, absolute goals for their process measures (eg, "95% completion of all processes") while linking absolute goals for outcome measures to national benchmarks. Second, teams can set goals relative to baseline performance (eg, "reduce the time required to process refill prescription requests by 50%"). This can be particularly effective when baseline performance is poor. When the outcomes being measured are rare (eg, "pediatric codes outside the ICU"), goals can be conceptualized in terms of time between events (eg, "reach 6 months with no pediatric codes outside the ICU"). Finally, goals can be a combination of the above strategies, as well as staged over time (eg, "reduce wait time for well child appointments to half of present wait time within 6 months, and to less than 2 days within 12 months"). In the authors' experience, whether they are staged or not, it is usually preferable to use absolute goals rather than relative goals because they are more tangible and meaningful to teams and stakeholders.

Planning for Sustainability

Sustainability is a key component of measurement development, and should be considered from the earliest phases. Quality improvement efforts that are sustained over long periods are usually those in which sustainability is considered early in the program's design and implementation, including the measurement strategy. What may seem like a reasonable measurement strategy when viewed in the lifespan of a QI project (eg, "review 10 medical records each week to determine the percentage of children receiving recommended hemoglobin screening") may seem burdensome when extended beyond the project period. If data collection is considered "extra" work to the involved staff or is performed by an external research team or a team that will not operate at the completion the project, long-term sustainability of the measurement process will be unlikely. Conversely, if data collection is integrated into the everyday responsibilities of frontline staff, the likelihood of sustained data collection will increase. Successful teams often reduce the frequency of measurement (eg, from weekly to monthly or monthly to quarterly) after goal performance has been reached, as well as strive to "hard-wire" data collection into standard practice operations. The authors provide further discussion about implementing the sustainability plan later in this article.

PRINCIPLES OF QUALITY IMPROVEMENT FEEDBACK

Quality improvement measures not only document progress in QI efforts but also serve as strong motivators for improvement. However, in order for these data to resonate with and motivate frontline clinicians and staff, both the message and the messenger must be thoughtfully considered. Bradley and colleagues[27] recently identified seven themes essential to effective feedback of data in QI projects (**Box 1**). Six of the seven themes relate directly to the message of the data feedback, and the remaining theme relates to the messenger.

The Message: Is it Believable?

The importance of the perceived validity of the feedback is highlighted in three themes: (1) data must be viewed as valid to motivate change; (2) it takes time to develop data credibility; and (3) the source and timeliness of data feedback are critical to perceived validity. Discharge diagnosis codes, for example, can be an excellent means of identifying cases of a given illness in administrative data. However, if clinicians are skeptical about the accuracy of discharge diagnosis coding, inferences drawn from such data may garner little traction for improvement. Likewise, year-old data leave room for clinicians to assert, "things have changed since then," whereas real-time data are more difficult to dismiss.

The Message: Is it in the Proper Context and can it be Sustained?

As previously discussed, feedback can be framed in ways that enhance its effectiveness. Comparison of local data to national or other benchmarks can provide motivation for improvement. Similarly, clinician-level data documenting each individual's performance in relation to the group's performance can be valuable, though considerable care is needed to avoid creating a punitive atmosphere. Lastly, just as the sustainability of any measurement strategy must be considered in its development, the sustainability of the feedback system is equally important and must be formally integrated into the standard operating procedure of an organization if it is to persist.

Box 1
Key themes for effective quality improvement measurement feedback

Data must be perceived by [clinicians] as valid to motivate change

It takes time to develop the credibility of data within [an organization]

The source and timeliness of data are critical to perceived validity

Benchmarking improves the meaningfulness of the data feedback

[Clinician] leaders can enhance the effectiveness of data feedback

Data feedback that profiles an individual [clinician's] practices can be effective but may be perceived as punitive

Data feedback must persist to sustain improved performance

Data from Bradley EH, Holmboe ES, Mattera JA, et al. Data feedback efforts in quality improvement: lessons learned from US hospitals. Qual Saf Health Care 2004;13(1):26–31.

The Message: Does it Effectively Convey the Underlying Information?

Valid and actionable data are most effective when they are presented to frontline users in visually compelling ways.[28,29] A complex table of data may provide all the necessary information, but this display of data may make it difficult to determine whether improvements are being made. In contrast, an annotated run chart, which plots data over time, can more readily provide answers to questions such as, "how far have we progressed toward our goal?", "how much further do we have to go?", "have we sustained our gains?" and "what change, if any, resulted in an improvement?" Annotating run charts to indicate key events (eg, time the project team started or new change introduced) and applying statistical process control limits to distinguish random (noise) from nonrandom variation (signal) add useful detail to the visual display of performance data. These enhancements help distinguish true changes in processes or outcomes from the expected variation seen in stable systems over time.

The Messenger

Respected leaders, often described as "champions," are frequently the most effective messengers for delivering performance data to frontline clinicians and staff.[27,30] For example, when physician leaders provide feedback to other physicians, it provides validation that the data came from colleagues with shared interests in promoting, as well as shared barriers to providing, optimal clinical care. In contrast, when data originate from an external body, such as a QI department or payer, clinicians may be more likely to view the data as invalid, punitive, or simply irrelevant. The importance of identifying messengers who can convey the feedback in honest and motivational ways cannot be overstated and is consistent with the literature on the effectiveness of academic detailing (the use of clinical expert outreach visits to physician practices).[31]

ASSURING SUSTAINABILITY OF ONGOING MEASUREMENT

Achieving sustainability of QI projects depends on continuing to measure key processes and outcomes. For QI teams, measurement provides a source of learning during implementation and a method of maintenance after implementation. Some of the measures developed and used in testing and implementation should be considered for ongoing use in the organization when the QI team disbands. However, the measures may be reported and analyzed less frequently during this ongoing monitoring phase. Measuring over time allows an organization to determine whether it is continuing to get the desired results and whether those results can be predicted to continue in the future. This process addresses the question, "Is there a need to update the process or make new changes?"

To prepare for this continued use of key measures, the QI team should consider strategies such as these:

- Incorporate measurement with another existing work activity;
- Use existing data collection systems or develop easy-to-use data collection forms;
- Build measurement into EMRs, registries, or other data systems so that it is easy for administrative staff and clinicians to use as part of usual clinical care;
- Clearly define roles and responsibilities for ongoing data collection after the QI project is complete;
- Set aside time to review data with those who collect it before completion of the QI project. This will help everyone understand how the data is being used, and provide reinforcement for their efforts.

Although run charts of the key measures are effective for learning during an improvement project, plotting key measures on a statistical process control chart is more useful for maintaining a change. These charts provide signals to detect whether the process is beginning to deteriorate (eg, staff reverts to practices used before the improvements were made). In addition, control charts allow teams to predict future expected performance. Statistical process control charts can be maintained for the key measures used in any improvement effort. **Fig. 2** shows an example of a control chart[32] for a measure of harm during hospital admission. These maintenance charts will provide signals if the process ever begins to deteriorate, or, in this example, if data exceeds the upper control limit.

MEASUREMENT FOR SUPPORTING ORGANIZATIONAL PERFORMANCE

Just as measures are used to identify performance gaps and set priorities for improvement at the project level, health care organizations, including clinical practices, networks, hospitals, and health systems, also need a balanced set of system-level measures to track progress toward their strategic goals. Measures guide the direction and focus of QI efforts across the organization and should complement other system-level performance measures (eg, finance, use).[33] Collectively, this set of measures should serve as both a gauge of current performance and as input into the future direction of the organization.[34] Leaders and governing boards need to be actively involved in selecting and developing a dashboard of quality measures that reflects the culture and mission of their organization.[30,35] To improve quality at the system-level, senior leadership needs to be committed and accountable to improving (or maintaining) performance on these measures, and prepared to build the will needed to drive change throughout the organization.[30,36]

Organizational performance measures should help leaders understand their progress toward accomplishing their mission. Leadership should identify a limited set of approximately 10 to 20 high-level measures that are focused on what the organization

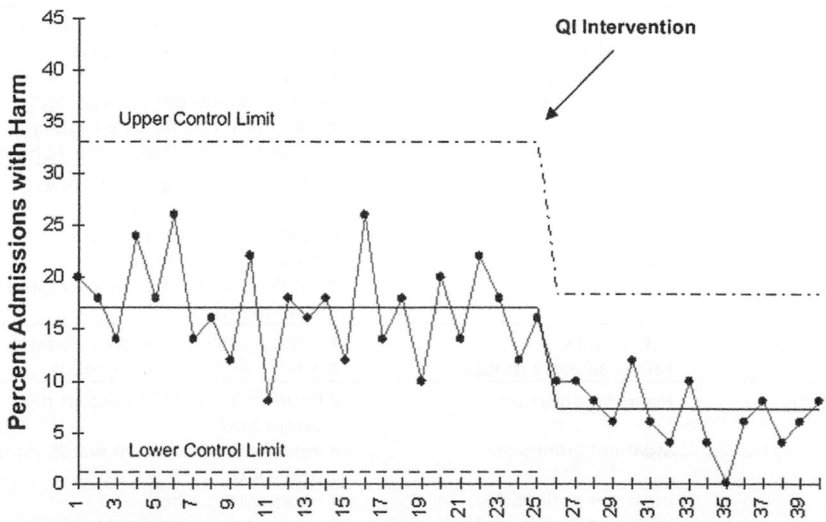

Fig. 2. Statistical process control chart showing an improved process that can be monitored for sustainability. The chart has an annotation marking the beginning of the QI intervention.

wants to accomplish and are balanced from the perspective of organization stakeholders. Dashboard measures should endure year to year; however, the strategic priorities of the organization will often focus on one or two measures each year.

This dashboard of measures should include operational definitions that can be easily understood at all levels of the organization, from the leadership to front-line clinicians and staff (see **Table 3** for an example of a children's hospital dashboard). Like project measurement, organizational measurement must be timely (no more than a month's lag between data and review) and it should not require excessive data collection, which hinders sustainability. The data should be extracted and graphed to show patterns and trends so that improvements can be tracked over time.[30,37] Following these principles ensures that leaders and the governing board of the health care system can continuously monitor and respond to data, and keep the organization moving toward meeting its goals.

Another question that system-level performance measures should help to answer is: "How do we compare with others?" Unlike the mission question stated above, which should be asked at every leadership and board meeting, this question should be addressed annually when reevaluating the organization's strategic goals.[38] Benchmarking against peer organizations can help determine how the system is comparatively performing and it can identify opportunities for learning from other best practices.[37]

Table 3
An example of a children's hospital dashboard, which tracks the organization's performance.

Strategic Category	Measure	Operational Definition
People	New hire nursing turnover	% nurses leaving within 12 months of hire
	Faculty overall satisfaction	% rating "very good"
	Staff overall satisfaction	% rating "very good"
Service	Patient/family overall satisfaction	% recommending UNC
Clinical Quality	Adverse events	Adverse drug events per 1000 doses
	Hospital associated infections	# infections per 1000 pt days
	Raw mortality	# inpatient deaths
	Cardiac arrests	# cardiac arrests per 1000 pt days
	Chronic care management	# patients in chronic care registry
	Readmission rate	# patients readmitted within 72 hours
Finance	Payor mix	% distribution of gross revenues across insurance plans
	Gross charges	Actual cash collection on bills
	Fundraising	Amount of gifts per year
	RVU	# relative value units (inpatient and outpatient)
Innovation	Publications	# faculty publications per quarter
	Family advisory groups	# active family advisory groups
Growth	Hours on diversion	# hours PICU unable to accept new admissions
	Inpatient admissions	# inpatients admitted to wards, PICU and NICU
	Inpatient patient days	# inpatients in a bed
	Inpatient length of stay	Average # days patients stay in hospital

Courtesy of North Carolina Children's Hospital, Chapel Hill, NC; with permission.

Tracking organizational performance on quality measures is increasingly relevant to the financial security of practices, networks, hospitals, and health systems. These measures are being incorporated into federal data reporting standards, such as The Joint Commission and the CMS Core Measures. CMS will link hospital reimbursement to organizations' performance on the core measures, a strategy known as "pay for performance," an approach that numerous payors have adopted or will soon adopt.[39,40]

SUMMARY

Measurement and feedback are fundamental aspects of QI. The authors have described a pragmatic approach to measurement and feedback for QI efforts in local health care settings, including hospitals and clinical practices. The authors included evidence-based strategies from health care and other industries, augmented by their collective practical experience designing measurement and feedback strategies. The authors also described an approach to developing, testing, and implementing measurement and feedback strategies during the stages of a typical QI project.

The process as described here will assist health care professionals in knowing how to measure the effects of their QI projects and how to use these data to improve care. Health care professionals will need to understand and know how to apply the principles that are summarized in this article in order for hospitals and clinical practices to meet the growing demand to dramatically improve their performance.

ACKNOWLEDGMENTS

The authors are grateful for the thoughtful review and feedback provided by John B. Anderson, MD, MPH; Virginia (Ginna) Crowe, RN, EdD; Michael Steiner, MD; Jayne M. Stuart, MPH; and Jane Taylor, EdD.

REFERENCES

1. Institute of Medicine. Crossing the quality chasm: a new health system for the 21st century. Washington, DC: National Academy Press; 2001.
2. Nelson EC, Mohr JJ, Batalden PB, et al. Improving health care, part 1: the clinical value compass. Jt Comm J Qual Improv 1996;22:243–58.
3. Solberg LL, Mosser G, McDonald S. The three faces of performance measursmement: improvement, accountability and research. Jt Comm J Qual Improv 1997; 23(3):135–47.
4. Codman EA. A study in hospital efficiency (1917). Reprinted by the Joint Commission on Accreditation of Healthcare Organizations. Illinois: Oakbrook Terrace; 1996.
5. Shewhart WA. The economic control of quality of manufactured product (1931). Milwaukee (WI): Reprinted by ASQC; 1980.
6. Deming WE. Out of the crisis. Cambridge (MA): Massachusetts Institute of Technology; 1986.
7. Donabedian A, Bashshur R. An introduction to quality assurance in health care. New York: Oxford University Press; 2003.
8. Kenney C. The best practice: how the new quality movement is transforming medicine. New York: Public Affairs; 2008.
9. Forrester J. Principles of systems. Cambridge (MA): Productivity Press; 1986.
10. Nolan TW. Understanding medical systems. Annals of Internal Medicine 1998; 128(4):293–8.

11. Deming WE. The new economics for industry, government, and education. 2nd edition. Cambridge (MA): Massachusetts Institute of Technology; 1994. p. 92–115.
12. Senge P. The fifth discipline: the art & practice of the learning organization. New York: Doubleday; 1994.
13. Langley G, Nolan K, Nolan T, et al. The improvement guide: a practical approach to enhancing organizational performance. San Francisco (CA): Jossey-Bass Pub; 1996.
14. Shewhart WA. In: Deming WE, editor. Statistical method from the viewpoint of quality control (1939). New York: Dover Press; 1986. p. 1–15.
15. Joint Commission on Accreditation of Health Care Organizations. Attributes of core performance measures and associated evaluation criteria. 2008. Available at: http://www.jointcommission.org/PerformanceMeasurement/PerformanceMeasurement/. Accessed November 18, 2008.
16. NQMC Agency for Healthcare Research and Quality. National quality measures clearinghouse. 2008. Available at: http://www.qualitymeasures.ahrq.gov/. Accessed November 18, 2008.
17. Association of Public Health Observatories. The good indicators guide: understanding how to use and choose indicators. NHS Institute for Innovation and Improvement. 2008. Available at: http://www.apho.org.uk/resource/item.aspx?RID=44584. Accessed November 18, 2008.
18. Christakis DA, Wright JA, Zimmerman FJ, et al. Continuity of care is associated with well-coordinated care. Ambul Pediatr 2003;3(2):82–6.
19. National Quality Forum. 2008. Available at: http://www.qualityforum.org/. Accessed November 18, 2008.
20. Institute for Healthcare Improvement. 2008. Available at: http://www.ihi.org. Accessed November 18, 2008.
21. National Initiative for Children's Healthcare Quality. 2008. Available at: http://www.nichq.org. Accessed November 18, 2008.
22. American Academy of Pediatrics Steering Committee on Quality Improvement and Management and Committee on Practice and Ambulatory Medicine. Principles for the development and use of quality measures. Policy statement. Pediatrics 2008;121:411–8.
23. Nolan T, Berwick DM. All-or-none measurement raises the bar on performance. JAMA 2006;295(10):1168–70.
24. Reeves D, Campbell S, Adams J, et al. Combining multiple indicators of clinical quality: an evaluation of different analytic approaches. Med Care 2007;45(6):489–96.
25. Nelson EC, Splaine ME, Plume SK, et al. Good measurement for good improvement work. Qual Manag Health Care 2004;13(1):1–16.
26. Pronovost PJ, Nolan T, Zeger S, et al. How can clinicians measure safety and quality in acute care? Lancet 2004;363:1061–7.
27. Bradley EH, Holmboe ES, Mattera JA, et al. Data feedback efforts in quality improvement: lessons learned from US hospitals. Qual Saf Health Care 2004;13(1):26–31.
28. Carey RG, Lloyd RC. Measuring quality improvement in healthcare: a guide to statistical process control application. Wisconsin: Quality Press; 2001. p. 43–150.
29. Tufte ER. The visual display of quantitative information. 2nd edition. Cheshire (CT): Graphics Press; 2001.
30. Denham CR. Leaders need dashboards, dashboards need leaders. J Patient Saf 2006;2(1):45–53.

31. O'Brien MA, Rogers S, Jamtvedt G, et al. Educational outreach visits: effects on professional practice and health care outcomes. Cochrane Database Syst Rev 2007;4:CD000409. DOI: 10.1002/14651858.
32. Lloyd R. Quality health care: a guide to developing and using indicators. Boston: Jones & Bartlett Publishers; 2004.
33. Martin LA, Nelson EC, Lloyd RC, et al. Whole system measures. IHI innovation series white paper. Cambridge (MA): Institute for Healthcare Improvement; 2007.
34. Provost L, Leddick S. How to take multiple measures to get a complete picture of organizational performance. Natl Prod Rev 1993;12(4):477–90.
35. Kroch E, Vaughn T, Koepke M, et al. Hospital boards and quality dashboards. J Patient Saf 2006;2(1):10–9.
36. Conway J. Getting boards on board: engaging governing boards in quality and safety. Jt Comm J Qual Patient Saf 2008;34(4):214–20.
37. Reinertsen JL, Pugh MD, Bisognano M. Institute for Healthcare Improvement. IHI innovation series. Seven leadership leverage points for organization-level improvement in health care. Cambridge (MA): Institute for Healthcare Improvement; 2005.
38. Reinertsen JL. From the top: getting the board on board. IHI conference: boards, dashboards, and data. Boston. 2007. Available at: http://www.ihi.org/IHI/Topics/LeadingSystemImprovement/Leadership/EmergingContent/BoardsDashboardsData.htm. Accessed November 10, 2008.
39. The Joint Commission. Performance measurement initiatives. Available at: http://www.jointcommission.org/PerformanceMeasurement/PerformanceMeasurement/default.htm. Accessed November 10, 2008.
40. Kaiser Daily Health Policy Report. Medicare stops paying for 10 reasonably preventable medical errors. Available at: http://www.kaisernetwork.org/daily_reports/rep_index.cfm?hint=3&;DR_ID=54758. Accessed October 1, 2008.

GLOSSARY

Balanced set of measures: A set of measures which, taken together, reflect as much of a system as possible without duplication, overlap or gaps.[17]

Benchmark: An externally agreed-upon comparator to compare performance between similar organizations or systems.[17]

Composite indicator: An aggregation of numerous indicators that aims to give a one-figure indicator in order to summarize measures further.

Control charts: A graphical tool for displaying the results of statistical process control.

Control limits: Define the area representing random (also called "common cause") variation on either side of the centerline, plotted on a control chart.

Dashboard: A tool used for collecting and reporting data on system-level measures that demonstrate the overall quality of a health system over time. Dashboards provide a quick summary of structural, process and outcome performance.

Plan-Do-Study-Act (PDSA) Cycle: A quality improvement method consisting of four repetitive steps for learning and improvement. Plan: develop a plan to learn, test, or implement a change; Do: execute the plan; Study: compare predictions to results and document learning; Act: make changes based on learning and set up next cycle. Most changes require several PDSA cycles.

Run chart: A time series graph where the X-axis represents time longitudinally and the measure value is on the Y-axis. Run charts often include a median for the data points and can be augmented by inserting comments (annotations) at the point in time where process changes are made by the improvement team or other changes occur that could affect the data (outside of those made by the improvement team, such as a sudden loss of several staff members in a clinic).

Statistical process control (SPC): Statistical analysis and display (eg control charts), which helps distinguish normal, everyday, inevitable variation ("common cause variation") from nonrandom ("special cause variation") variation. The latter indicates something special is happening which could be caused by an improvement project or something that warrants a fuller understanding and investigation.[17]

Modifying the Toyota Production System for Continuous Performance Improvement in an Academic Children's Hospital

F. Bruder Stapleton, MD[a,*], James Hendricks, PhD[a,b],
Patrick Hagan, MHSA[a], Mark DelBeccaro, MD[a,c]

KEYWORDS

- Quality Improvement
- CPI (or Continuous Performance Improvement)
- TPS (or Toyota Production System) • Safety
- Efficiency • Waste

Imagine a patient arriving at a clinic and waiting in line for registration, sitting in the waiting room for 30 minutes beyond the appointment time, finding that the previsit laboratory tests were lost and the letter describing the clinic visit never arrived at the referring pediatrician's office. How could this happen? In fact, the above scenarios occur at every interface of our health care system. How did we develop such a tolerance for errors, waste, and poor service? Imagine that the same patient arrived at the hospital's outpatient ambulatory center and after sitting in the waiting room for 5 minutes beyond the appointment time, a yellow light began blinking and the clinic administrator immediately appeared to discuss why the patient was not in the room seeing a physician. If by 10 minutes, the patient was still not in the examining room, the hospital's COO and head of nursing immediately appeared to determine how this could happen and to prevent it from happening to any other patient in the future?

[a] Department of Pediatrics, University of Washington School of Medicine, Seattle Children's Hospital, 4800 Sand Point Way NE T0211, Seattle, WA 98105, USA
[b] Seattle Children's Research Institute, 1900 9th Avenue, Seattle, WA 98101, USA
[c] Children's Hospital and Regional Medical Center, 4800 SandPoint Way NE Mail Stop B5520, Seattle, WA 98105, USA
* Corresponding author.
E-mail address: bruder.stapleton@seattlechildrens.org (F.B. Stapleton).

Pediatr Clin N Am 56 (2009) 799–813
doi:10.1016/j.pcl.2009.05.015
pediatric.theclinics.com

Is this imaginable? It is the type of response that occurs in a Toyota Production System (TPS) environment for every process step in One Piece Flow. In such a system, there is NO tolerance for errors or waste.

The reports of the Institute of Medicine of the past 10 years on hospital errors and medical quality shortfalls have added substance to the steady decline in public opinion of hospitals and health care professionals. Sadly, the reality of health care in America today, in many respects, is deserving of such low opinion. Clinical errors remain with us and are generally more the subject of debate about definition and data than about how to prevent them. These results are produced at a national cost of $2.4 trillion, which in 2007 equated to 17% of the United States gross domestic product.[1] We've all heard this before. Yet, we also know that the American health care system is composed of very bright and talented people providing the best care they can, but doing so within dysfunctional systems.

Seattle Children's Hospital has embraced the goal of having the "best" quality of care for our patients and families. Being the "best" translates into having a system of care in an academic environment that is unsurpassed in quality. To accomplish this goal, our physicians, nurses, administrators, and staff have adopted the principles of TPS[2] in a program called Continuous Performance Improvement (CPI), as we began a journey to improve the quality of care for our patients. This article describes the principles of CPI and offers examples of how an academic children's hospital has applied these principles in our missions of clinical care, education, and research.

PRINCIPLES OF CONTINUOUS PERFORMANCE IMPROVEMENT

The philosophy of Continuous Performance Improvement (CPI) recognizes that the continuous improvement of an organization's performance is a long-term generational effort. The CPI organization serves its customers first, vigorously supports its people in their work, and with rigor and discipline applies the scientific method to the iterative improvement of its practices. In so doing the organization recognizes the inter-relationship of Quality, Cost, Delivery, Safety, and Engagement. Successfully implemented CPI yields improvement in Quality of care and service, reduction in Cost, improvement in the Delivery of care and service, improvement in patient and staff Safety, and the Engagement of faculty and staff in improving the organization's care and service. A successful CPI program requires tenacity and patience from the organization's leaders. As important as it is for the organization's leaders to espouse and require this philosophical approach, it is more important that the faculty and staff be provided with effective principles and methods (the "tools" of CPI) to enable improvement at the bedside and wherever patient service is provided or supported. The effective use of these tools requires that improvement efforts focus on enhancing the experience of the patient via use of the "Value Stream," and focus on the removal of waste from processes that affect the patient, faculty, and support staff.

The Value Stream

The primary focus of CPI is the patient. The definition of value and conversely the definition of waste are seen through the eyes of the patient. In manufacturing, value for the customer is seen only when an action changes or transforms the shape or character of the product. From the perspective of the customer all other actions are waste. The "Value Stream" is the sequence of actions that occur from the moment the customer orders the product until the customer receives the product. The objective of any company should be to continuously improve its performance to reduce the amount of time between customer order and product delivery by eliminating waste from its processes and systems.

If you watch the flow of products on an assembly line it is relatively easy to see where and how a "product" is being changed and transformed as it moves down the line. You can see how worker movements, worker waiting, and worker searching (for tools, supplies, and so forth) may seem important to the assembly of the product, but in fact are extraneous steps and examples of waste. In health care it is more difficult to see the "flow" of patients through our processes and therefore more challenging to see if our actions are wasteful or provide value. The value stream approach requires that we understand the health care experience from the perspective of the patient. An excellent way to understand the value stream in health care is to map the process of a patient presenting for diagnosis, therapy, and care until medical care is completed—from the patient's perspective. With CPI, value stream maps are drawn by multidisciplinary clinical teams that include patients and families. The results of the mapping effort are complex, confounding, and overwhelming, accurately reflecting our patients' experience.

Once the health care value stream map is drawn, it quickly becomes a remarkable tool for identifying wasteful steps and events a patient experiences in the course of diagnosis and treatment. Examples of waste are identified as "opportunities for improvement" and the tools of CPI are used to reduce and eventually eliminate the waste. Let's use the waste of "waiting" as an example. Without the value stream approach and seeing value and waste from the patient's perspective, waiting is accepted as an unavoidable part of the health care experience. In fact, we design hospital and clinic facilities by building the most welcoming spaces possible to enable restful waiting. Instead, these design efforts should start with the premise that waiting is waste and seek to eliminate it. On the value stream map the reasons for waiting can be clearly seen and addressed through CPI. The value stream map is the tool that gets the improvement process started.

Waste

The definition of "waste" in the context of CPI is often viewed as extreme, and even wrong, by most who encounter the definition—at first. Why? Because the CPI definition of waste shows that virtually 95% of what we do in health care *is waste* from the perspective of the patient. The opposite of waste is value, and value from the patient perspective is defined as "an activity which changes the form or function of a product or service in a way that enhances value from a *patient's perspective*."[3] Expressed in another way, value is "an activity that the patient would be willing to pay for."[3] Waste in health care includes processing, correction (re-work), searching, transportation, underused staff, poorly used space, inventory, complexity, and waiting. The waste of processing is best exemplified by form or signature redundancy; correction is related to any and all errors; searching occurs when information, materials, or equipment are not immediately at hand; transportation involves any unnecessary movement of staff, goods, or patients; the poor or underuse of people and space occurs because of unnecessary peaks and valleys in patient or other activity; excess inventory occurs because of unnecessary variation in activity; complexity relates to the lack of reliable methods and standard work in health care; and waiting is caused by, or is a symptom of, all the other types of waste.

Some waste is *necessary*. Some regulatory requirements are examples of necessary waste. CPI aims to *eliminate* the unnecessary work of no value to the patient, to reduce the necessary work of no value to the patient, and to improve the value-added work we provide patients.

Standard Work

Standard work is required for CPI, although hard to establish in health care. It is impossible to improve any process unless it has been standardized.[4] Creating Standard Work requires identifying the repeatable elements of a process, assessing the best way to perform those elements, developing a reliable method to ensure the performance of those elements, and then performing the reliable method according to a calculated time that meets customer demand. Physicians often express skepticism that because patients are unique and highly variable, standard work is not possible in health care. It is precisely because patients are unique and highly variable that everything else in health care needs to be reliable and standard, so that the variability of a patient's condition can be isolated and not compounded in complexity by the variability in our "system" processes. An example is hospital teaching rounds. When the rounding method is known to all team members and is the same regardless of day of the week or attending physician, the wastes of searching and waiting (for people, information, patients, and so forth) are greatly diminished because physicians and nurses to know what to expect, what to do, and when to do it. With waste reduction, rounds take less time, leaving more time for thinking about the patient, teaching, conducting research, or going home on time.

Just-in-time

Another key CPI principle is "Just-In-Time" (JIT). It simply means that one does one's work only when it is demanded by the customer and, whenever possible, one step at a time (One Piece Flow). Although these two principles are often seen as having to do only with supplies and inventory, there is great application for clinical or administrative practice. When we do not have Just-in-Time or One Piece Flow in clinical practice; we tend to "batch" our work (ie, save up a great quantity of similar work, such as charting or orders), as opposed to doing that work one patient at a time (one piece flow). Going back to rounds, a sound Reliable Method would include the time and means by which all work associated with each patient is completed before the Team moves on to the next patient. When rounds are over, the work is done. The other benefit to one piece flow and JIT is that batching tends to obscure waste and errors. When work is being completed or delivered one at a time the existence of variation or error is easier to spot and prevent from passing on to the next step in the process.

Built-in Quality

The CPI principle of Built-in Quality has its roots in the simple admonition to "do it right the first time." Our challenge is to "error proof" our processes or, failing that, implement self-inspection and other "check" steps to ensure that errors do not get passed on. When variation and complexity are reduced through the development of reliable methods and standard work, process auditing and especially automated fail-proof controls can help prevent errors or at least keep errors from moving to the next step. A good example is the development of reliable methods in automated medication ordering through Electronic Medical Records systems or, short of automation, monitoring and auditing closely in real time. Beyond Built-in Quality, another advantage of reliable methods in order writing (*and* Patient Rounds) is that the pharmacy is better able to project medication inventory and pharmacist workload, aiding in its effort to provide needed materials Just-In-Time.

Rapid Process Improvement Workshop

An excellent CPI tool used for developing and implementing these types of changes is the rapid process improvement workshop (RPIW). RPIWs are designed to educate the participants in CPI principles and methods applicable to the task at hand, and to enable them to redesign and implement a process change in 5 days' time. In many respects it epitomizes the practical application of the scientific method to clinical and administrative practice. To be successful, the RPIW requires data collection and analysis, problem assessment and workshop planning, leadership sponsorship and resource deployment, qualified workshop facilitation and support, and a representative multidisciplinary (including patients and families) workshop team.

In the RPIW, facts and data drive decisions, and opinions and professional titles get "checked at the door." Individuals intent on power plays must be managed respectfully but effectively and quickly. The RPIW Sponsor is responsible for approving the "Charter" (**Fig. 1**) for the workshop, keeping the workshop within scope and on track, and ensuring that barriers and obstacles to the team's success (like power players) are mitigated or eliminated.

An RPIW Team usually includes an executive or faculty leader as Sponsor (one per workshop), key executives and faculty leaders as members of a Management Guidance Team, an "on-the-ground" leader as "Process Owner" (usually only one), and

PROCESS NAME: General Medicine Discharge Criteria SPONSOR: MD	PROCESS OWNER: MD CPI TEAM: (2)	
Boundaries *Starting Point*: Patient admitted *Ending Point*: Patient discharged *Sub-processes included*: Identification and modification of criteria, Documentation/communication of criteria, Incorporation of information into rounds, Education of Residents	**Team Members (10):** **Staff RN** **Staff RN** **Care Coord** **CPI** **R1** **Community MD** **Charge RN** **Sr. Resident** **MD** **Patient/Family rep**	**Management Guidance Team (10):** **COO** **RN** **RN** **MD** **MD** **RN** **RN** **MD** **MD** **MD**
Current Situation *(includes baseline data):* Criteria for discharge inconsistently documented, in various places *85% of charts reviewed did not document discharge criteria • Criteria for discharge inconsistently discussed during rounds *No standard format currently exist for discussing discharge criteria during rounds • Team & Families not always aware of discharge criteria prior to discharge *RN = 1.3 at 24 hours of admission *Family = 3.0 at 24 hours of admission	**Resource Representatives:** Communications MD Pharmacist Social Work Family Resource Health Info and Privacy	**Stakeholders:** **Sub-Specialties** **MCC**
Targets: Discharge criteria will be defined, documented and made visual to Team & Families • (Goal of 65% at 30 Days; 85% at 60 Days w/ Stretch Goal of 100%) Discharge criteria will be communicated to Team & Family within 24 hours of admission Discharge criteria will be updated and communicated daily		
RPI Theme: Reliable method design and implementation, Visual display	**Administrative Support**	**Measurement Specialists**
	Replications Needs & Resources: Sub-Specialties MCC All inpatient units	

Fig. 1. An example of a team RPIW charter.

Team members selected from representative groups affected by the process under consideration. The RPIW Team that redesigned General Medicine patient rounds included the Hospital COO as Sponsor; the Pediatrics Chairman, the Chief Nursing Officer, and Chief Medical Officer as members of the Management Guidance Team; the chief hospitalist and hospital nurse leader as Process Owners; and faculty, nurses, residents, parents, and unit coordinators as team members.

RPIW Teams are expected to develop proposed design changes (ie, hypotheses) and then share them with affected "stakeholders" during the workshop week. By the end of the week a new design is implemented after which it will be audited on a 30-, 60-, and 90-day basis to determine both whether the new process is being followed and whether it is having the desired result. This is the stage at which the application of the "Deming Cycle" of Plan Do Check Act (PDCA)[2] is important to the organization in the short and long term. In the short run, PDCA provides the means by which improvement work is evaluated in real time, and for the long term it is the means by which the organization remains credible in its commitment to continuous improvement. Through the RPIW tool and its evaluation with PDCA, an organization can bring the practical application of the scientific method to the improvement of clinical and administrative practice.

CONTINUOUS PERFORMANCE IMPROVEMENT PRINCIPLES ADAPTED TO CLINICAL PRACTICE

Many of the process changes are designed and implemented using the RPIW methodology. During the workshop, the team goes to the actual clinical site and watches the actual process. To expose the many forms of waste it is important to follow a series of standard steps when looking at a process. The team maps and quantifies the actual steps involved, the time for each step, and the distance traveled with each step, then determines which steps add value and designs and implements the improved process during the week. While the ideal state is identified, our philosophy is that 50% improvement in a process, continued measurement, and further cycles of improvement are more important than attempting perfection. The following examples will illustrate how CPI methodology was used to improve quality, remove waste, and improve flow.

Central Line Process Improvements

We used the CPI methodology in a multipronged set of improvements aimed at reducing central line infections. These interventions were specifically targeted at the overuse and complexity in the use and ordering of peripherally inserted central catheters (PICC).[5] Overutilization in itself is a form of waste and contributes to an increased risk of infection. Our existing ordering process was nonstandard, confusing, error prone, and wasteful. Orders for PICC line placement could be sent to interventional radiology, anesthesia, or the registered nurse (RN) line placement team. There also were no specific criteria to determine the need for the PICC or the method of placement. These issues were the basis of a RPIW.

A series of three RPIW events for line placement were completed over a 9-month period. Participants in this RPIW included a multidisciplinary group of MDs, RNs, residents, and nurse practitioners. Workshops occurred over 3 to 5 days with participants being relieved from all other duties. The first workshop identified the elements of standard rounding to ensure that central lines are included as part of the daily discussion during morning patient rounds. This work was started on the medicine service (model line) and then replicated to surgical and other services and was dubbed the "6th Vital Sign." The subsequent workshops identified the criteria for

PICC line placement and the design of the vascular access service to centralize the process. To error proof these design elements (and avoid the waste of complexity and rework), the steps were "hard wired" in an RPIW event to use our computerized provider order entry (CPOE) system with order sets and linked electronic forms. The new process required steps to screen for appropriate need of the line placement and to ensure that the vascular access service had the necessary information (avoid rework) to schedule placement. The electronic order form also served a secondary purpose by supplying information at the point of use for the provider. This is both a mistake-proofing adjunct and a JIT teaching moment for our residents. These last steps were not put in place until the prior three workshops had standardized the process steps. This is an important concept—do not leap to automation until the process is worked out.

Each event also had a series of outcome measures that included provider satisfaction and the use of PICC lines.[5] Following the workshops there has been a sustained drop in PICC line use for over 3 years, as well as improved provider satisfaction. Although it cannot be shown to be causally related, this probably has also been a factor in our institution's decrease in central line infections during the same time period. The PICC line work illustrates multiple CPI concepts: reduce unnecessary variation, mistake/error proof, reduce waste (complexity, rework-correction, search time), multiple iterative improvements, and reliable methods (order set and form make it easy to do the right thing).

Surgical Site Infections

Prevention of surgical site infections is a national priority. Prior efforts at Seattle Children's had not led to a reliable method for dosing and re-dosing of antibiotics during surgical procedures. Our infection rates were above 4/100 high-risk procedures (cardiac and spine cases). Using CPI methodology we developed and implemented the following interventions: created cardiovascular and spinal surgery guidelines of care for perioperative antibiotic usage, which included antibiotic choice, dosage, timing, and accountabilities (standard work); added antibiotic orders to the preop order set; ensured correct doses go with the patient and chart to the OR (reliable method); designed standard preop bathing processes that included chlorhexidine bath at home by families and a chlorhexidine wipe down the morning of surgery by families (standard work); updated inpatient order set to include preop bathing (reliable method); and removed all razors from the facility so that preop hair removal, if done, must be done with clippers (error-proof, reliable method).

Following the above set of interventions we have sustained dosing and re-dosing (> 97%) and infection rates below 2 of 100 cases. Although these are neither perfect nor adequate, they do show the concept of at least 50% improvement with a commitment to return, reevaluate, and improve the process.

Emergency Department Throughput

The emergency department (ED) at Seattle Children's has used CPI methods for a number of years to improve the quality of care and specifically to address wait time to see a provider, length of stay, and the number of patients leaving without being seen (LWBS). Early RPIWs mapped the movements of the providers against an architectural room layout of the ED creating a "spaghetti" diagram. The time required to travel in the ED was also quantified. These measurements of movements and times allowed the providers to see the waste of movement. This waste did not mean the providers were not working hard, but were wasting their time and skills on movement.

The RPIW and subsequent workshops led to formation of work units designed to more closely match the ability of the team to match the patient arrival demand and to begin to institute a system that pulls patients into the ED. The ED LWBS rate, which fluctuated as high as 4.5%, has now remained below 1% for 3 years.

A more recent ED RPIW used a multidisciplinary team to look at flow and charting to redesign the ED chart into a multidisciplinary chart that also encourages charting at the patient bedside. Charting at the bedside is an example of one piece flow as opposed to traditional charting, which is often batched away from the patient, sometimes long after the patient is gone. Traditional workflows have been based on the belief that running from patient to patient is more efficient and moves patients faster. Using the CPI methodology and strict measuring of time, distance, rework, handoffs, seek time, and other forms of waste actually shows the work is completed more rapidly and with higher quality using one piece flow (complete each task as you go).

CONTINUOUS PERFORMANCE IMPROVEMENT IN THE ACADEMIC TEACHING SETTING

As described previously, a culture of CPI with participation of the entire hospital community is required for success. In a teaching hospital, clinical care is provided in a supervised educational process with a team of resident physicians and medical students. The daily teaching rounds have been described as a mobile one-room school house. Early in our journey with CPI, we developed a philosophy of including a resident or residency director in most clinical improvement processes. This approach prevented us from creating improvements that would diminish our outstanding education programs. To ensure that sufficient numbers of residency representatives were available for this program, we increased the number of chief residents from two to three and provided CPI leadership training for each of the three chiefs. Having residents participate as members of improvement workshops provided essential knowledge of the daily clinical processes, as well as opportunities for residents to feel ownership of changes in the daily work at the hospital, and pride in achieving improved patient outcomes.

Selected examples of improvement workshops and targets for improvement in which residents provided essential guidance were: reducing errors in total parenteral nutrition orders, creating a model of care in the ED, reducing errors in formula orders, reducing pharmacy order turnaround time, ensuring medication reconciliation, eliminating dangerous abbreviations, improving transfer of patients from the ED to the inpatient service, and designing the medically complex child inpatient service. Many of these improvement processes required changes in how residents did their daily work. The residents who participated in these improvement workshops facilitated acceptance of change within the residency program by communicating the rationale for the changes and providing positive leadership.

Teaching rounds have been a continuing focus of our CPI program. The introduction of the 80-hour work week, a growing patient census, implementation of the electronic medical record, and moving into a new inpatient hospital wing offered many challenges to the teaching and clinical care programs. CPI proved invaluable in meeting these challenges. As a result of our CPI work, teaching rounds moved out of the conference rooms and became truly family centered. Team communication with families by the entire team, including nurses and interpreters, occurred at the bedside. Parent satisfaction has increased dramatically with each new improvement in our teaching rounds. Surprisingly, after 3 years of CPI focus on the inpatient teaching rounds, we discovered from our regular residency satisfaction surveys that what had been the most popular resident hospital experience—the senior inpatient resident team—had become the least popular resident rotation. This discovery provided us a unique opportunity to apply CPI principles to a teaching process.

A Unique Rapid Process Improvement Workshop: Improving the Experience of the Senior Inpatient Resident

First we had to ascertain the causes of resident dissatisfaction with this rotation. We learned that with the time constraints in the existing resident schedule, the senior resident was able to examine only approximately 25% of the patients on the service and had to rely on the intern and attending examinations to make patient decisions. Another concern was that family-centered rounds were becoming so lengthy that there was insufficient time to discuss all the assigned patients before the noon conference and departure of the residents to continuity clinics. This situation seemed to be an outstanding opportunity for CPI. A 5-day RPIW was planned. The Chair of the Department of Pediatrics served as the sponsor and supported the Process Owners, the residency directors, and a chief resident. The CPI office staffed the initial design discussions and began to measure the problem by collecting data to inform the goals of the RPIW.

Pre-RPIW work found that residents actually spent 3 to 4 hours rounding, when the block of time allotted for teaching rounds was 2.5 hours. During the mean 3 to 4 hours of rounding, 17% to 20% of the time was spent waiting for attendings and 12% to 13% of rounding time was spent traveling around the hospital. Each team received an average of 20 phone call interruptions during the teaching rounds and 45% of the senior residents examined fewer than 25% of their patients each day. The senior resident satisfaction score for the inpatient team was 2.85 out of 5.00, with 5.00 being most satisfied.

The RPIW sponsor and leadership group concluded that the desired outcomes for the event were to reduce phone call interruptions during rounds, increase the percentage of patients examined by the chief residents, increase attendance at morning report and noon teaching conferences, and increase resident satisfaction. In addition to the sponsor, process owners, and the CPI staff, the RPIW project team included three residents, a unit clerk, a patient care coordinator, a floor nurse, an attending hospitalist, a pediatric specialty attending, a patient's family representative, and a community physician. The management group that offered feedback during the RPIW included more residents, the floor nursing supervisor, the hospital Chief Operating Officer, the Chief Nursing Officer, and hospital medical leadership.

One of the most unique aspects of this project was that unlike **every** other RPIW, it was not the patient and family who were seen as the customer, but rather the senior resident. This different focus was actually somewhat uncomfortable for the residents, and the conversations during the event continually came back to what was best for the patients. Many of the participants in this project did not have experience with CPI methods. For this reason, the core concepts of standard work, waste reduction, and error proofing were provided during the first day of the event. The second day was spent observing team rounds with stopwatches, pedometers, and evaluation forms. The number of phone interruptions were recorded, as well as the distance in team walking, the average time required to complete family-centered rounds and answer parent questions, and the time and reasons for waiting or revisiting patient rooms. A process map of where the team traveled was created. The findings were eye-opening. The team traveled over a mile during rounds. The path that the teams traveled was redundant and chaotic; the average time to meet with families, discuss patient findings, and create the daily plan was 8 minutes. Telephone calls were a constant source of interruption and distraction and rounds were almost never completed by noon.

On day 3, changes were proposed based on the data and input that the team received. What were the interventions? Nurses and consultants agreed not to phone during rounds unless it was an emergency, and phone calls during rounds were converted to text messages. This had an immediate and profound positive effect on rounds. A new 30-minute team work time was created at the beginning of the morning. Part of this work time was used to determine how many patients needed to be seen and if there was sufficient time for the entire team to see all the patients during rounds, using the average cycle time of 8 minutes. A visual board was set up to alert the team of excessive census and the team would divide in order to see the patients, with one team being led by a senior resident. Noon conferences were changed to start at 12:15 PM rather than noon so that residents could more predictably attend. Morning report was moved to 8:00–8:30 AM. Attendings agreed to be available promptly at assigned times and specialty service attendings were assigned specific times to interface with the team on their patients. These changes were implemented on day 4.

The new system was generally well received and tolerated by residents and faculty. PDCA cycles made selected changes for one team owing to the nature of the specialty patients, and the timing of morning report was moved to 8:30 to allow the 30-minute team work time to occur at 8:00 AM. The introduction of the new system was delayed for a week so that all teams initiated the new system on the day that the new attendings assumed responsibility for the services. The head of the hospital service held a special preparatory session for the new attendings to explain the new design.

One week following the implementation of the new design, phone call interruptions had declined by nearly 50% (**Fig. 2**). The average number of patients examined by the senior residents increased from 43% to 53%. Attendance at morning report increased by 15%, at noon conferences by 30%, and at Grand Rounds by 20%. Senior resident satisfaction increased from 2.87 to 3.46 with these changes. Minor modifications of these changes have been required, but the gains in the metrics have been sustained and increased over a 2-year period. Residents who participate in CPI activities become enthusiastic advocates for change and improvements. This has led to

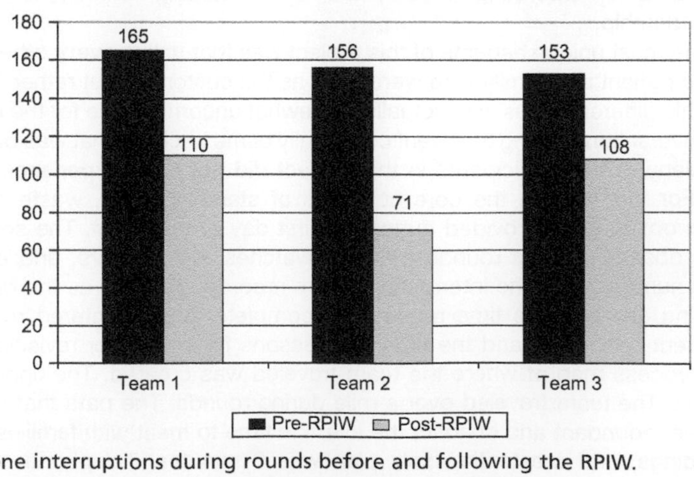

Fig. 2. Phone interruptions during rounds before and following the RPIW.

improved morale during heavy workloads, as the organization has confidence that solutions will be developed to ensure patient flow, safety, and quality care.

RESEARCH APPLICATIONS

The past decade has been marked by rapid advances in technology that have transformed the conduct of biomedical research and accelerated the pace of scientific discovery. These advances have been fueled largely by funding from the National Institutes of Health (NIH). Having doubled between 1998 and 2003, the NIH budget has stagnated in recent years. The current economic crisis exigencies threaten the NIH budget, and with it, the pace of scientific discovery. Rather than implementing cost-reduction strategies aimed solely at "weathering the current storm," it is time for research institutions to adopt a long-term, sustainable approach to cost control. When applied rigorously and throughout the research enterprise, CPI can have a dramatic affect on productivity, cost, and quality.

Because the scientific method is embedded in the tools and techniques of CPI, it is particularly amenable to the research enterprise. Despite this fact, the leadership of Seattle Children's Research Institute (SCRI) recognized that creating a lean culture would require a strong commitment from investigators. To secure that commitment, it was decided to focus initial efforts on maximizing value and eliminating waste from core processes (value streams) in which the investigator was considered the "customer." This initial focus on supporting business lines included Institutional Review Board approvals, animal care services, and other core services.

Institutional Review Board

Institutional review boards (IRBs) are generally regarded by investigators as a "necessary (albeit important) hurdle" to conduct clinical research. IRB requirements are considered overwhelming, and the review process unnecessarily slow. IRBs face unwieldy federal requirements, mountains of paperwork and a burgeoning workload, and suffer from high levels of work-in-progress, a volatile workload, long and variable lead times, and the absence of standard work. These characteristics provide a burning platform for change.

The tools of the CPI Management System make it possible to examine the IRB review process as a set of action steps, each of which must be accomplished in such a way to attain the key value step—application approval. Lean methodologies relentlessly focus on the customer; however, identifying the primary customer may prove difficult. In the IRB CPI implementation, investigators viewed themselves as the IRB's primary customer, whereas the IRB community viewed prospective research participants as their customer. The IRB community viewed the IRB as serving the interests of research participants, not facilitating the work of investigators. They were concerned that defining the investigator as customer could compromise the independence of the IRB. Research leadership emphasized the distinction between the IRB and the staff that support the IRB application process. IRB support staff are charged with moving applications through the review and approval process, working as a conduit between investigators and the IRB. Because support staff are not voting members of the IRB, the staff serves investigators as the primary (external) customer and the IRB as a secondary (internal) customer. Reaching consensus on this issue helped to establish roles for future CPI workshops. The administrative director of Children's Office of Institutional Assurances was appointed workshop leader. Workshop teams consisted of investigators and IRB support staff.

The first RPIW was conducted in early 2006. As the first step in CPI, in fiscal year (FY) 2004, the IRB began collecting turn-around-time (TAT) data for several rate-limiting steps identified in a full-review process analysis (**Fig. 3**A). As shown in **Fig. 3**B, the average TAT for full IRB review was 70 days in FY 2004 and 86 days in

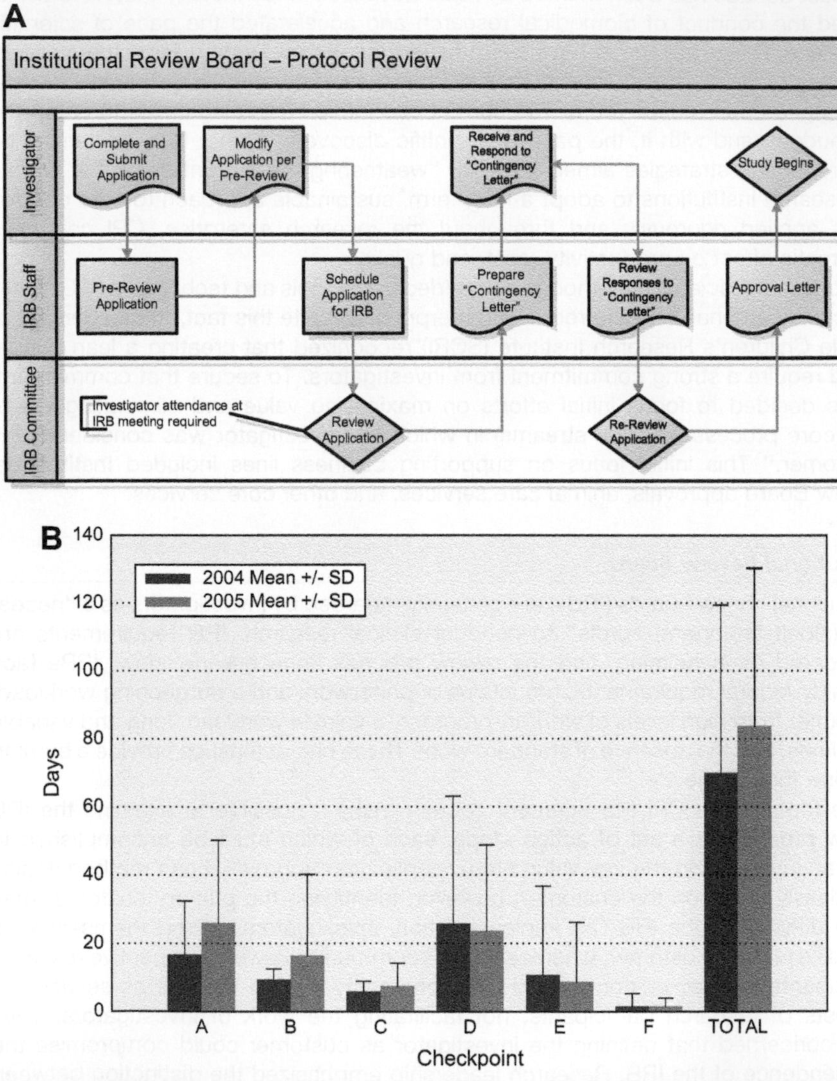

Fig. 3. Assessment of "current state" for full IRB review process. (*A*) Process analysis to identify rate-limiting steps involving investigator, IRB support staff, and the IRB committee. (*B*) Checkpoint summary for full IRB review in FY 2004 and FY 2005. Checkpoint A, date of application receipt to date pre-review completed; checkpoint B, date pre-review completed to date of first IRB meeting; checkpoint C, date of first IRB meeting to date Investigator notification of contingencies; checkpoint D, date investigator notification of contingencies to date response received by IRB; checkpoint E, date response received from Investigator to date contingencies finally removed (may involve subsequent IRB meetings); checkpoint F, date contingencies removed to date IRB chair signs approval letter.

FY 2005. The greatest contributors to the total TAT time were checkpoints A (date of application receipt to date prereview completed) and Checkpoint D (date investigator notification of contingencies to date contingency response received). The workshop was led by a member of Seattle Children's CPI Department and involved a team consisting of two IRB staff members, two investigators, the IRB Chairman, and an IRB manager from a partner institution. The workshop team began by mapping the IRB review process in its current state, including the flow of information and people throughout the process. Each step of the process was evaluated for value from the perspective of the customer, as well as waste. **Table 1** shows process data that came out of the RPIW for the current and future states. A total of 22 steps were eliminated from the process. Significant reductions in the waste associated with handoffs, check-steps, and queues were also achieved. Target TATs for each checkpoint were established, along with a target total TAT of 60 days. In an effort to notify management of potential process problems, a visual management signboard listing days in process for each application was prominently displayed in the IRB office. Any application exceeding the target approval time for each checkpoint in the process activated a formal troubleshooting review. As a result of the RPIW, the total TAT for full-review applications was reduced from 86.0 days to 46.5 days. This reduction has been maintained for more than 2 years.

Animal Care Services

Animal research facilities provide a centralized resource for the efficient delivery of high-quality humane animal care. Under cost principles set forth by the Office of Management and Budget, all costs associated with animal research must be recovered as direct costs on grants and contracts. Animal research facilities develop animal per diem rates based on cost accounting data. Although most research institutions subsidize per diem rates to some extent, biomedical research inflation requires frequent revisions to the animal per diem rate. In multiyear research projects, these revisions can prove problematic if the institution is unable to increase its subsidy. In the current economic climate, cost containment has become a priority. The tools of CPI provide a strategy for reducing costs without compromising quality, and can be applied effectively to animal research operations.

We conducted several CPI events aimed at improving efficiency and reducing waste in its operations. These events have focused primarily on equipment processing and material handling.

Good animal husbandry practices require the frequent washing and sanitation of cages. SCRI processes an average of 230 cages per day in its murine-specific pathogen-free animal facility. This represents a significant volume of work, and has proven

Table 1
Institutional Review Board process data collected during the rapid process improvement workshop for current and future state of full review by the Institutional Review Board

Measure	Current State	Future State
No. steps	57	35
No. value-added steps	5	5
% Value-added steps	9%	14%
No. handoffs	54	19
No. check-steps	28	8
No. queues	25	8

a useful target for CPI efforts. As published elsewhere,[6] an RPIW focused on cage washing activities resulted in a 34% reduction in processing time and increased staff safety by reducing repetitive bending and twisting motions. Significant reductions in processing times contributed to reduced costs, improved production predictability, and increased customer service.

In traditional "batch" animal operations management, a cage buffer inventory is maintained to offset variation in cage processing caused by demand forecast inaccuracies and machine downtime. In CPI JIT animal operations management, however, customer demand dictates production, reducing the need for inventory. The SCRI animal facility implemented a simple visual management system as a customer demand signal. The signal for cleaning consisted of a cart onto which dirty cages were placed by the staff. The wall behind the cart was taped off at a level consisting of 72 cages, the maximum capacity of the cage washer. As soon as the cart was filled, cage-washing production was initiated. By implementing this system, the animal facility was able to decrease its buffer inventory by 51%.[7] A small buffer inventory was maintained in the event of equipment failure.

In an RPIW focused on further reductions in the frequency of cage changes, the workshop team suggested using rodent feces as a "biologic signal." The team noted that all cages were changed at 7 days regardless of the number of occupants. The team initiated an Institutional Animal Care and Use Committee (IACUC)-approved trial designed to measure bedding conditions in cages containing from one to five mice

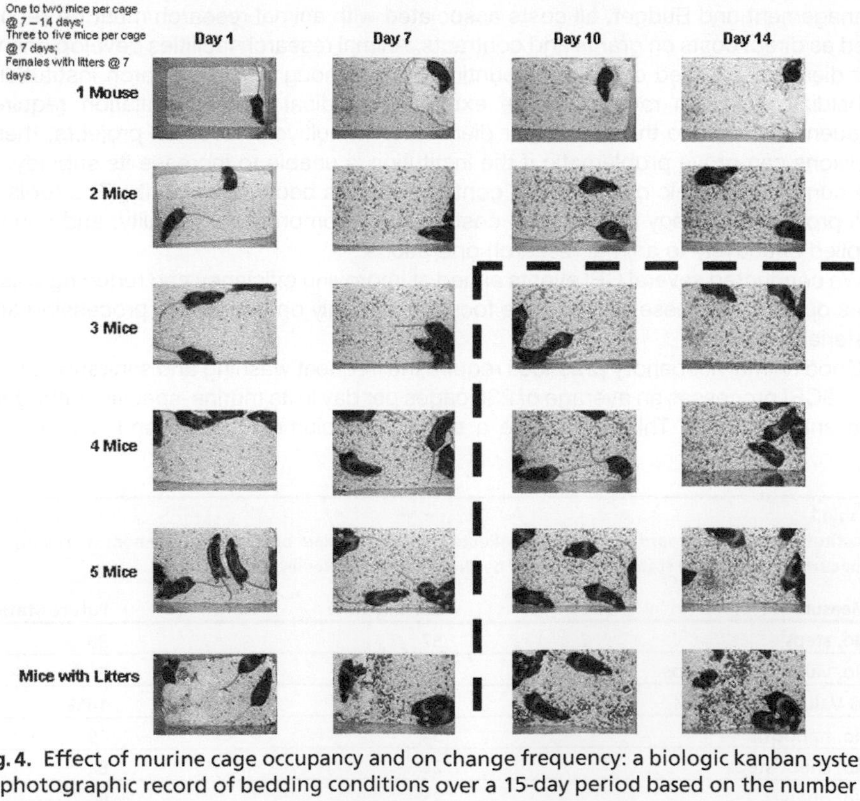

Fig. 4. Effect of murine cage occupancy and on change frequency: a biologic kanban system. A photographic record of bedding conditions over a 15-day period based on the number of cage occupants.

maintained for a period of 14 days without a cage change. A photographic record of bedding conditions at days 1, 7, 10, and 14 are shown in **Fig. 4**. Based on this study, the team concluded that cages containing a single mouse could be changed at 14 days; cages containing two to three mice could be changed at 10 days, and cages containing four to five mice or litters must be changed at 7 days. By matching the frequency of cage changes with the number of cage occupants, our animal facility was able to further enhance operating efficiencies aimed at reducing costs.

SUMMARY

Continuous performance improvement based on the principles of the Toyota Production System can be successfully adapted to improve the quality of medical care and academic processes. Seattle Children's has been evolving along this journey for a number of years. We believe the improved quality, safety, efficiencies, and cost savings examples shown in this article are the tip of the iceberg for clinical, administrative, and academic programs. Since 2005, there have been well over 200 CPI events using these tools at our institution that have improved nearly every aspect of our academic health environment. Patience, persistent education, and commitment from the administrative, academic, and clinic leadership is critical to fully engage faculty and to reach the tipping point of a cultural change in which mistakes, waste, and planning silos are eliminated.

REFERENCES

1. National Coalition on Health Care. Health insurance costs. Available at: http://www.nchc.org/facts/cost.shtml. Accessed January 30, 2009.
2. Liker JK. The Toyota way. New York: McGraw-Hill; 2004. p. 23–4.
3. Wellman J. Excerpt from "Waste module: lean leader training/rapid process improvement" copyright. Seattle, WA: Joan Wellman & Associates, Inc.; 2005.
4. Ohno T. Toyota production system: beyond large scale production. New York: Productivity Press; 1988. p.130.
5. Migita D, Postetter B, Hagan P, et al. Governing peripherally inserted central venous catheters by combining continuous performance improvement and computerized physician order entry. Pediatrics 2009;123:1155–61.
6. Khan N, Umrysh B. Improving animal research facility operations through the application of lean principles. ILAR J 2008;49:15–22.
7. Kahn N, Daniel C. Improving access to lab services through the implementation of lean principles. Clin Leadersh Manag Rev 2007;21(4).

Approach to Improving Quality: the Role of Quality Measurement and a Case Study of the Agency for Healthcare Research and Quality Pediatric Quality Indicators

Kathryn M. McDonald, MM

KEYWORDS

• Quality assurance • Quality indicators • Health care
• Pediatrics • Comparative reporting

A 1-year-old undergoes abdominal surgery, and her parents are relieved it is over, start to relax, and make plans for returning home. Three days later, their baby returns to the operating room for reclosure of postoperative disruption of the abdominal wall. A 7-year-old complains loudly to his mother about sharp belly pains in his lower right side; she calls the pediatrician's office and is told to come right in. Lacking transportation, she does not make it in with the boy, and no one calls to see why. That night, he is writhing and they take a cab to the emergency room from where he is rushed to the operating room to remove his rupturing appendix.

These two stories hit us in the gut, quite literally. Anecdotes of suboptimal care make us ask what could have been done to avoid the bad outcome for that child. But how do we know how well the health care system is doing on a larger scale? Data and well-constructed measures can quantify the scale of the problem and

The author is funded by the Agency for Healthcare Research and Quality (AHRQ), Rockville, MD, for the continued support and refinement of the AHRQ Pediatric Quality Indicators. The author reports no conflict of interest.
Center for Primary Care and Outcomes Research, Stanford University, Stanford, CA 94305-6019, USA
E-mail address: kathy.mcdonald@stanford.edu

Pediatr Clin N Am 56 (2009) 815–829
doi:10.1016/j.pcl.2009.05.009 pediatric.theclinics.com

thereby direct efforts to make improvements. From 2000 to 2003, the rate of wound dehiscence requiring a return to the operating room during the same hospitalization remained steady at 0.76 cases per 1000 abdominopelvic surgeries, and the rate of perforated appendix was also unchanged, but much higher, at 31% of appendectomies.[1]

A clarion call has sounded for children's health care[2] to develop interventions to improve outcomes of care, develop comparative quality reports for decision making and accountability, and create incentives that pay for performance. Each of these three goals requires data and measures. This article describes the context for measurement in pediatrics, provides a case study of the development of an indicator set using routinely collected hospital discharge data, and addresses considerations for selecting and using measures in various circumstances.

THE CURRENT MEASUREMENT LANDSCAPE AND PEDIATRICS

Many researchers, governmental agencies at the federal and state levels, provider organizations, and health care payers have instituted quality measurement aimed at performance improvement. In 2006, the Institute of Medicine published "Performance Measurement: Accelerating Improvement," a report from their Committee on Redesigning Health Insurance Performance Measures, Payment, and Performance Improvement Programs.[3] This report highlighted the incredible proliferation of measures and consequent need for standardization to mitigate the potential burdens of excessive measurement and reporting requirements. Because the report resulted from a congressional mandate oriented toward the Medicare program, there was scant coverage of children's health, but there was a clear message that measurement is important to quality improvement.

Measure development in children's health is at an earlier stage compared with adult medicine, with a need for more measures across all settings of care.[4,5] At some stage in the future, though, the same problem of a plethora of measures and insufficient standardization could emerge for children's health. An obstacle to rational measurement in pediatrics—development of the right number of measures, covering the right areas, available at the right moment—may be the fragmented payment terrain and, thus, a lack of a single entity or program (eg, Medicare) that can provide the necessary incentives to make health care quality measurement and underlying information infrastructures as crucial as they are becoming for adult care.[6,7]

Nevertheless, motivation for quality measurement in pediatrics is increasing because reports show that quality gaps exist in pediatric ambulatory, emergency room, and hospital care that are similar to those demonstrated in adult settings.[8–11] Simply applying adult indicators to younger age ranges is insufficient in many situations. Specific challenges arise from the "four Ds" that distinguish children from "little adults:" differential epidemiology, dependency, demographics, and development.[4,12] Whether developing child health indicators from scratch or based on adult analogs, measure developers must consider the implications of each of these factors to produce robust indicators and comprehensive measure sets (**Table 1**). Although there are special challenges in pediatrics, many of the approaches to indicator development, assessment, and application are similar regardless of age of the patient population of interest.

Numerous frameworks exist for assessing indicators and measure sets, and vary somewhat with regard to the purpose of measurement (eg, comparative reporting among countries,[13] national consensus measures for use in public reporting and quality improvement,[14] and inclusion in a clearinghouse of measures[15]). In addition,

Table 1
Special considerations for pediatric measures

Children's Health Consideration	Description	Implication for Measurement
Differential epidemiology (versus adult care)	Relatively healthy Seldom have multiple illnesses Special populations	Measure preventive care Risk adjustment is simpler Targeted indicators are needed
Dependency	Parents or other adults involved in financing, decisions, care	Care evaluation depends on information derived from more sources
Demographics	From neonate to adolescent More poverty More ethnically/racially diverse	Sample sizes vary by group Risk adjustment potentially more complex
Development	Constantly changing physically, emotionally, and cognitively	Different measures by age group or development stage

composite measures that combine similar measures are becoming more prevalent in health care. Through their consensus process, the National Quality Forum (NQF) is currently reviewing a composite pediatric patient safety measure[16] and developing criteria to assess such composites.[17]

The American Academy of Pediatrics' Steering Committee on Quality Improvement and Management and Committee on Practice and Ambulatory Medicine published a policy statement in early 2008 on "Principles for the Development and Use of Quality Measures." They noted, "measures are an important component of improving quality," believing that "the primary purpose of quality measurement should be to identify opportunities to improve patient care and outcomes, including health status and satisfaction."[18] **Box 1** summarizes their recommendations for measure development and compares these to the NQF framework.[19] The NQF currently leads a national effort aimed at improving American health care through the endorsement of consensus-based standards. In pediatrics, diverse stakeholders have centralized around these efforts, including national, state, and regional groups representing clinicians and health care professionals, consumers, private and public employers, hospitals, and research organizations and institutions (eg, the Agency for Healthcare Research and Quality [AHRQ], the National Association of Children's Hospitals and Related Institutions [NACHRI], Child Health Corporation of America, the Alliance for Pediatric Quality, and the Hospital Quality Alliance).

Despite increasing measurement-related activities, there remain a limited number of indicators available in pediatrics, particularly for care that crosses settings and for ambulatory care. Additional indicator development is needed to feed into endorsement and reporting processes aimed at catalyzing performance improvement. Development efforts geared to specific areas provide the greatest opportunity to provide meaningful measures. For example, in 2003, the Joint Commission spurred activity on inpatient asthma measures for inclusion in their ORYX performance measurement initiative. As a result, the Pediatric Data Quality Systems Collaborative Measures Workgroup formed and focused first on asthma

Box 1
Criteria for measure development (American Academy of Pediatrics) versus Endorsement (National Quality Forum)

American Academy of Pediatrics Recommendations for Quality Measurement

Important issues for children

- Addresses discrepancy between current and ideal practice and the potential for substantial impact
- Enables assessment of disparities for vulnerable populations

Appropriateness

- Takes into consideration the unique characteristics of pediatric populations

Scientific validity

- Evidence-based, transparent, and accurately and reliably assesses what it is intended to measure
- Risk adjustment or stratification as appropriate

Feasibility

- Should not cause any undue burden on clinician, patient, or family, with attention to clear specification instructions, minimal resource use for data collection, adequate sampling
- Tailored to use in proposed practice setting
- Easily interpretable by users—includes use of methods to allow a focus on causes of variation and benchmarks

Improved quality of care

- Focuses on issues that clinicians and health systems can influence

NQF Evaluation Criteria for Endorsement Process

Importance of measuring and reporting

- Targets making gains in quality (safety, timeliness, effectiveness, efficiency, efficiency, equity, patient centeredness) and outcomes where performance varies or is poor

Requirements for consideration

- Available publicly and maintained by a responsible entity
- Fully developed and tested against NQF criteria

Scientific acceptability

- Produces reliable, valid results about quality of care

Feasibility

- Required data are available (retrievable without undue burden) and can be implemented for performance measurement

Usability

- Intended audiences can understand the results of the measure and are likely to find them useful for decision making

care and more recently on the pediatric ICU environment, vetting numerous potential indicators and ultimately seeking and receiving endorsement for several measures for each clinical situation.[20] Two of the asthma measures are already available in "Hospital Compare"[21] for consumer decision making in hospital selection.

CASE STUDY: DEVELOPMENT OF THE AGENCY FOR HEALTHCARE RESEARCH AND QUALITY PEDIATRIC QUALITY INDICATORS

Another major recent effort, the AHRQ Pediatric Quality Indicators (PDIs), offers an example of measure development that builds on previous efforts and uses a standardized methodology to develop a full set of indicators.[1,22] The approach to the development of the AHRQ PDIs mirrored that used for earlier AHRQ indicator modules, originally developed by the University of California San Francisco–Stanford Evidence-Based Practice Center, with collaborators from other institutions including the University of California Davis and Battelle Memorial Institute.[23] Indicators from previous AHRQ sets provided the candidate list for the initial pediatric module to keep the task manageable within the resources available and to limit the sets to those that could be implemented with routinely collected hospital discharge data. This data source is ubiquitous, providing the ability to make comparisons between individual hospitals or among similar types of hospitals (eg, nonspecialized community hospitals, children's specialty hospitals). On the other hand, administrative discharge data lack important clinical details, making risk adjustment for accurate quality assessment and fair comparisons more challenging.

The team's indicator set development process for the PDIs and other AHRQ indicator modules is serial and iterative, as shown in **Fig. 1**. The first task is to identify all of the possible indicators from multiple sources. Consulting the research literature and seeking ideas from key informants about indicators in use but not reported in the literature result in a candidate list of indicators for a given purpose. The goal for the candidate list is to identify as many potential indicators as possible for the anticipated use. Sometimes there will be areas of clinical significance for which no indicators exist. In these cases, new indicators could be developed by using quality concepts from Donabedian's classic framework of structure, process, and outcome of care.[24] Is there a structural element of care, such as neonatal ICU level, that has been shown to correspond to quality? Is there a process of care, such as weight checks every 2 weeks on patients who have eating disorders, that has not been adopted in a measure but emanates from a clinical guideline or standard of care? Is there an outcome, such as disease-free survival in patients who have acute lymphocytic leukemia, that might vary from one setting to another on the basis of quality of care? Looking at clinical guidelines, practice standards, trigger tools from the patient safety literature, and other evaluations showing a connection between something that might be measured and high-quality care is a more time-intensive approach to identifying potential indicators.

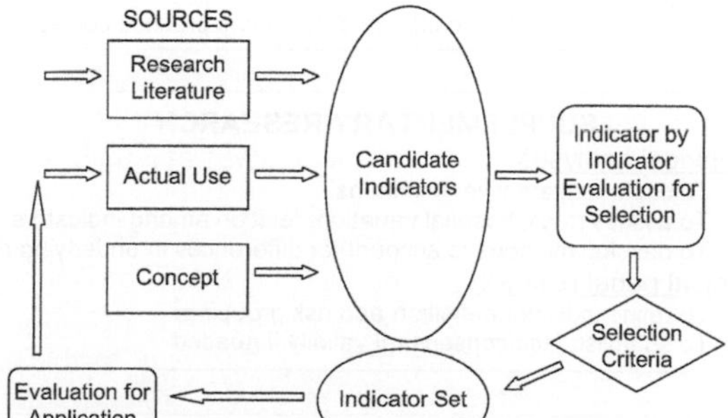

Fig. 1. Quality indicator set development process. This figure shows the major activities undertaken to develop and continually refine indicator sets.

After a candidate list of indicators is assembled, the team's process requires a thorough review of each indicator drawing from published literature, external input, and further research (**Fig. 2**). The overall review is guided by a series of questions relating to the scientific soundness and usability of the indicator (**Fig. 3**). When evidence from the readily available sources is inconclusive, the evaluation process requires a clinical panel review.

This structured review by a multidisciplinary group of clinicians establishes consensual validity, which "extends face validity from one expert to a panel of experts who examine and rate the appropriateness of each item."[25] For the PDIs review, 19 national organizations nominated 125 individuals, from which 45 panelists were selected to create four panels with applicable and diverse membership in terms of setting (eg geographic region, community hospital, children's hospital, and ambulatory care) and field of practice (eg, adolescent medicine, allergy/immunology, cardiology, cardiothoracic surgery, critical care medicine, emergency medicine, endocrinology, family medicine, general pediatrics, general surgery, hematology/oncology, hospital medicine, infectious diseases, pulmonology, neonatology, neurosurgery, nursing, radiology, and urology).

Adapting the RAND/UCLA Appropriateness Method,[26] the process for clinical panel assessment consists of sending each panelist a packet of background information and a questionnaire for each indicator, reviewing each panelist's ratings and comments, and using areas of disagreement to develop an agenda for moderated discussion by way of telephone with all panel members, followed by final independent assessment by clinician panelists using the same questionnaire. For the PDIs, a previous clinical panel review questionnaire was modified to seek input on different indicator applications, specifically comparative reporting among hospitals and quality improvement within a hospital. In earlier work on the AHRQ Patient Safety Indicators, quality indicators were mostly used for quality improvement, and comparative

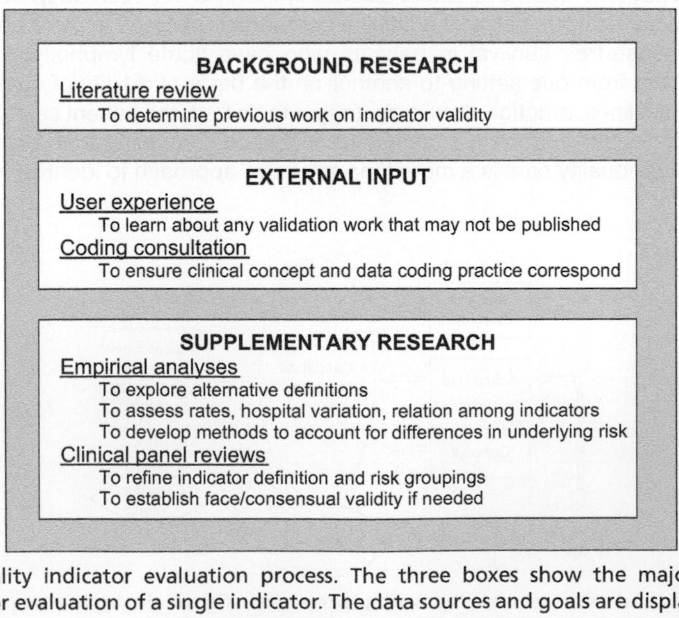

Fig. 2. Quality indicator evaluation process. The three boxes show the major activities required for evaluation of a single indicator. The data sources and goals are displayed within each box.

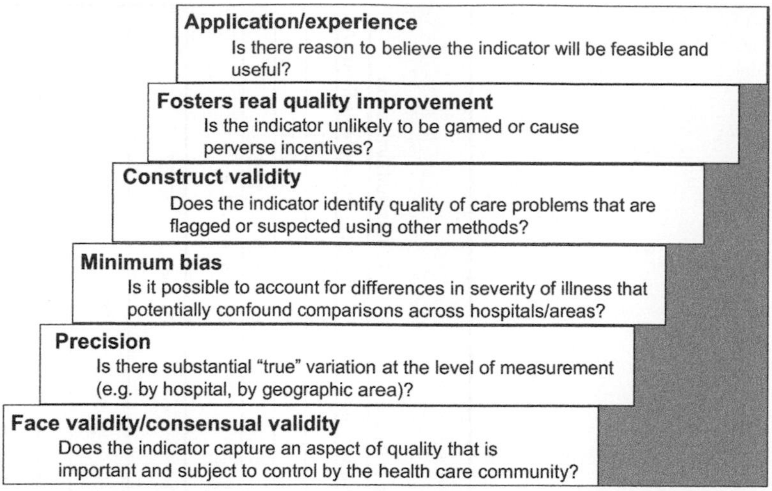

Fig. 3. Evaluation criteria and guiding questions. The figure presents the building blocks to assessing individual indicators for scientific soundness, unintended consequences of use, and potential acceptability.

reporting applications were rare. Additional indicators for the PDIs set included rates of potentially avoidable hospitalization, which required a different set of questions about threats to validity than those used for patient safety metrics.[22,27] Given the changes in the measurement environment, future indicator assessments could also evaluate usefulness for pay-for-performance applications.

Of the 30 indicators in the AHRQ Quality Indicators that were potentially applicable to pediatrics, 18 indicators were selected for inclusion in the PDIs module.[1] Some were removed from consideration prior to panel review because of issues raised by empiric analyses. For example, pneumonia mortality is too rare in children to be used as a reliable measure. Input from users and unpublished chart reviews led to elimination of the failure-to-rescue indicator. Some indicators were eliminated or changed based on clinical panel review. The clinical review results for the final set of indicators are shown in **Table 2**.

Selection is relative, in that an indicator set attempts to bring in the best indicators at the time that meet a reasonable level of credibility in response to the quality indicator validity framework (see **Fig. 3**). As indicator sets are made available, further research and actual use of the indicators provides additional data regarding validity. As shown in **Fig. 1**, this information also can feed back into the process of indicator refinement, may suggest potential revisions to the set as a whole, and expand knowledge for interpreting indicator results in practice. The AHRQ Quality Indicator program provides ongoing support and access to the research team (by way of e-mail to www.support@qualityindicators.ahrq.gov), making technical assistance and this feedback loop seamless.

APPLICATION OF THE AGENCY FOR HEALTHCARE RESEARCH AND QUALITY PEDIATRIC QUALITY INDICATORS

An important early application of the AHRQ PDIs module is research.[28–30] More in-depth study may guide appropriate use and interpretation. For example, NACHRI supported a chart review study of cases flagged by 11 indicators from the PDIs set at

Table 2
Indicators selected for inclusion in the Agency for Healthcare Research and Quality Pediatric Quality Indicators

		Panel Usefulness Rating		76-hospital Evaluation	
PDIs	Age Range[a]	Internal QI	Comparative Reporting	PPV Range[b]	Preventable Events/y
Accidental puncture or laceration	0–17 y	Yes (–)	No	32.4–68.0	286–601
Decubitus ulcer	0–17 y	Yes (–)	Yes (–)	51.4–78.9	157–241
Foreign body left in during procedure	0–17 y	Yes	Yes	44.4–80.0	14–26
Iatrogenic pneumothorax (in neonates at risk)	<28 days, birth weight of 2500 g or less	Yes	Yes (–)	10.0–20.0	2–4
Iatrogenic pneumothorax (in nonneonates)	0–17 y, excludes those who have a birth weight of 2500 g or less	Yes	Yes (–)	29.0–64.2	50–111
Pediatric heart surgery mortality rate	<18 y, excludes those <30 d with PDA closure only	Yes	Yes	n/a	n/a
Pediatric heart surgery volume	Same as above	n/a	n/a	n/a	n/a
Postoperative hemorrhage and hematoma	0–17 y	Yes	Yes	12.9–57.1	18–79
Postoperative respiratory failure	0–17 y	Yes	Yes (–)	13.9–39.8	106–305
Postoperative sepsis	0–17 y, neonates excluded	Yes (–)	No	25.6–66.9	177–464

Postoperative wound dehiscence	0–17 y	Yes	Yes	34.1–75.0	10–22
Selected infection due to medical care	0–17 y	Yes (–)	No	40.0–80.7	605–1221
Transfusion reaction	0–17 y, neonates excluded	Yes	Yes (–)	0.0–20.0	0–1
Area-level potentially preventable hospitalizations					
Asthma	2–17 y	Yes	Yes (–)	n/a	n/a
Diabetes short-term complications	6–17 y	Yes	No	n/a	n/a
Gastroenteritis	3 mo–17 y	Yes (–)	No	n/a	n/a
Perforated appendix	1–17 y	Yes (–)	Yes (–)	n/a	n/a
Urinary tract infection	3 mo–17 y	Yes (–)	No	n/a	n/a

The notation "Yes (–)" reflects a rating with less concordance among panelists than a simple "Yes" without the minus sign.

Abbreviations: n/a, not accessed; PPV, positive predictive value; QI, quality indicator.

[a] All indicators have specific inclusion, exclusion, and risk adjustment defined in detail elsewhere.[22] All exclude neonates who had birth weight less than 500 g, obstetric patients, and normal newborns (if applicable).

[b] PPV for preventable cases relative to all cases flagged by indicator, after excluding cases present on admission. Low estimates more certain and high estimates possible, depending on clinical interpretation.

Data from McDonald K, Romano P, Davies S, et al. Measures of pediatric health care quality based on hospital administrative data: the pediatric quality indicators. Rockville (MD): Agency for Healthcare Research and Quality (AHRQ); 2007; and Scanlon MC, Harris JM, Levy F, et al. Evaluation of the Agency for Healthcare Research and Quality Pediatric Quality Indicators. Pediatrics 2008;121(6):e1723–31.

76 children's hospitals. The study quantified the effect of missing information from the administrative data source about whether a complication of care was present on admission.[27] Three indicators had high rates of flagged cases present prior to the hospital admission: decubitis ulcer (40%), postoperative sepsis (40%), and selected infections caused by medical care (43%). With new requirements for hospital administrative data sets to distinguish whether a complication occurred during the hospital stay, and with modifications to the PDI software to use this information, the accuracy of finding cases of potentially preventable complications will improve. The study also examined the preventability of complications experienced by patients, calculating positive predictive values for finding preventable complications relative to all complications uncovered by the PDI (see **Table 2**). The assessment of preventability depends on the individual clinician evaluating the chart and the state of medical science at the time. A complication that is not preventable today may be amenable to strategies developed in the future to reduce its occurrence.

Similarly to the NACHRI study, hospitals can run (or have another organization analyze) the entire PDIs set with their data to efficiently produce a subset of cases, and then drill down with chart review and additional data capture to guide quality improvement efforts. In the NACHRI review that started with 1.7 million hospitalizations, approximately 25,000 discharges (1.5%) were flagged for further study. Alternatively, a hospital quality program officer might use specific indicators that line up with particular quality improvement initiatives and monitor indicator results over time. These and other applications to quality improvement may benefit from comparison to national data on the PDIs, which are available by query from the Healthcare Cost and Utilization Project (HCUP) Web site (www.HCUPnet.ahrq.gov).[31] Any comparative use of a quality indicator necessitates appropriate risk adjustment to the extent feasible with the given data source. The AHRQ PDIs have this capability built into the software.

Figs. 4 and **5** are based on the HCUP Nationwide Inpatient Sample extracted from HCUPnet and show national estimates for adjusted rates for 3 years—2001, 2003, and 2005—for the four area-level indicators with population denominators (see **Fig. 4**) and for the hospital-level indicators that netted at least 100 potentially preventable complications per year among the 76 hospitals in the NACHRI study (see **Fig. 5**). Rates have not changed much over the period, indicating opportunity for improvements in the future.

In addition to uses by researchers and hospitals, the PDIs are under review or already implemented in several state reports.[32,33] Some reports are not officially mandated and are made available by the research community, such as an analysis of 2005 state data for Tennessee of the five area-level PDIs that identify potentially avoidable pediatric hospitalizations (PAPH).[34] This report's application of the PDIs found 6725 PAPH discharges that cost hospitals a total of $17.6 million in 2005. Of note, the diabetes short-term complication rate was much higher than the national average, indicating a useful starting point for delving into potential barriers to high-quality primary care for those diabetic children who were hospitalized. Texas, like some other states, has ongoing mandates for comparative public reporting of hospital data. With the availability of the AHRQ PDIs, the Texas data organization considered potential inclusion of the indicators in its annual reports. A collaborative developed between hospitals and the state's representatives to anticipate and address each other's needs in the short- and long-range.[35] Selected AHRQ PDIs were incorporated and released at the end of 2007 and are available for comparison of hospitals.[36] Meanwhile, the collaborative is working toward incorporating other sources of data and indicators into public reports.[35] The ongoing challenge of these efforts is finding publicly available, clinically rich data collected in a standardized fashion in all relevant settings.

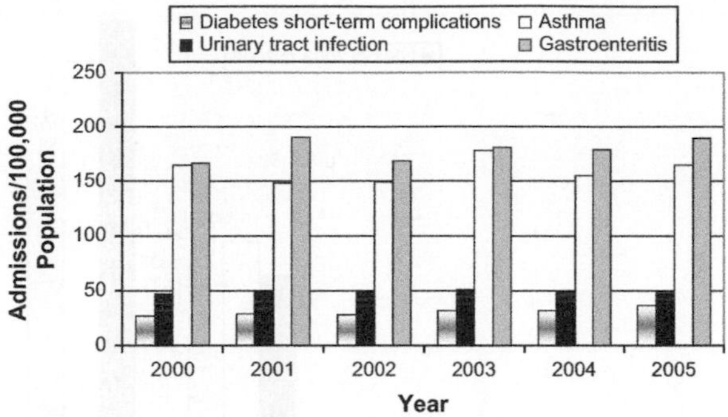

Fig. 4. Area-level PDI rates. The graph presents the risk-adjusted rates of four indicators from the AHRQ PDIs. Diabetes short-term complications admissions include ketoacidosis, hyperosmolarity, or coma in children aged 6 to 17 years. Urinary tract infection admissions include children aged 3 months to 17 years, and exclude patients who have disorders of the kidneys or urinary tract and patients in an immunocompromised state. Asthma admissions for children aged 2 to 17 years exclude patients who have cystic fibrosis or respiratory system anomalies. Gastroenteritis admissions for children 3 months to 17 years exclude patients who have gastrointestinal abnormalities or bacterial gastroenteritis. All area-level indicators exclude patients transferred from another institution. Each indicator is calculated and risk adjusted according to detailed specifications available at: www.qualityindicators.ahrq.gov, and is derived from the HCUP Nationwide Inpatient Sample for the given year and Version 3.1 of the AHRQ PDIs software.

CHALLENGES IN INDICATOR SELECTION AND USE

As with the Texas experience and that of others, real stumbling blocks exist in selecting and using measures. If we wait for ideal data sources, then progress will be slow on the path toward quality improvement; however, in using data sources that are missing some of the information that would make assessments more meaningful, we risk misinterpretation. This risk can be mitigated if we consider the use of a particular measure and apply it appropriately, benefiting from the indicator's strengths and carefully accommodating its deficiencies.

Quality measurements are part of the diagnostic toolbox for understanding what ails the health care system at a given point in time. As with patient care, interpreting a diagnostic test result is a function of the likelihood of the patient having a disease and the performance characteristics of the test. We have mounting evidence about gaps in quality, and so measures that are "good enough" and not necessarily as high performing on sensitivity and specificity as we might ultimately want can move us toward directing quality improvement activities to good effect.

But thinking about any adverse consequences to treating prematurely or empirically in a given context merits careful consideration. If quality indicators are applied directly to quality improvement, then adverse consequences or overinspection of the indicators' shortcomings may distract providers from investigating and treating potential clinical and organizational sources of suboptimal care that could relate to the indicator finding, if true. Thus, the assumption that the indicator result is pointing to a deficiency could be followed up with an assessment about which interventions might reduce the likelihood of poor performance on the metric. Empiric therapy would result in implementing the interventions and seeing whether improvement in the indicator follows.

If the quality indicators are used for public comparative reporting, then adverse consequences of a false positive include patients choosing a hospital they think is

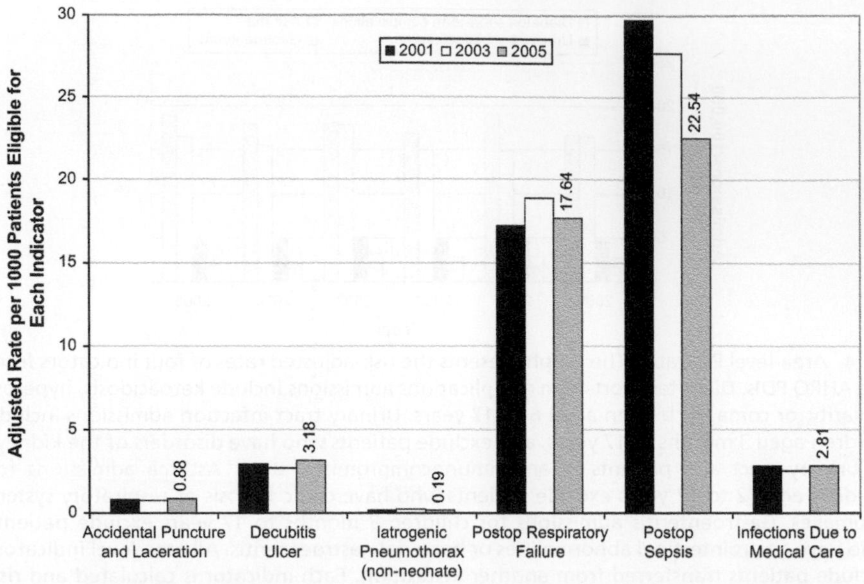

Fig. 5. Selected hospital-level AHRQ PDIs. The graph presents the risk-adjusted rates for six indicators from the AHRQ PDIs. All indicators rely on secondary diagnosis coding to count a complication of care for the numerator (after excluding patients in whom the complication is unlikely to be preventable to the extent feasible with administrative data) and use patients at risk for the complication as the denominator. For example, postoperative sepsis is defined as the number of patients who have sepsis (secondary diagnosis for septicemia, septic shock, inflammatory response attributable to infectious process, and so forth) per 1000 eligible admissions (all surgical patients aged 0–17 years, except with a principal diagnosis of sepsis or infection, neonates, and stays under 4 days). Each indicator is calculated and risk adjusted according to detailed specifications available at: www.qualityindicators.ahrq.gov, and is derived from the HCUP Nationwide Inpatient Sample for the given year and Version 3.1 of the AHRQ PDI software. Postop, postoperative.

better, when in fact it is not, and having a worse outcome from their care. In addition, the hospitals and care providers measured will expend lots of time and energy to support their credible claim that the measure is giving an incorrect reading on the actual quality delivered. Thus, public exposure argues for more robust measures and a good system of conveying the confidence interval reflecting the measurement error. If, however, comparative reporting is used in hospital consortiums and away from the public's eye, then the situation and thresholds for "good enough" measurement are more akin to those in the quality improvement application.

Finally, measure use for reimbursement is becoming commonplace. This movement offers the possibility of rewarding systems and providers who offer the best quality of care. This newer territory, however, makes the need for high-fidelity measures more pressing. Potential adverse consequences of using less refined measures depend on the specific deficiencies in measurement and the particular circumstance but could include (1) changing practice behavior to avoid taking care of sicker patients (eg, "cherry-picking") if risk adjustment is inadequate, (2) giving less attention to that which is not measured but may be vital clinically, and (3) moving the focus to the measures as opposed to the actual care of the children and support of their families. As with other applications, the issue is not only the measurement's performance characteristics but also what steps are taken on the basis of results from the measure. Even pay-for-performance could use less developed measures if the initial results were followed by careful audits and efforts to supplement the data and analysis to assure fairness.

SUMMARY

With a large pipeline of measures for potential NQF endorsement, with the recent developments to not pay for some iatrogenic complications (for Medicare patients), and with public knowledge about quality variation, measures are here to stay. They can cause some distress, given the exposure of both accurate and inaccurate findings about quality of care. The pediatric field has some advantages compared with the adult counterpart, as it enters more deeply into measurement territory. The smaller number of patients makes the world of pediatrics cozier and potentially more collaborative, and more lessons are available from the intense scrutiny in the adult-care arena. These factors offer an opportunity to the pediatrics community to view the development and application of measures from the perspective of an evolutionary process of continuous quality improvement. Past history has shown that criticism of measures will not obviate the need for this vital tool for quality improvement. Instead, critiques can make the measures better. Within this context, measures and their uses are best approached the same way we think about quality itself—through a continuous cycle of improvement.

ACKNOWLEDGEMENTS

I thank Sheryl Davies, Corinna Haberland, Jeffrey Geppert, Patrick Romano, and Olga Saynina for their ongoing teamwork and contributions to quality measure research and continuous improvement of the AHRQ PDIs. Thanks also to Kristin Cox for administrative assistance and help with background research.

REFERENCES

1. McDonald KM, Davies SM, Haberland CA, et al. Preliminary assessment of pediatric health care quality and patient safety in the United States using readily available administrative data. Pediatrics 2008;122(2):e416–25.
2. Perrin JM, Homer CJ. The quality of children's health care matters—time to pay attention. N Engl J Med 2007;357(15):1549–51.
3. Committee on Redesigning Health Insurance Performance Measures, Payment, and Performance Improvement Programs. Performance measurement: accelerating improvement. Washington DC: National Academies Press; 2005.
4. Beal AC, Co JP, Dougherty D, et al. Quality measures for children's health care. Pediatrics 2004;113(1 Pt 2):199–209.
5. Dougherty D, Simpson LA. Measuring the quality of children's health care: a prerequisite to action. Pediatrics 2004;113(1 Pt 2):185–98.
6. Shaller D. Implementing and using quality measures for children's health care: perspectives on the state of the practice. Pediatrics 2004;113(1 Pt 2):217–27.
7. Menachemi N, Struchen-Shellhorn W, Brooks RG, et al. Influence of pay-for-performance programs on information technology use among child health providers: the devil is in the details. Pediatrics 2009;123(Suppl 2):S92–6.
8. Mangione-Smith R, DeCristofaro AH, Setodji CM, et al. The quality of ambulatory care delivered to children in the United States. N Engl J Med 2007;357(15):1515–23.

9. Knapp JF, Simon SD, Sharma V. Quality of care for common pediatric respiratory illnesses in United States emergency departments: analysis of 2005 National Hospital Ambulatory Medical Care Survey Data. Pediatrics 2008;122(6): 1165–70.
10. Miller MR, Zhan C. Pediatric patient safety in hospitals: a national picture in 2000. Pediatrics 2004;113(6):1741–6.
11. Woods D, Thomas E, Holl J, et al. Adverse events and preventable adverse events in children. Pediatrics 2005;115(1):155–60.
12. Simpson L, Dougherty D, Krause D, et al. Measuring children's health care quality. Am J Med Qual 2007;22(2):80–4.
13. Kelley E, Hurst J. Health care quality indicators project conceptual framework paper. OECD Health Working Paper. 2006. Available at: http://www.oecd.org/dataoecd/1/36/36262363.pdf. Accessed January 29, 2009.
14. NQF Measure Evaluation Criteria. Available at: http://www.qualityforum.org/about/leadership/measure_evaluation.asp. Accessed January 29, 2009.
15. National Quality Measures Clearinghouse Inclusion Criteria. Available at: http://www.qualitymeasures.ahrq.gov/submit/inclusion.aspx. Accessed January 29, 2009.
16. NQF Candidate Consensus Standards as of October 29, 2008. Available at: http://www.qualityforum.org/pdf/tblcandidatemeasurescurrent.xls. Accessed January 29, 2009.
17. Kaplan S, Normand S. Conceptual and analytical issues in creating composite measures of ambulatory care performance. Standardizing Ambulatory Care Performance Measures Project (Phase 3). Available at: http://www.qualityforum.org/pdf/projects/CEF/5%2024%2007%20Kaplan-Normand.pdf. Accessed January 29, 2009.
18. Hodgson ES, Simpson L, Lannon CM. Principles for the development and use of quality measures. Pediatrics 2008;121(2):411–8.
19. The National Quality Forum Measure Evaluation Criteria. Available at: http://www.qualityforum.org/about/leadership/tbEvalCriteria2008-08-28Final.pdf. Accessed February 1, 2009.
20. Pediatric Data Quality Systems (Pedi-QS) Collaborative Measures Workgroup. Available at: http://www.pediqs.com/home.html. Accessed January 29, 2009.
21. Hospital Compare. A quality tool provided by medicare. Available at: http://www.hospitalcompare.hhs.gov/Hospital/Static/About-HospQuality.asp?dest=NAV%7CHome%7CAbout%7CQualityMeasures. Accessed January 29, 2009.
22. McDonald K, Romano P, Davies S, et al. Measures of pediatric health care quality based on hospital administrative data: the pediatric quality indicators. Rockville (MD): Agency for Healthcare Research and Quality (AHRQ); 2007.
23. AHRQ quality indicators. Available at: http://qualityindicators.ahrq.gov/general_faq.htm. Accessed January 29, 2009.
24. Donabedian A. Evaluating the quality of medical care. Milbank Mem Fund Q 1966;44(3 Suppl):166–206.
25. Green L, Lewis F. Measurement and evaluation in health education and heath promotion. Mountain View (CA): Mayfield Publishing Company; 1998.
26. Fitch K, Bernstein S, Aguilar M, et al. The RAND/UCLA Appropriateness Method user's manual. Santa Monica (CA): RAND; 2001.
27. McDonald K, Romano P, Geppert J, et al. Measures of patient safety based on hospital administrative data—the patient safety indicators. Technical Review 5 (Prepared by the University of California San Francisco-Stanford Evidence-based Practice Center under Contract No. 290-97-0013). AHRQ Publication

No. 02-0038. Rockville (MD): Agency for Healthcare Research and Quality; 2002.
28. Scanlon MC, Harris JM, Levy F, et al. Evaluation of the agency for healthcare research and quality pediatric quality indicators. Pediatrics 2008;121(6): e1723–31.
29. Herrod HG, Chang CF. Potentially avoidable pediatric hospitalizations as defined by the Agency for Healthcare Research and Quality: what do they tell us about disparities in child health? Clin Pediatr (Phila) 2008;47(2):128–36.
30. Smith RB, Cheung R, Owens P, et al. Medicaid markets and pediatric patient safety in hospitals. Health Serv Res 2007;42(5):1981–98.
31. HCUPnet, Healthcare Cost and Utilization Project. Agency for Healthcare Research and Quality. Available at: http://hcupnet.ahrq.gov. Accessed January 29, 2009.
32. State of New Jersey. Department of Health and Senior Services: Office of Health Care Quality Assessment. Available at: http://www.state.nj.us/health/healthcarequality/index.shtml. Accessed January 24, 2009.
33. Community engagement. Iowa Healthcare Collaborative. 2008 Iowa Report. Available at: http://www.ihconline.org/iowareport/2008/documents/IowaReport2008.pdf. Accessed January 24, 2009.
34. Chang C, Herrod H, Steinberg S. Potentially avoidable pediatric hospitalizations in Tennessee, 2005. Memphis (TN): Methodist LeBonheur Center for Healthcare Economics, The University of Memphis; 2008.
35. Levy FH, Henion JS, Harris JM. Journey toward meaningful pediatric quality metric reporting: the Texas experience. J Healthc Qual 2008;30(3):36–42, 50.
36. Quality of Children's Care in Texas Hospitals, 2006. Center for Health Statistics, Texas Health Care Information Collection. Available at: http://www.dshs.state.tx.us/THCIC/Publications/Hospitals/PDIReport/PDIReport.shtm. Accessed January 29, 2009.

Quality Improvement, Clinical Research, and Quality Improvement Research—Opportunities for Integration

Peter Margolis, MD, PhD[a,*], Lloyd P. Provost, MS[b], Pamela J. Schoettker, MS[c], Maria T. Britto, MD, MPH[d]

KEYWORDS

- Quality improvement • Quality improvement research
- Implementation sciences • QI

Society's investments in biomedical research have produced an explosion of new discoveries, and it is widely anticipated that advances will be translated into much more effective medical care and better health outcomes for patients. Yet the medical community is still slow to implement most new discoveries or to ensure reliable delivery of known effective treatments.[1,2] Studies have demonstrated significant variation in health outcomes across providers and communities in the use of appropriate care and in the safety and quality of care.[3–6] For example, investigators at the RAND Corporation showed that adults in the United States receive only 50% to 60% of recommended acute, chronic, and preventive health care.[3,4] Using the same methodology, they found that children receive only 47% of recommended care.[7]

The National Institutes of Health Roadmap initiative recognizes the need for much greater emphasis on research that spans the trajectory from discoveries in the laboratory, though the evaluation of new therapies at the bedside, to their application in routine medical practice.[8] The conversion of discoveries in the laboratory into

[a] Center for Health Care Quality, Division of Health Policy and Clinical Effectiveness, Cincinnati Children's Hospital Medical Center and University of Cincinnati College of Medicine, 3333 Burnet Avenue, Mail Location 7014, Cincinnati, OH 45229-3039, USA
[b] Associates in Process Improvement, 115 East Fifth Street, Suite 300, Austin, TX 78701, USA
[c] Division of Health Policy and Clinical Effectiveness, Cincinnati Children's Hospital Medical Center, 3333 Burnet Avenue, Mail Location 7014, Cincinnati, OH 45229-3039, USA
[d] Divisions of Adolescent Medicine and Health Policy and Clinical Effectiveness, Cincinnati Children's Hospital Medical Center and University of Cincinnati College of Medicine, 3333 Burnet Avenue, Cincinnati, OH 45229-3039, USA
* Corresponding author.
E-mail address: peter.margolis@cchmc.org (P. Margolis).

Pediatr Clin N Am 56 (2009) 831–841
doi:10.1016/j.pcl.2009.05.008
pediatric.theclinics.com
0031-3955/09/$ – see front matter

widespread clinical care has been called translational research. Although initially conceived as the research necessary to move from discovery in the laboratory to the validation of laboratory findings at the bedside, translational research also embodies studies that go beyond the testing of what care works to the changes required to get effective treatments into widespread clinical practice.[9]

Health services research examines how people get access to health care, how much care costs, and what happens to patients as a result of this care. The goals of health services research are to identify the most effective ways to organize, manage, finance, and deliver high-quality care, to reduce medical errors, and to improve patient safety.[10] Among the most important contributions of health services research have been the identification and description of gaps in care. But describing gaps is different than closing gaps. Fixing the problems in health care delivery will require more intervention-oriented activities aimed at helping redesign the health care delivery system. The need to understand how to change clinical practice to incorporate new knowledge increases the relevance of quality improvement (QI) methods.

Other articles within this issue provide an overview of QI methods and measurement approaches. In this article, some of the opportunities for and challenges of integrating QI and more traditional forms of clinical research to achieve broad improvements in medical care are described. The authors suggest that such integration would include more active experimentation in the health care delivery system and that the application of QI methods offers a rational, effective, and reasonably fast method to support the learning required to adapt new knowledge to specific practice environments and to create and test innovations needed to improve systems of care delivery.

WHAT IS QUALITY IMPROVEMENT?

A July 2006 special report by The Hastings Center[11] defined QI in health care as systematic, data-guided activities designed to bring about immediate, positive changes in the delivery of health care in particular settings. While QI uses a wide variety of methods, they all involve deliberate actions to improve care, guided by data reflecting the effects. Depending on the activity, QI can look like a type of practical problem solving, an evidence-based management style, or the application of a theory-driven science of how to bring about system change. Introducing QI methods often means encouraging people in the clinical care setting to use their daily experience to identify promising ways to improve care, implement changes on a small scale, collect data on the effects of those changes, and assess the results. The goal is to find interventions that work well, implement them more broadly, and thereby improve clinical practice.

The report goes on to suggest that QI is more than the implementation of discrete projects and includes an ongoing process of "self-conscious change, undertaken as a natural consequence of health care providers' ethical responsibility to serve the interests of their patients."[11] This makes QI different from research, which is aimed at addressing a specific question and takes place over a discrete period. The report also makes a distinction between QI and clinical and managerial innovation and adaptation that may take place as part of the normal work of leaders, managers, and workers, without the use of data or formal application of tests of changes.

Box 1 lists a number of additional characteristics of QI in health care. QI methods can be applied to (1) fixing problems in care delivery to become more effective, safe, or efficient; (2) improving processes, products, and services; and (3) designing new processes, products, services, and systems.[12] To date, most QI activity in health care has focused on the first two types of applications. For example, a multidisciplinary

Box 1
Characteristics of health care quality improvement

Contextual factors (background variables or confounders in research) are a major focus.

The initial intervention (changes to the system) is adapted and modified as study progresses.

Involves measuring over time (improvement is temporal).

Includes graphic analysis using statistical process control methods and presentation.

There is involvement of local expertise in conducting the project.

Includes multiple experimental cycles for quick feedback and learning.

Employs multifactor experiments to learn from complex systems that have nonlinear and dynamic cause-and-effect relationships.

Building reliability of the interventions can be a major part of the effort.

Sustainability is a consideration, often from the beginning of the project.

team at Cincinnati Children's Hospital Medical Center (CCHMC) implemented an evidence-based pediatric-specific bundle of care strategies in the pediatric ICU to reduce rates of ventilator-associated pneumonia (VAP).[13] The bundle consisted of a number of elements designed to prevent bacterial colonization of the oropharynx, stomach, and sinuses and prevent aspiration of contaminated secretions. Following implementation of the bundle, the VAP rate was reduced from 5.6 infections per 1000 ventilator days at baseline to 0.3 infections per 1000 ventilator days.

WHAT IS THE SCIENCE OF QUALITY IMPROVEMENT?

Deming[14] described the science of improvement as a body of knowledge that he called a "system of profound knowledge: the interplay of the theories of systems, variation, knowledge, and psychology." Deming believed that it was not necessary to be an expert in all of these areas to participate in QI, but that leaders of QI should understand the basic theories, how the different areas interrelate, and why they are important for any improvement effort. He considered the concept of profound knowledge a lens through which to view organizations and believed that, when combined with appropriate subject matter knowledge, the use of this lens could result in innovative approaches to improving health care processes and systems.

From a scientific standpoint, QI methods emphasize (1) the value of standardization as a means of learning and improving outcomes, (2) a forward-looking analytic framework designed to enable learning from each sequential data point, (3) explicit characterization of prior knowledge, and (4) testing theories about organizational processes and systems through experimentation and replication to produce a detailed understanding of factors affecting system performance. Seeking to understand multiple complex system interactions, rather than controlling or eliminating them, distinguishes QI interventions from therapeutic trials.

The application of QI is particularly useful in understanding the nonlinear, multitiered nature of relationships between processes and outcomes in complex organizational systems. This systems perspective implies that changes in the processes of care may take place at one or more levels within or outside a health care organization. For example, the user's manual[15] for the Institute of Medicine's report on "Crossing the Quality Chasm"[16] proposed a systems framework that identifies the potential influence of multiple layers of the health care system on the outcomes of health care for patients and families. Changes aimed at improving care can be made at the levels of patients and communities; the small work units (microsystems) that provide the care that patients experience; the functioning of larger organizations such as hospitals or health systems that house or otherwise support the microsystems (macrosystems); and the environment (eg, policy, payment, and regulation) that shapes the behavior, interests, and opportunities of organizations. Appreciation of the multitiered nature of organizational systems is useful when guiding the design of interventions or changes. The potential for significant nonlinear effects within complex systems is great, making prediction more difficult. The difficulty of prediction in complex systems increases the importance of experimentation and replication as a basis of learning and theory development.

Reducing unintended variation through standardization is an important strategy in QI. Care standardization itself may significantly improve the quality of care and outcomes by eliminating errors. Indeed, much of the recent emphasis of QI in medicine has concentrated on the benefits that can be achieved by standardizing care. Changes produced by QI efforts typically take place over time. Changes are tested first on a small scale before implementing them widely, on the basis of data being collected as part of the improvement process itself. Thus, the application of QI makes extensive use of interrupted time series or repeated measures designs because of the significant time-related effects. Statistical process control methods,[17] which have been widely used in many industries for nearly 75 years, provide the analytic basis for studying the impact of interventions while they are ongoing so that they can be refined depending on emerging information.

A project to improve influenza vaccination rates for high-risk children and adolescents is an example of the use of QI methods described here. Diffusion of innovation theory[18] was used to scale up to a much larger population a series of evidence-based immunization strategies that resulted in an increase in the proportion of high-risk patients who received the influenza vaccination at seven clinics within the CCHMC.[19] Participating practices included five Ohio regional cystic fibrosis centers, the original seven CCHMC clinics, four additional CCHMC clinics treating high-risk children, and 164 physicians in 39 community-based pediatric practices in the greater-Cincinnati area.[20] The team at each participating site was presented with a tool kit containing supporting literature, sample goals, and communication strategies. The improvement strategies presented to each site were grounded in the previous initiative and modified on the basis of what was learned from that project. The strategies included (1) increased communication through reminder postcards sent to all families, (2) improved access through influenza shot clinics, (3) a standard influenza order set, (4) a Web-based registry and tracking system to identify and follow at-risk patients, (5) in-clinic reminders to patients and health care providers, (6) preplanning with suppliers to obtain vaccine, (7) posting weekly vaccination rates, (8) recall phone calls, and (9) a designated leader at each site. Each site was encouraged to adapt and customize the improvement strategies to meet its specific culture and needs. The intervention targeted 18,866 high-risk children, and 49.7% received the influenza vaccination. The community-based practices that actively participated in the scale-up effort reported using significantly more intervention strategies and achieved higher immunization rates than nonparticipating practices.

WHAT IS QUALITY IMPROVEMENT RESEARCH?

Although QI involves the structured application of the scientific method, it is not research per se for the reasons outlined previously. The authors define QI research as the *design, development, and evaluation* of complex interventions to produce *generalizable* new knowledge related to creating and sustaining improvement in health care delivery in real world settings. This definition emphasizes the importance of producing generalizable knowledge as a feature of QI research.

QI research involves two types of studies: studies of interventions that apply QI methods to redesign care delivery and evaluate the effectiveness of the intervention, and studies focused on evaluating the efficacy of QI methods themselves.[11] The authors' work on improving preventive services delivery in primary care practices is an example of research that incorporates the application of QI. In this randomized trial, the authors evaluated the effectiveness of a QI-based continuing medical education intervention on rates of preventive services delivery in pediatric and family practices.[21] Research evaluating QI might include, for example, a study of different techniques to apply QI methods to affect change, or a study of the impact of various contextual factors such as leadership, incentives, teamwork, and QI knowledge on the effectiveness of QI.

INTEGRATING QUALITY IMPROVEMENT AND RESEARCH

To date, the application of QI in medicine has emphasized reducing errors and achieving more consistent and reliable care delivery. This emphasis has resulted in numerous studies of the process of care delivery. It is not enough to simply change the process and assume that improvements in outcomes will accrue unless those process changes have previously been shown to also improve outcomes. As public demand to redesign the health care delivery system grows, there is an increasing need to create entirely new systems of care delivery and to put new discoveries into practice more rapidly. Therefore, the use of QI methods could be an important part of ongoing health care research.

In the authors' view, greater use of QI methods offers the potential to contribute to the design, conduct, and analysis of health care research. Incorporating these methods may facilitate the design and development of new interventions, may enable greater use of studies of variation to understand organizational behavior and to identify innovations, and may support experimentation in the health care delivery system to better understand the importance of changes to care delivery in specific settings.

Campbell and colleagues[22] described the design and testing of complex interventions in care delivery as proceeding through a number of stages, including developing the theoretic and system models to be tested, defining intervention components, assessing the feasibility of interventions on care delivery, using formal experiments to test the intervention, and performing ongoing study of the intervention as it is disseminated into practice. **Box 2** outlines these phases of research implementation that are based on the framework developed by Campbell and colleagues[22] and describes the contributions of QI.

To illustrate how QI methods might support each of these stages, the authors use the example of designing and testing a care process to improve the management of children who have pain secondary to extremity injury in the emergency department (ED). Pain is the most common reason for seeking care in the ED, making up 48% to 72% of the presenting complaints of all patients.[23] Yet, despite its high prevalence, pain has been poorly managed in ED settings.[24,25] Pain management is particularly poor for children, who are approximately 33% to 50% less likely than adults to receive medication to relieve pain.[24,26]

Numerous QI tools and methods are applicable to the studies required to create a theoretic model and to define intervention components. For example, the Model

Box 2
Phases of research implementation and the contributions of quality improvement

Developing the theoretic and system models to be tested

Understanding the needs of the consumer (Kano survey method)

Process for intervention planning (Model for Improvement)

Relating changes to outcomes (key driver model)

Defining intervention components

Creativity methods and change concepts

Process and system mapping

Use of statistical process control to identify and learn from special causes

Assessing the feasibility interventions on care delivery

Quasi-experimental designs

Statistical process control charts

Using formal experiments to test the intervention

Multifactor experiments

Use of blocking to incorporate background variables in test design

Performing ongoing study of the intervention as it is disseminated into practice

Collaborative improvement methods

for Improvement[12] provides a framework to support the process of specifying outcomes goals and relating changes in the process of care to desired outcomes. Structured methods to incorporate patient perspectives in defining important outcomes of care delivery can take advantage of tools such as the Kano method or conjoint analysis, both of which are formal methods of eliciting the preferences and perspectives of patients.[12] Identifying and documenting current care processes using process mapping can uncover unexpected opportunities for reorganizing care delivery. The application of statistical process control methods can facilitate the study variations in care delivery within a single ED to uncover reasons for inadequate pain management.

The use of industrial benchmarking techniques to study how different EDs handle pain management provides a means to extend studies of variation to learn from the performance of outliers. Statistical process control and other recently developed methods[27] are useful to compare care sites and to support studies of variation across health care delivery settings. Unlike biologic systems, the organizational systems in which QI takes place are largely under the control of the organization's management. In health care, the process of care delivery, therefore, reflects changes in the behavior of the caregivers themselves. Research involving individuals must use epidemiologic tactics such as careful selection of patients and randomization to allow for the variation in biologic response to treatment. Organizational systems such as health care delivery systems permit much greater potential for investigators to understand the organization's rationale for specific care delivery processes. Study designs that combine quantitative and qualitative methods (known as mixed methods studies) offer the opportunity to uncover innovations in care delivery that are associated with better health care outcomes. Thus, QI methods are applicable to unraveling the many factors that result in different levels of performance of certain health care organizations or locations. By engaging care providers, these methods also offer the opportunity for more direct feedback into the research process itself.

QI methods are particularly applicable to testing the feasibility of an intervention and to estimating the magnitude of effect. For example, annotated statistical process control charts[28] can be used to identify and quantify the impact of specific changes in care delivery with improved outcomes.

A particular challenge in QI efforts is that the unit of analysis is often the clinical care site, and changes that are made in care delivery are typically applied to many patients or significant subpopulations at a site. Testing interventions at a single site may limit the ability of investigators to have a comparison group. Quasi-experimental methods such as the interrupted time series design and its variations[29] provide a basis for studies in such settings. These designs are useful in excluding the presence of secular trends but cannot overcome the limitations of generalizability that occur when experiments are conducted in a single setting. For this reason, some QI research can best be conducted using multisite studies. Broader testing of care delivery system interventions across diverse clinical settings would produce better evidence about how to apply new knowledge. From a methodologic standpoint, this type of testing requires that investigators use well-established methods for the analysis of clustered data.[30]

To be useful, research about new treatments must provide information about how to apply new treatments in different types of patients in different types of care settings. EDs caring for children differ significantly in many ways that are related to the success of an intervention to control pain. The types of patients seen (pediatric versus combined children and adults), the training of physicians and staff, and the volume and severity of illness all influence the likelihood of being able to implement a new approach to care delivery. The randomized trial provides information about the average effects of therapies. More advanced experiments using factorial designs are better suited to understanding how to implement components of a new complex intervention in different environments. For example, multifactorial experiments, a method to study multiple components of a system at once,[31] are common in other industries but have seen limited use in clinical research. For example, an initial experiment to understand the factors of pain medication, the use of a dedicated pain treatment room, and a new pain monitoring scale might use a complex (23-1 fractional factorial) design to simultaneously test the importance of these changes in controlling pain in children who have obvious deformities and in those who do not have deformities.

Other advantages of QI methods include their value for research execution. Standardizing care can improve outcomes by reducing variability. Care standardization also offers significant advantages to those interested in experimentation because of the potential to increase study power and lower sample sizes, thereby detecting intervention effects.

WHAT RESOURCES AND INFRASTRUCTURE ARE NEEDED TO COMBINE QUALITY IMPROVEMENT AND RESEARCH?

A more effective system for learning about how to improve health care delivery must address barriers that inhibit studies about how to improve care delivery more effectively. First, institutions and organizations must develop systems to address ethical and human subjects issues related to QI, especially QI that uses experimental methods. The Hastings report suggested procedures for ensuring the ethical conduct of QI, regardless of whether it meets criteria as human subjects research.[11] Although understanding and guidance regarding the gray areas between QI and research are evolving quickly, some general agreement has emerged. Efforts to incorporate accepted standards of care such as evidence-based practice guidelines do not require human subjects review. On the other hand, projects involving randomization or in which patients may receive nonstandard care should be reviewed by human subjects boards. Intent to publish does not automatically imply the need for human subjects review. The institutional review boards at some leading children's hospitals have begun to provide specific, practical guidance regarding QI and human subjects.[32,33] Second, the unit-of-analysis problem (ie, interventions applied to populations rather than to individual patients) means that multiple sites may be needed to produce the sample size required to generate new knowledge about the effectiveness of novel approaches to care delivery. Third, there are limited numbers of children who have adverse outcomes or chronic diseases. Even large children's hospitals may not have enough patients to determine whether specific changes in care delivery are associated with better outcomes. Fourth, to be able to study the effectiveness of changes in care delivery means that health care "laboratories" are needed at which care can be redesigned. The ability to study the effectiveness is especially important in an era of rapidly emerging technologies and that emphasizes more personalized medicine. The authors conclude by outlining the unique role for academic centers in redesigning care delivery.

As more advanced applications of QI methods take place, there will be an emphasis on the use of active experimentation in the health care delivery setting, requiring the capacity to deliver care and conduct complex experiments at the same time and overcoming the traditional barriers between clinical care, education, and research. There is an opportunity for health care organizations to improve practice by becoming hubs of innovation and transformation, with linkages across the entire spectrum of

Box 3
Features of a redesigned health care laboratory

Infrastructure for improvement and quality improvement research

Leadership

Use of quality improvement methods to achieve stable and reliable care delivery

Sites for developing and testing new ideas

Appropriate teams and skills

Scientific tools and resources

Health services and outcomes research capacity

Institutional review board familiarity with quality improvement methods and research

Real-time data management capable of collecting data during care delivery and of rapidly analyzing data

Application of advanced quality improvement methods for experimentation

Appropriate staff skills

Frontline staff capable of conducting improvement and research

Ongoing development of managerial and academic leaders through training in improvement methods and quality improvement research

Multidisciplinary project teams spanning translational steps (bench-bedside-community)

research—from basic science to application of new knowledge. The features of such a redesigned health care laboratory will include a greater capacity throughout the health care organization to apply QI methods; an appropriate array of scientific tools and resources, including well-developed health services and outcomes research capacity; and knowledgeable staff (**Box 3**). Some health care organizations, such as the Veteran's Administration, Kaiser Permanente, and CCHMC, have recognized the potential value of integrating their resources in this way, and it is likely that more organizations will do so in the future. For example, CCHMC has developed a chronic illness care innovation laboratory where physicians, staff, and patients work together to conduct experiments in care delivery. CCHMC has also developed a disease-specific outcomes and innovation program aimed at linking discovery-oriented research with the redesign of care delivery around specific conditions such as cystic fibrosis. In addition, CCHMC participates in networks of subspecialty care sites such as inflammatory bowel disease practices to conduct multisite improvement and research.

In summary, the opportunity to mobilize linkages between QI and research is at an early stage. Some of the opportunities and challenges that may be involved are outlined in this article. The authors believe that better integration of QI and research methods offers the possibility of more rapid learning and improvement of care delivery simultaneously.

ACKNOWLEDGMENTS

The authors thank Dr. Srikant Iyer for providing details of his research on improving the management of children who have pain secondary to extremity injury in the emergency department.

REFERENCES

1. Cabana M, Rand C, Powe N, et al. Why don't physicians follow clinical practice guidelines? A framework for improvement. J Am Med Assoc 1999;282(15): 1458–65.
2. Grol R, Wensing M. What drives change? Barriers to and incentives for achieving evidence-based practice. Med J Aust 2004;180(6 Suppl):S57–60.
3. Kerr E, McGlynn E, Adams J, et al. Profiling the quality of care in twelve communities: results from the CQI study. Health Aff (Millwood) 2004;23(3):247–56.
4. McGlynn E, Asch S, Adams J, et al. The quality of health care delivered to adults in the United States. N Engl J Med 2003;348(26):2635–45.
5. Asch S, Kerr E, Keesey J, et al. Who is at greatest risk for receiving poor-quality health care? N Engl J Med 2006;354(11):1147–56.
6. Schuster M, McGlynn E, Brook R. How good is the quality of health care in the United States? Milbank Q 1998;76(4):517–63.
7. Mangione-Smith R, DeCristofaro A, Setodji C, et al. The quality of ambulatory care delivered to children in the United States. N Engl J Med 2007;357(15):1515–23.
8. U.S. Department of Health and Human Services, National Institutes of Health, Division of Program Coordination P, and Strategic Initiatives (DPCPSI). NIH roadmap for medical research: overview of the NIH roadmap. Available at: http://nihroadmap.nih.gov/overview.asp. Accessed December 23, 2008.
9. Dougherty D, Conway P. The "3T's" road map to transform US healthcare: the "hows" of high-quality care. JAMA 2008;299(19):2319–21.
10. U.S. Department of Health and Human Services, Agency for Healthcare Research and Quality. What is AHRQ? AHRQ Pub. No. 02–0011, February

2002. Available at: http://www.ahrq.gov/about/whatis.pdf. Accessed December 29, 2008.
11. Baily M, Bottrell M, Lynn J, et al. The ethics of using QI methods to improve health care quality and safety. Garrison (NY): The Hastings Center; 2006. Available at: www.thehastingscenter.org/Publications/SpecialReports/Detail.aspx?id=1342. Accessed December 23, 2008.
12. Langley G, Nolan K, Nolan T, et al. The improvement guide. A practical approach to enhancing organizational performance. San Francisco (CA): Jossey-Bass; 1996.
13. Bigham M, Amato R, Bondurrant P, et al. Ventilator-associated pneumonia in the pediatric intensive care unit: characterizing the problem and implementing a sustainable solution. J Pediatr 2009;154(4):582–7.
14. Deming W. The new economics for industry, government, education. Cambridge (MA): Massachusetts Institute of Technology, Center for Advanced Engineering Study; 1993.
15. Berwick D. A user's manual for the IOM's 'Quality Chasm' report. Health Aff (Millwood) 2002;21(3):80–90.
16. Institute of Medicine. Committee on Quality Health Care in America: crossing the quality chasm—a new health system for the 21st century. Washington, DC: National Academy Press; 2001.
17. Shewhart W. Economic control of quality of manufactured product. New York: Van Nostrand; 1931.
18. Rogers E. Diffusion of innovations. 4th edition. New York: Free Press; 1995.
19. Britto M, Pandzik G, Meeks C, et al. Combining evidence and diffusion of innovation theory to enhance influenza immunization. Jt Comm J Qual Patient Saf 2006; 32(8):426–32.
20. Britto M, Schoettker P, Pandzik G, et al. Improving influenza immunization for high-risk children and adolescents. Qual Saf Health Care 2007;16(5):363–8.
21. Margolis P, Lannon C, Stuart J, et al. Practice based education to improve delivery systems for prevention in primary care: randomised trial. BMJ 2004; 328(7436):388.
22. Campbell M, Fitzpatrick R, Haines A, et al. Framework for design and evaluation of complex interventions to improve health. BMJ 2000;321(7262):694–6.
23. Cordell W, Keene K, Giles B, et al. The high prevalence of pain in emergency medical care. Am J Emerg Med 2002;20(3):165–9.
24. Petrack E, Christopher N, Kriwinsky J. Pain management in emergency department: patterns of analgesic utilization. Pediatrics 1997;99(5):711–4.
25. Todd K, Ducharme J, Choiniere M, et al. Pain in the emergency department: results of the pain and emergency medicine initiative (PEMI) multicenter study. J Pain 2007;8(6):460–6.
26. Brown J, Klein E, Lewis C, et al. Emergency department analgesia for fracture pain. Ann Emerg Med 2003;42(2):197–205.
27. Schulman J, Spiegelhalter D, OParry G. How to interpret your dot: decoding the message of clinical performance indicators. J Perinatol 2008;28(9):588–95.
28. Amin S. Control charts 101: a guide to health care applications. Qual Manag Health Care 2001;9:1–27.
29. Speroff T, O'Connor G. Study designs for PDSA quality improvement research. Qual Manag Health Care 2004;13(1):17–32.
30. Campbell M, Donner A, Klar N. Developments in cluster randomized trials and statistics in medicine. Stat Med 2007;26(1):2–19.
31. Moen RD, Nolan TW, Provost LP. Quality improvement through planned experimentation. 2nd edition. New York: McGraw-Hill; 1999.

32. Children's Hospital Boston. The Clinical Investigation Policy and Procedure Manual. Guidance: what quality improvement and education/competency evaluation activities are considered research and subject to Committee on Clinical Investigation Review. Available at: http://www.childrenshospital.org/cfapps/research/data_admin/Site2206/Documents/cipp_081_014_qi_vs_rsrch.doc. Accessed April 1, 2009.
33. Institutional Review Board for the Research Foundation, Cincinnati Children's Hospital Medical Center. Available at: http://www.cincinnatichildrens.org/research/administration/irb/default.htm. Accessed April 1, 2009.

The Pediatric Quality of Life Inventory: Measuring Pediatric Health-Related Quality of Life from the Perspective of Children and Their Parents

James W. Varni, PhD[a,b,*], Christine A. Limbers, MS[c]

KEYWORDS

- Pediatric Quality of Life Inventory
- Health-related quality of life
- Pediatrics • Health • Children

The past decade has evidenced a dramatic increase in the development and use of pediatric health-related quality of life (HRQOL) measures in an effort to improve pediatric patient health and determine the value of health care services.[1,2] HRQOL is a multidimensional construct, consisting at the minimum of the physical, psychological (including emotional and cognitive), and social health dimensions delineated by the World Health Organization.[3] A number of authors have argued that improving

---

Dr. Varni holds the copyright and the trademark for the PedsQL and receives financial compensation from the Mapi Research Trust, which is a nonprofit research institute that charges distribution fees to for-profit companies that use the Pediatric Quality of Life Inventory.

The PedsQL is available at http://www.pedsql.org.

[a] Department of Pediatrics, College of Medicine, Texas A&M University, College Station, TX 77843, USA

[b] Department of Landscape Architecture and Urban Planning, College of Architecture, Texas A&M University, 3137 TAMU, College Station, TX 77843-3137, USA

[c] Department of Psychology, College of Liberal Arts, Texas A&M University, 4235 TAMU, College Station, TX 77843-4235, USA

* Corresponding author. Department of Landscape Architecture and Urban Planning, College of Architecture, Texas A&M University, 3137 TAMU, College Station, TX 77843-3137.

E-mail address: jvarni@archmail.tamu.edu (J.W. Varni).

Pediatr Clin N Am 56 (2009) 843–863
doi:10.1016/j.pcl.2009.05.016

quality of life is the ultimate goal of health care.[4] Although the term "quality of life" (QOL) is sometimes used interchangeably with HRQOL, QOL is actually a broader construct that encompasses aspects of life which are not amenable to health care services. Thus, HRQOL has emerged as the most appropriate term for QOL health dimensions that are within the scope of health care services.[5]

During the past several years, legislative changes including the Pediatric Exclusivity Provision of the Best Pharmaceuticals for Children Act (BPCA) and the Pediatric Research Equity Act (PREA) have created both voluntary and mandatory guidelines for drug studies in children, resulting in a substantial increase in pediatric clinical trials. Nevertheless, although the above pediatric initiatives have opened the opportunity for children to be included in clinical trials, pediatric patients have not been afforded the right to self-report on matters pertaining to their health and well-being when evaluating the health outcomes of treatments in most pediatric clinical trials to date.[6] This fact stands in sharp contrast to the recent Food and Drug Administration (FDA) Draft Guidance for Industry for evaluating patient-reported outcome (PRO) instruments as health outcomes in clinical trials in which the FDA is quite definitive in stating that "some treatment effects are known only to the patient."[5] Thus, what has been an obvious recognition in clinical trials for adult patients, that is, that PROs are *patient self-reported* outcomes, has not received the same level of recognition in clinical trials for pediatric patients.[6]

PATIENT-REPORTED OUTCOMES

By definition, PROs are self-report instruments that directly measure the patient's perceptions of the impact of disease and treatment as clinical trial end points.[5] PROs include multi-item health-related quality of life (HRQOL) instruments, as well as single-item symptom measures (eg, pain visual analog scale [VAS]).[7–9]

It has been extensively documented in the PRO measurement of children with chronic health conditions and healthy children that information provided by proxy-respondents is not equivalent to that reported by the child.[10,11] The findings on the *proxy problem* "indicate that parent reports cannot be substituted for child self-reports"[12] and evaluations of pediatric patients' perspectives regarding treatment outcomes should be included in pediatric clinical trials given the documented differences between child and parent report.

THE ROLE FOR PARENT PROXY-REPORT

Although pediatric patient self-report should be considered the standard for measuring perceived HRQOL,[13] there may be situations when the child is too young, too cognitively impaired, or too ill or fatigued to complete an HRQOL instrument, and parent proxy-report may be needed in such cases. Further, it is typically parents' perceptions of their children's HRQOL that influences health care use.[14,15] Thus, HRQOL instruments should be chosen that measure the perspectives of both the child and parent because these perspectives may be independently related to health care use, risk factors, and quality of care. Ideally, parent and child HRQOL instruments should measure the same constructs with parallel items to make comparisons between self and proxy report more meaningful.[16]

GENERIC AND DISEASE-SPECIFIC HEALTH-RELATED QUALITY OF LIFE INSTRUMENTS

Although there are a number of disease-specific instruments available, there are potential benefits of integrating generic and disease-specific approaches.[17–19]

Disease-specific measures may enhance measurement sensitivity for health domains germane to a particular chronic health condition, while a generic HRQOL measurement instrument enables comparisons across pediatric populations and facilitates benchmarking with healthy population norms. Thus, there is an emerging perspective that for pediatric chronic health conditions, both generic and disease-specific HRQOL measures should be administered so as to gain a more comprehensive evaluation of the patient's HRQOL.

PEDIATRIC QUALITY OF LIFE INVENTORY MEASUREMENT MODEL

Consistent with the measurement paradigm that generic and disease-specific HRQOL measures should be administered so as to gain a more thorough evaluation of the patient's HRQOL, the Pediatric Quality of Life Inventory (PedsQL) Measurement Model was designed as a modular approach to measuring pediatric HRQOL, developed to integrate the relative merits of generic and disease-specific approaches.[19] Although other pediatric HRQOL instruments exist, including generic measures and disease-specific measures,[2,20] it has been an explicit goal of the PedsQL Measurement Model[19] to develop and test brief measures for the broadest age group empirically feasible, specifically including child self-report for the youngest children possible.[13] The items chosen for inclusion were initially derived from the measurement properties of the child self-report scales, whereas the parent proxy-report scales were constructed to directly parallel the child self-report items. Thus, the development and testing of the PedsQL as a pediatric PRO explicitly emphasizes the child's perceptions. The PedsQL includes child self-report for ages 5 to 18 and parent proxy-report for ages 2 to 18.[21,22] For ages 8 to 18, the PedsQL is self-administered. For ages 5 to 7, the PedsQL is interviewer-administered.

The PedsQL 4.0 Generic Core Scales were designed for application in both healthy and patient populations,[21–23] whereas the PedsQL Disease and Condition Specific Modules were designed to measure HRQOL dimensions specifically tailored for pediatric patients with chronic health conditions.[24–31]

PEDIATRIC QUALITY OF LIFE INVENTORY 4.0 GENERIC CORE SCALES

The PedsQL 4.0 Generic Core Scales have resulted from an extensive iterative process over the past 25 years, involving numerous patient and parent focus groups and individual focus interviews, item generation, cognitive interviewing, pre-testing, and subsequent field testing following standardized protocols,[32–35] with international data on more than 35,000 healthy children and children with numerous pediatric chronic health conditions published or in press in more than 345 peer-reviewed journals since 2001. (A full listing of the updated peer-reviewed journal publications is available at www.pedsql.org.)

The PedsQL 4.0 Generic Core Scales distinguish between healthy children and children with pediatric chronic health conditions, have demonstrated sensitivity to disease severity and responsiveness through patient change over time, and evidence significant intercorrelations with disease-specific symptom scales (based on the conceptualization of disease-specific symptoms as causal indicators of generic HRQOL[36]).[21,22,25–28,31,37–49] Further, the PedsQL 4.0 has shown an impact on clinical decision making, demonstrating significant associations with quality of health care, barriers to health care, and prediction of health care costs over time.[40,50–52]

The items selected for the PedsQL 4.0 Generic Core Scales reflect those that are of universal concern across childhood age groups. Attempts were made to keep wording, and thus the content, as similar as possible across parallel forms, while being sensitive to developmental differences in cognitive ability. For instance, the only differences between child and adolescent self-report is the use of "kids" for items in the Social Functioning Scale in the child self-report version and "teens" for those items in the adolescent self-report version, and "It is hard to keep up with my peers" for the adolescent self-report version rather than "It is hard to keep up when I play with other kids" for the child self-report version. Additionally, parent proxy-report for the toddler age range (ages 2–4) includes only three age-appropriate items for the School Functioning Scale and developmentally appropriate wording for some items in the other scales (eg, "Participating in active play or exercise" rather than "Participating in sport activity or exercise"; "Bathing" rather than "Taking a bath or shower by him or herself"; "Worrying" rather than "Worrying about what will happen to him or her"). This scale construct consistency facilitates the evaluation of differences in HRQOL across and between age groups, as well as the tracking of HRQOL longitudinally. The PedsQL 4.0 Generic Core Scales is the only empirically validated generic pediatric HRQOL measurement instrument that we are aware of to span ages 2 to 18 for parent proxy-report and ages 5 to 18 for child self-report while maintaining item and scale construct consistency. Recent research with the PedsQL 4.0 Generic Core Scales has extended the age range to ages 19 to 25, with additional research in progress on the PedsQL Infant Scales for ages 1 to 24 months.

INTERNATIONAL TRANSLATIONS

There are now more than 65 international translations of the PedsQL 4.0 Generic Core Scales (see www.pedsql.org). Many of these translations were conducted by the Mapi Research Institute in Lyon, France, with the remaining translations conducted by research teams in countries worldwide. The Mapi Research Institute's translations are "official" PedsQL translations,[53] whereas the individual research teams' translations are considered preliminary national translations until further validated by the Mapi Research Institute's translation team.

PEDIATRIC QUALITY OF LIFE INVENTORY DISEASE- AND CONDITION-SPECIFIC MODULES

The PedsQL Disease and Condition-Specific Modules were designed to measure HRQOL dimensions specifically tailored for pediatric chronic health conditions, and currently include the PedsQL Asthma,[27,39] Arthritis/Rheumatology,[28] Brain Tumor,[29] Cancer,[26] Cardiac,[31,54] Cerebral Palsy,[24] End-Stage Renal Disease,[30] and Diabetes Modules,[25] as well as the generic PedsQL Multidimensional Fatigue Scale,[26,38] Pediatric Pain Questionnaire,[55] Family Impact Module,[56] and the Healthcare Satisfaction Module.[57,58] The PedsQL Module Scales were developed through focus groups, cognitive interviews, pre-testing, and field testing measurement development protocols.[32–35] New PedsQL Disease- and Condition-Specific Modules currently in various phases of development and testing include the PedsQL Organ Transplantation Module, Neuromuscular Module, and Sickle Cell Disease Module, with other modules in the planning and early development stages.

The PedsQL Disease- and Condition-Specific Modules are composed of parallel child self-report and parent proxy-report formats, exactly like the PedsQL 4.0 Generic Core Scales. This exact matching format greatly facilitates the integration of the generic and disease-specific scales as originally envisioned in the PedsQL Measurement Model. Each Module contains disease-specific scales that are scored individually, and used as required to achieve the goals and objectives of a particular study. For instance, in a randomized clinical trial testing a new pharmaceutical intervention for pediatric asthma, the 11-item PedsQL Asthma Module Asthma Symptoms Scale would be integrated with the 23-item PedsQL 4.0 Generic Core Scales when the intent of the intervention is to improve asthma symptom control and overall generic HRQOL. In this hypothetical study, for example, it would not be required, nor advised, to include all of the other Asthma Module Scales, such as the Worry and Communication Scales, as these constructs were not the primary objective of the intervention, although the Asthma Treatment Problems Scale might be indicated if barriers to medication adherence were of empiric interest. Thus, the primary outcome measures in this hypothetical randomized clinical trial would be the Asthma Symptoms Scale and the Generic Core Total Scale Score, with the individual Scale Scores from the generic core instrument as secondary outcomes.

This strategy of selecting individual Module Scales depending on the intent of the randomized clinical trial serves to reduce respondent burden and the costs of the trial, and may increase "statistical efficiency" by empirically determining the number of patients needed in a clinical trial through examining subscale intercorrelations, standard deviations, and predicted relative effects.[59] Vickers[59] has delineated a useful strategy for determining the statistical implications of selecting an individual subscale or a combination of subscales as the primary outcome in a randomized trial. When subscales measure distinctly different constructs, the cost/benefit ratio of combining them into a composite score must be carefully considered given the potentially significant implications for respondent burden, the number of patients needed given a specified effect size, and the associated costs. Thus, in the case of the Asthma Module, for example, although there may be a rationale for combining the Asthma Symptoms Scale and the Asthma Treatment Problems Scale into a single composite score, Vickers' statistical efficiency strategy might inform the decision-making process by demonstrating the relative effect sizes for either the Scales individually or as a combined subscale composite score based on the existing data from these Asthma Module Scales. It is likely that for a clinical trial concerned with asthma symptom control, using the Asthma Symptoms Scale as the primary outcome would be more conceptually precise and demonstrate greater statistical efficiency rather than creating a composite score by combining two subscales.

In sum, the PedsQL Disease- and Condition-Specific Modules have been developed to provide disease- and condition-specific Scales that can be individually used for a particular randomized trial, rather than necessitating the costs and respondent burden of requiring that all of the Scales in a particular Module are included. This flexibility is meant to increase the efficiency of determining the efficacy and effectiveness of an intervention with an integrated set of generic and disease-specific HRQOL constructs and scales. Greater detail on the measurement properties of each of the Modules is contained in the published peer-reviewed journal articles cited in the reference list, including age-specific findings. These Modules are briefly described next.

PEDIATRIC QUALITY OF LIFE INVENTORY ASTHMA MODULE

The 28-item PedsQL Asthma Module encompasses 4 Scales[27,39]: (1) Asthma Symptoms (11 items), (2) Treatment Problems (11 items), (3) Worry (3 items), and (4) Communication (3 items). The Asthma Symptoms Scale includes such items as "It is hard to take a deep breath"; "I feel wheezy"; "My chest hurts or feels tight"; "I cough"; "I get out of breath." The Treatment Problems Scale includes such items as "My medicines make me feel sick"; "I have trouble using my inhaler"; "I forget to take my medicines"; "I don't like to carry my inhaler."

PEDIATRIC QUALITY OF LIFE INVENTORY ARTHRITIS/RHEUMATOLOGY MODULE

The 22-item PedsQL Arthritis/Rheumatology Module Scales encompass[28]: (1) Pain and Hurt (4 items), (2) Daily Activities (5 items), (3) Treatment (7 items), (4) Worry (3 items), and (5) Communication (3 items). The Arthritis/Rheumatology Module Scales include such items as "I ache or hurt in my joints and/or muscles"; "I have trouble eating with a fork and knife"; "My medicines make me feel sick"; "I worry about my illness."

PEDIATRIC QUALITY OF LIFE INVENTORY BRAIN TUMOR MODULE

The 24-item PedsQL Brain Tumor Module encompasses 6 Scales[29]: (1) Cognitive Problems (7 items), (2) Pain and Hurt (3 items), (3) Movement and Balance (3 items), (4) Procedural Anxiety (3 items), (5) Nausea (5 items), and (6) Worry (3 items). The Brain Tumor Module Scales include such items as "It is hard for me to learn new things"; "I get headaches"; "It is hard for me to keep my balance"; "It is hard for me to pay attention to things."

PEDIATRIC QUALITY OF LIFE INVENTORY CANCER MODULE

The 27-item PedsQL Cancer Module encompasses 8 Scales[26]: (1) Pain and Hurt (2 items), (2) Nausea (5 items), (3) Procedural Anxiety (3 items), (4) Treatment Anxiety (3 items), (5) Worry (3 items), (6) Cognitive Problems (5 items), (7) Perceived Physical Appearance (3 items), and (8) Communication (3 items). The Cancer Module Scales include such items as "I hurt a lot"; "I become sick to my stomach when I have medical treatment"; "I get scared when I have to have blood tests"; "I worry about the side effects from medical treatments"; "It is hard for me to pay attention to things"; "I don't like other people to see my scars."

PEDIATRIC QUALITY OF LIFE INVENTORY DIABETES MODULE

The 28-item PedsQL Diabetes Module encompasses 5 Scales[25]: (1) Diabetes Symptoms (11 items), (2) Treatment Barriers (4 items), (3) Treatment Adherence (7 items), (4) Worry (3 items), and (5) Communication (3 items). The Diabetes Module Scales include such items as "I feel thirsty"; "I get irritable"; "It is hard for me to take insulin shots"; "It is hard for me to exercise"; "I worry about long-term complications from diabetes."

PEDIATRIC QUALITY OF LIFE INVENTORY CARDIAC MODULE

The 27-item PedsQL Cardiac Module encompasses 6 Scales[31,54]: (1) Heart Problems and Treatment (7 items), (2) Treatment II (5 items), (3) Perceived Physical Appearance (3 items), (4) Treatment Anxiety (4 items), (5) Cognitive Problems (5 items), and (6) Communication (3 items). The Cardiac Module Scales include such items as "My chest hurts or feels tight when I do sports activity or exercise"; "I wake up at night with trouble breathing"; "My heart medicine makes me feel sick"; "It is hard for me to remember what I read."

PEDIATRIC QUALITY OF LIFE INVENTORY CEREBRAL PALSY MODULE

The 35-item PedsQL Cerebral Palsy Module encompasses 7 Scales[24]: (1) Daily Activities (9 items, eg, "It is hard for me to button my shirt"), (2) School Activities (4 items, eg, "It is hard for me to use a mouse for the computer"), (3) Movement and Balance (5 items, eg, "It is hard for me to move one or both of my legs"), (4) Pain and Hurt (4 items, eg, "I ache or hurt in my joints and/or muscles"), (5) Fatigue (4 items, eg, "I feel tired"), (6) Eating Activities (5 items, eg, "It is hard for me to eat with a spoon and/or fork"), and (7) Speech and Communication (4 items, eg, "It is hard for other people to understand my words").

PEDIATRIC QUALITY OF LIFE INVENTORY MULTIDIMENSIONAL FATIGUE SCALE

The 18-item PedsQL Multidimensional Fatigue Scale encompasses 3 Scales[26,38]: (1) General Fatigue Scale (6 items, eg, "I feel tired"; "I feel too tired to do things that I like to do"), (2) Sleep/Rest Fatigue Scale (6 items, eg, "I feel tired when I wake up in the morning"; "I rest a lot"), and (3) Cognitive Fatigue Scale (6 items, eg, "It is hard for me to keep my attention on things"; "It is hard for me to think quickly").

RESPONSIVENESS OF THE PEDIATRIC QUALITY OF LIFE INVENTORY

Improvement in HRQOL is a primary goal in the management of acute and chronic health conditions. As such, determining a HRQOL measure's capacity to detect change in clinical trials and intervention studies is important. Responsiveness is the psychometric property associated with an instrument's ability to measure meaningful or important change.[60] The responsiveness of a measurement instrument is demonstrated through a longitudinal analysis of changes within patients in whom a change is anticipated as a result of, for example, an intervention of known or expected efficacy.[61,62] Responsiveness is a particularly important issue when selecting an HRQOL measure, because instruments that are highly responsive allow clinical trials and intervention studies to be conducted with fewer patients.[63]

The PedsQL has demonstrated responsiveness to evidenced-based interventions and access to health care. **Table 1** illustrates examples of the published data on responsiveness of the PedsQL 4.0 Generic Core Scales and Disease-Specific Modules.

As an example, the PedsQL Generic Core Scales and Asthma Module have demonstrated responsiveness to evidence-based chronic disease management. Specifically, Mangione-Smith and colleagues[64] conducted a national effectiveness trial in pediatric asthma following the Chronic Care Model and the Breakthrough Series collaborative team approach. The Chronic Care Model identifies 6 elements of the health care system such as organization/leadership, patient self-management, delivery system design, health care provider decision support, informational technology, and links to community resources that can be used to optimized chronic disease care.[64] The Breakthrough Series collaborative process emphasizes a team approach to continuous quality improvement in patient chronic disease management.[64] In this effectiveness study,[64] pediatric patients with asthma receiving care from clinics participating in the collaborative intervention had significant improvements in processes of care variables, such as monitoring their peak flows and having a written asthma action care plan. Patients in the intervention group demonstrated higher generic and asthma-specific scores on the PedsQL Generic Core Scales and the PedsQL Asthma Module. This real-world effectiveness trial suggests the potential utility of the PedsQL as a HRQOL outcome measure in clinical practice settings.

The PedsQL 4.0 Generic Core Scales has also demonstrated responsiveness to access to health care.[65] As part of a 2-year, prospective cohort study of enrollees in the California State Children's Health Insurance Program, parents and children completed the PedsQL 4.0 Generic Core Scales at enrollment and after 1 and 2 years in the program.[65] Realized access to care and forgone care were assessed through parents' reports of problems getting necessary care ("In the last 12 months, how

Table 1
Published studies demonstrating responsiveness of the PedsQL 4.0 Generic Core Scales and Disease-Specific Modules

Study	Patient Population/Treatment Condition	PedsQL Outcome(s)	Findings
Varni et al. (2002)[28]	34 pediatric patients with rheumatologic conditions ages 5–18 years receiving clinical care provided by a pediatric rheumatologist; the pediatric rheumatologist evaluated the child for the first time (ie, first visit as a new patient), with treatment then initiated at this visit (Visit 1), with two subsequent follow-up visits (Visits 2 and 3).	PedsQL 4.0 Generic Core Scales PedsQL 3.0 Rheumatology Module	For child self-report and parent proxy-report, the PedsQL Generic Core Total and Summary Scale Scores increased progressively from Visit 1 through Visit 3, with larger effect sizes at Time 3. Effect sizes were in the small range at Time 2, and in the medium to large effect size range at Time 3. The PedsQL 3.0 Rheumatology Module Scales demonstrated improvement over time primarily for Pain and Hurt, with small to medium effect sizes at Time 2, and large effect sizes at Time 3.
Varni et al. (2002)[40]	47 children ages 5–18 years presenting at a pediatric orthopedic clinic for the treatment of fractures	PedsQL 4.0 Generic Core Scales	The PedsQL 4.0 demonstrated responsiveness in the orthopedic clinic sample, with statistically significant changes in scores from the initial clinic visit for the treatment of a fracture to the subsequent follow-up (mean duration follow-up 7.53 months). At the follow-up evaluation, the recovered patients as a group demonstrated a return to health when compared with the healthy children scores.
Sallee et al. (2004)[73]	2968 children ages 6–12 years with a DSM-IV diagnosis of attention-deficit hyperactivity disorder participating in a prospective, open-label trial in which the baseline stimulant treatment regimen of immediate-release methylphenidate was converted to an approximately equivalent once-daily dose of extended-release mixed amphetamine salts	PedsQL 4.0 Generic Core Scales	For parent proxy-report, mean PedsQL 4.0 Generic Core Total Scale score at baseline was 74.5 compared with 81.0 ($P < .01$) after 7 weeks of treatment with extended-release mixed amphetamine salts (child self-report was not assessed in this study).

Mangione-Smith et al. (2005)[64]	385 asthmatic children receiving care at an intervention clinic and 126 receiving care at a control clinic (all children ages 2–17 years); intervention consisted of three 2-day educational sessions for quality improvement teams from participating sites followed by 3 "action" periods over the course of a year	PedsQL 4.0 Generic Core Scales PedsQL 3.0 Asthma Module	The overall process of asthma care improved significantly in the intervention group but remained unchanged in the control group ($P < .0001$); patients in the intervention group were more likely than patients in the control group to monitor their peak flows ($P < .0001$) and to have a written action plan ($P = .001$); patients in the intervention group had better PedsQL 4.0 Generic Core Total Scale scores (80 versus 77, $P = .05$) and asthma-specific quality of life related to treatment problems (89 versus 85, $P < .05$).
Schwimmer et al. (2005)[74]	Single-arm open-label pilot study of metformin 500 mg twice daily for 24 weeks in 10 obese nondiabetic children with biopsy-proven nonalcoholic steatohepatitis ages 8–17 years	PedsQL 4.0 Generic Core Scales	Participants self-reported a significant ($P < .01$) improvement in the mean PedsQL 4.0 Generic Core Total Scale score from baseline (69.00) to following treatment (81.00) at 24 weeks (only child self-report scores reported in manuscript).
Connelly and Rapoff (2006)[75]	40 children with a recurrent headache syndrome ages 7–12 years participating in a 4-week self-directed cognitive-behavioral pain management program	PedsQL 4.0 Generic Core Scales	At 3-month follow-up, participants receiving the self-directed cognitive-behavioral pain management intervention demonstrated significant improvements on the PedsQL 4.0 Generic Core Total Scale score ($P < .01$), Physical Functioning Scale ($P < .01$), and Psychosocial Summary score ($P = .01$; only child self-report scores reported in manuscript).
Felder-Puig et al. (2006)[76]	68 patients receiving allogeneic bone marrow or stem cell transplantation ages 4–18 years	PedsQL 4.0 Generic Core Scales PedsQL 3.0 Cancer Module	In all analyzed PedsQL domains on the Core and Cancer Module for child self-report and parent proxy-report (except for pain), PedsQL scores were significantly better ($P < .01$) at 1 year post transplant compared with the two measurement time points before bone marrow transplant.

(*continued on next page*)

Table 1
(continued)

Study	Patient Population/Treatment Condition	PedsQL Outcome(s)	Findings
Razzouk et al. (2006)[77]	Anemic patients ages 5–18 years receiving myelosuppressive chemotherapy for nonmyeloid malignancies, excluding brain tumors, received intravenous epoetin alfa (EPO) 600 units/kg to 900 units/kg (n = 111) or placebo (n = 111) once weekly for 16 weeks	PedsQL 4.0 Generic Core Scales	EPO-treated patients had greater increases in hemoglobin (Hb) overall ($P = .002$) and were more likely to be transfusion free after 4 weeks (38.7% versus 22.5%; $P = .010$); change in Hb was correlated with change in PedsQL 4.0 Generic Core Total Scale score in the EPO group ($r = 0.242$; $P = .018$), but was not in the placebo group ($r = 0.086$; $P = .430$). Young children ages 5–7 years had the greatest Hb response (92.3% of 5- to 7-year-olds in the EPO group were Hb responders); consistent with these findings, mean patient-reported PedsQL 4.0 Generic Core Total Scale scores at the final visit were significantly greater in the EPO group among patients 5 to 7 years of age (88.0 versus. 78.1; $P = .043$), but not among patients 8 years to 12 years of age or 13 years to 18 years of age.
Seid et al. (2006)[65]	4925 children ages 2–16 years enrolled in the California State Children's Health Insurance Program	PedsQL 4.0 Generic Core Scales	Foregone health care in the past 12 months and problems getting health care in the past 12 months significantly reduce parent proxy-report PedsQL scores by 3.5 and 4.5 points ($P < .001$) and child self-report PedsQL scores by 3.2 and 4.4 points ($P < .001$).

Cuomo et al. (2007)[78]	57 ambulatory children ages 5–15 years with cerebral palsy undergoing multilevel soft tissue surgery to correct sagittal imbalance	PedsQL 4.0 Generic Core Scales	Significant improvements in the PedsQL 4.0 Generic Core Total Scale score and Physical Functioning score were evidenced for parent proxy-report ($P < .001$) approximately 12 months postoperative.
Fullerton et al. (2007)[79]	80 sixth- and seventh- graders at-risk-for-overweight and overweight Mexican American children participating in 6 months of intensive weight management or self-help	PedsQL 4.0 Generic Core Scales	Children in the intensive weight management program condition achieved significantly greater weight loss (z BMI, −0.13; $P < .001$) and significantly greater PedsQL Physical Functioning improvements than those in the self-help condition at 6 months ($P < .05$). PedsQL Physical Functioning increases were associated with z BMI reduction ($P < .05$; only child self-report scores reported in manuscript).
Holterman et al. (2007)[80]	10 morbidly obese adolescents ages 14–17 years receiving laparoscopic adjustable gastric banding (LAGB)	PedsQL 4.0 Generic Core Scales	In the 8 patients with impaired HRQOL at baseline, the mean PedsQL 4.0 Generic Core Total Scale score rose from 62.6 at baseline to 75.6 ($P > .05$) 83.9 ($P = .03$), and 78.5 ($P = .06$) at 3, 6, and 9 months postoperative. For parent proxy-report, the mean PedsQL 4.0 Generic Core Total Scale score rose from 54.0 at baseline to 66.8 ($P < .002$) 74.8 ($P < .002$), and 72 ($P < .002$) at 3, 6, and 9 months postoperative.

(continued on next page)

Table 1
(continued)

Study	Patient Population/Treatment Condition	PedsQL Outcome(s)	Findings
Banks et al. (2008)[81]	29 pediatric oncology patients ages 2–18 years undergoing an intravenous chemotherapy cycle (intravenous chemotherapy given during week 1)	PedsQL 4.0 Generic Core Scales PedsQL 3.0 Cancer Module	From week 1 to week 4 for parent proxy-report, the PedsQL 4.0 Generic Core Total Scale score demonstrated a mean change of 17 points and the Cancer Module Total Scale score demonstrated a 12-point change (child self-report was not assessed in this study).
Cheuk et al. (2008)[82]	24 transfusion-dependent thalassemic patients who survived matched sibling hematopoietic (SCT) and 74 patients treated conventionally with transfusion and iron chelation	PedsQL 4.0 Generic Core Scales	PedsQL revealed posttransplant patients rated better for running ($P = .001$) and sports ($P = .038$) after adjustment for comorbidities.
de Vries et al. (2008)[83]	41 children ages 2–18 years with acute lymphoblastic leukemia undergoing dexamethasone treatment alternating 2 weeks on and 5 weeks off (6 mg/m^2/day)	PedsQL 3.0 Cancer Module	Halfway as well as at the end of treatment, parents rated their child's overall HRQOL to be more impaired during periods on dexamethasone as compared with periods off dexamethasone; at time 2 during dexamethasone, scores on the PedsQL were significantly lower for the subscales Pain ($P = .04$), Worry ($P = .02$) and Cognition ($P = .01$).
Nuboer et al. (2008)[84]	38 children ages 4–16 years with type 1 diabetes undergoing insulin pump treatment versus. four times daily injections lasting 3.5 months	PedsQL 4.0 Generic Core Scales	Pump treatment resulted in decreased symptomatic hypoglycaemia and lowered hemoglobin A1c by 0.22%; consistent with these findings, within-patient comparisons of the two treatment modalities showed significant improvement in PedsQL scores after pump treatment.

Parekh et al. (2008)[85]	25 patients ages 3–17 years with ureteropelvic junction obstruction undergoing pyeloplasty surgery	PedsQL 4.0 Generic Core Scales	6 weeks postoperative child Emotional Functioning (91.7) and Physical Functioning (90.3) improved significantly ($P < .05$) from preoperative scores; parent scores on Physical Functioning (88.4), Psychosocial Health (82.2), and Emotional Functioning (80.8) were significantly higher postoperative at 6 weeks.
Wade et al. (2008)[86]	Children and parents from 4 elementary schools with newly implemented school-based health centers and 4 elementary comparison schools	PedsQL 4.0 Generic Core Scales	There was a significant improvement in child self-reported HRQOL over the 3 years for school-based health center users compared with the comparison school group.
Yackobovitch-Gavan et al. (2008)[87]	71 obese adolescents ages 12–18 years participating in one of three 12-week diet regimens: low-carbohydrate low-fat, low-carbohydrate high-fat, or high carbohydrate low-fat diets	PedsQL 4.0 Generic Core Scales	A significant improvement in physical, emotional, school, and psychosocial functioning, as well as in the total PedsQL score was noted in the entire study population at the end of the interventions; a significant improvement in HRQOL was found in the low-carbohydrate low-fat group (emotional, school, and psychosocial functioning, and total PedsQL score) and in the high-carbohydrate low-fat group (physical, emotional, and psychosocial functioning, and total PedsQL score), but not in the low-carbohydrate high-fat group.

much of a problem, if any, was it to get care for your child that you or a doctor believed necessary?" and "In the past 12 months, has there been any time when you thought your child should get medical care, but did not?").[65] Realized access to care during the prior year was related to HRQOL for each subsequent year. Foregone care and problems getting care were associated with decrements of 3.5 and 4.5 points on the PedsQL for parent proxy report ($P < .001$) and with decrements of 3.2 and 4.4 points on the PedsQL for child self-report ($P < .001$). Improved realized access resulted in higher PedsQL scores, continued realized access resulted in sustained PedsQL scores, and foregone care resulted in cumulative declines in PedsQL scores over time.

MINIMAL CLINICALLY IMPORTANT DIFFERENCE

Related to responsiveness is the minimal clinically important difference (MCID), which has been defined as the smallest difference in a score of a domain of interest that patients perceive to be beneficial and that would mandate, in the absence of troublesome side effects and excessive costs, a change in the patient's management.[66] The Standard Error of Measurement (SEM)[67] has been linked to the MCID, in which one SEM identified the MCID in responsiveness in an HRQOL measure.[68] Excellent agreement between the SEM and MCID has been shown.[68] As an illustration in a population-based study, the MCID for the PedsQL 4.0 has been determined through calculating the SEM. A 4.4 change in the PedsQL 4.0 Total Scale Score for child self-report has been determined as a minimal clinically meaningful difference, whereas a 4.5 change in PedsQL4.0 Total Scale Score for parent proxy-report was determined as a minimal clinically meaningful difference.[22] Thus, the MCID can provide a metric for determining meaningful change in a clinical trial, or in the planning stages of a clinical trial to determine the sample size needed to detect a meaningful clinical difference.

CUT-POINT FOR AT-RISK STATUS

Scores approximating 1 standard deviation below the population mean have been proposed as a meaningful cut-off point score for an at-risk status for impaired HRQOL relative to population means.[1,2] As an illustration, cut-off points for at-risk status for impaired HRQOL have been examined for the PedsQL 4.0 using the 1 standard deviation below the mean of the total population sample.[22] For child self-report, the PedsQL 4.0 Total Scale Score cut-off point score was 69.7 (parent proxy-report score of 65.4). To provide the context for these cut-off scores, it is useful to examine PedsQL 4.0 Total Scale Scores for children with physician-diagnosed chronic health conditions. For example, pediatric oncology patients receiving chemotherapy and radiation therapy self-report a PedsQL 4.0 Total Scale Score of 68.9 (parent proxy-report score of 67.0).[26] Similarly, children with rheumatic conditions (eg, juvenile rheumatoid arthritis) self-report a PedsQL 4.0 Total Scale Score of 72.1 (parent proxy-report score of 71.).[28] Thus, scores approximating 1 standard deviation below the population sample mean represent PedsQL 4.0 Total Scale Scores similar to children with severe chronic health conditions.

SENSITIVITY OF THE PEDIATRIC QUALITY OF LIFE INVENTORY

Although the responsiveness of a measurement instrument provides the opportunity to determine changes in individual patients or patient groups over time (prospective or longitudinal analysis), measurement sensitivity facilitates the identification of differences among individual patients or patient groups at one point of time (cross-sectional analysis).[61,69] The sensitivity of a measurement instrument may be demonstrated through a cross-sectional analysis of differences between groups of patients with varying degrees of disease severity or through other group comparisons.[61] The PedsQL 4.0 Generic Core Scales has demonstrated sensitivity across disease severity for a number of pediatric chronic health conditions.[26,28,54,70,71] For example, Uzark and colleagues[54] conducted a cross-sectional analysis of health-related quality of life in children with varying severities of heart disease. Severity of heart disease was rated by a clinician blinded to the study outcomes and was categorized as (1) mild disease requiring no therapy or effectively treated nonoperatively (catheter therapy); (2) moderate disease surgically corrected (curative) or requiring no therapy; (3) surgical correction (one or more procedures) with significant residua or need for further surgery; (4) complex or severe disease, uncorrectable or palliated (includes single ventricle). Physical Functioning scores on the PedsQL 4.0 Generic Core Scales were significantly lower in children in disease category 3 or 4 compared with children in disease category 1 or 2 ($P < .01$) as rated by both children and parents. A significant difference in Psychosocial Health scores was demonstrated across disease severity categories ($P < .01$) with an incremental decrease in mean scores as disease severity increased.

PEDIATRIC QUALITY OF LIFE INVENTORY IN PEDIATRIC CLINICAL PRACTICE

Findings from the adult literature suggest that routine implementation of standardized HRQOL assessment may be a necessary but not sufficient condition for enhancing patients' HRQOL.[1] Incorporating specific resource management suggestions, such as appropriate referrals and tailored treatments are hypothesized to enhance the efficacy of HRQOL measurement by providing physicians and other health care professionals with viable options to identified problems.[1] In a recent study from the Netherlands,[72] adolescents with type I diabetes completed the PedsQL 4.0 Generic Core Scales and PedsQL Diabetes-Module on a computer before consultation with their pediatrician at three office visits within 12 months. PedsQL subscale scores were automatically calculated by a computer program and reports with the outcomes of the PedsQL were printed for the pediatrician and the adolescent to be discussed during the consultation.[72] Before beginning the study, pediatricians received a short training course on how to interpret and discuss PedsQL scores and were provided a small guide with instructions and a list of the individual items on the PedsQL subscale as a backup for discussing PedsQL scores. Pediatricians were instructed to start with discussing PedsQL 4.0 Generic Core scores, with Dutch norm scores as reference, and respectfully invite the adolescent to comment and discuss the outcomes.[72] Subsequently, the PedsQL Diabetes Module subscales were discussed, exploring possible solutions and actions.[72] At 12 months, mean scores on psychosocial well-being ($P < .001$), behavior ($P < .001$), mental health ($P < .001$), and family activities ($P < .001$) improved in the intervention group, except for adolescents with the highest A1C values.[72] Adolescents in the intervention group reported higher self-esteem at follow-up ($P = .016$), regardless of A1C, and were more satisfied with care ($P = .009$) than control subjects.[72]

SUMMARY

Health-related quality of life has been recognized as an important outcome, some contend *the* most important outcome for children's health care interventions.[4] The PedsQL Measurement Model was designed as a modular approach to measuring pediatric health-related quality of life, developed to integrate the relative merits of generic and disease-specific approaches. The PedsQL 4.0 Generic Core Scales have been translated into more than 65 languages, with published data on more than 35,000 children and adolescents in more than 345 peer-reviewed journals since 2001 in healthy children and numerous pediatric chronic health conditions. The PedsQL Disease- and Condition-Specific Modules were designed to measure HRQOL dimensions specifically tailored for pediatric chronic health conditions. The PedsQL has demonstrated feasibility, reliability, validity, sensitivity, and responsiveness for child self-report ages 5 to 18 years and parent proxy-report ages 2 to 18 years, and has been shown to be related to other key constructs in pediatric health care such as access to needed care, health care barriers, predictive of health care costs, and quality of primary care. Future advances in the PedsQL Measurement Model include Web-based electronic administration (ePedsQL), integration into the electronic medical record, further efficacy and effectiveness outcome trials, and the development of the generic PedsQL Infant Scales for ages 1 month to 24 months as well as additional disease- and condition-specific modules for other pediatric chronic health conditions such as solid organ transplants and sickle cell disease.

Finally, how can HRQOL outcomes become incorporated into health care to improve quality? We propose that the advent of the electronic medical record provides the opportunity for the integration of HRQOL outcomes as a quality indicator of the appropriateness and safety of the care provided. Perhaps the time will finally arrive in the next 5 years to consider pediatric patients' and parents' perceptions of the child's health and well-being as essential outcomes in the evaluation of the quality of care provided. We suggest that part of the process of improving the quality of health care includes measuring HRQOL outcomes from the perspective of children and their parents on a routine basis, consistent with a consumer-based health care system approach.

REFERENCES

1. Varni JW, Burwinkle TM, Lane MM. Health-related quality of life measurement in pediatric clinical practice: an appraisal and precept for future research and application. Health Qual Life Outcomes 2005;3(34):1–9.
2. Matza LS, Swensen AR, Flood EM, et al. Assessment of health-related quality of life in children: a review of conceptual, methodological, and regulatory issues. Value Health 2004;7:79–92.
3. World Health Organization. Constitution of the World Health Organization: basic document. Geneva, Switzerland: World Health Organization; 1948.
4. Kaplan RM. Quality of life in children: a health care policy perspective. In: Koot HM, Wallander JL, editors. Quality of life in child and adolescent illness: concepts, methods, and findings. East Sussex, Great Britain: Brunner-Routledge; 2001. p. 89–120.
5. FDA. Guidance for Industry. Patient-reported outcome measures: use in medical product development to support labeling claims. Rockville (MD): Center for Drug Evaluation and Research, Food and Drug Administration; 2006.
6. Clarke SA, Eiser C. The measurement of health-related quality of life in pediatric clinical trials: a systematic review. Health Qual Life Outcomes 2004;2(66):1–5.
7. Acquadro C, Berzon R, Dubois D, et al. Incorporating the patient's perspective into drug development and communication: an ad hoc task force report of the Patient-Reported Outcomes (PRO) harmonization group meeting at the Food and Drug Administration, February 16, 2001. Value Health 2003;6:522–31.

8. Willke RJ, Burke LB, Erickson P. Measuring treatment impact: a review of patient-reported outcomes and other efficacy endpoints in approved product labels. Control Clin Trials 2004;25:535–52.
9. Sherman SA, Eisen S, Burwinkle TM, et al. The PedsQL™ present functioning visual analogue scales: preliminary reliability and validity. Health Qual Life Outcomes 2006;4(75):1–10.
10. Upton P, Lawford J, Eiser C. Parent-child agreement across child health-related quality of life instruments: a review of the literature. Qual Life Res 2008;17: 895–913.
11. Eiser C, Morse R. Can parents rate their child's health-related quality of life? Results from a systematic review. Qual Life Res 2001;10:347–57.
12. Theunissen NCM, Vogels TGC, Koopman HM, et al. The proxy problem: child report versus parent report in health-related quality of life research. Qual Life Res 1998;7:387–97.
13. Varni JW, Limbers CA, Burwinkle TM. How young can children reliably and validly self-report their health-related quality of life? An analysis of 8,591 children across age subgroups with the PedsQL™ 4.0 generic core scales. Health Qual Life Outcomes 2007;5(1):1–13.
14. Campo JV, Comer DM, Jansen-McWilliams L, et al. Recurrent pain, emotional distress, and health service use in childhood. J Pediatr 2002;141:76–83.
15. Janicke DM, Finney JW, Riley AW. Children's health care use: a prospective investigation of factors related to care-seeking. Med Care 2001;39:990–1001.
16. Cremeens J, Eiser C, Blades M. Characteristics of health-related self-report measures for children aged three to eight years: a review of the literature. Qual Life Res 2006;15:739–54.
17. Patrick DL, Deyo RA. Generic and disease-specific measures in assessing health status and quality of life. Med Care 1989;27:S217–33.
18. Sprangers MAG, Cull A, Bjordal K, et al. The European Organization for Research and Treatment of Cancer. Approach to quality of life assessment: guidelines for developing questionnaire modules. Qual Life Res 1993;2:287–95.
19. Varni JW, Seid M, Rode CA. The PedsQL™: measurement model for the pediatric quality of life inventory. Med Care 1999;37:126–39.
20. Eiser C, Morse R. Quality of life measures in chronic diseases of childhood. Health Technol Assess 2001;5:1–158.
21. Varni JW, Seid M, Kurtin PS. PedsQL™ 4.0: reliability and validity of the Pediatric Quality of Life Inventory™ Version 4.0 generic core scales in healthy and patient populations. Med Care 2001;39:800–12.
22. Varni JW, Burwinkle TM, Seid M, et al. The PedsQL™ 4.0 as a pediatric population health measure: feasibility, reliability, and validity. Ambul Pediatr 2003;3:329–41.
23. Varni JW, Burwinkle TM, Seid M. The PedsQL™ 4.0 as a school population health measure: feasibility, reliability, and validity. Qual Life Res 2006;15:203–15.
24. Varni JW, Burwinkle TM, Berrin SJ, et al. The PedsQL™ in pediatric cerebral palsy: reliability, validity, and sensitivity of the generic core scales and cerebral palsy module. Dev Med Child Neurol 2006;48:442–9.
25. Varni JW, Burwinkle TM, Jacobs JR, et al. The PedsQL™ in type 1 and type 2 diabetes: reliability and validity of the Pediatric Quality of Life Inventory™ generic core scales and type 1 diabetes module. Diabetes Care 2003;26:631–7.
26. Varni JW, Burwinkle TM, Katz ER, et al. The PedsQL™ in pediatric cancer: reliability and validity of the Pediatric Quality of Life Inventory™ generic core scales, multidimensional fatigue scale, and cancer module. Cancer 2002;94: 2090–106.

27. Varni JW, Burwinkle TM, Rapoff MA, et al. The PedsQL™ in pediatric asthma: reliability and validity of the Pediatric Quality of Life Inventory™ generic core scales and asthma module. J Behav Med 2004;27:297–318.
28. Varni JW, Seid M, Knight TS, et al. The PedsQL™ in pediatric rheumatology: reliability, validity, and responsiveness of the Pediatric Quality of Life Inventory™ generic core scales and rheumatology module. Arthritis Rheum 2002; 46:714–25.
29. Palmer SN, Meeske KA, Katz ER, et al. The PedsQL™ brain tumor module: initial reliability and validity. Pediatr Blood Canc 2007;49:287–93.
30. Goldstein SL, Graham N, Warady BA, et al. Measuring health-related quality of life in children with ESRD: performance of the generic and ESRD-specific instrument of the Pediatric Quality of Life Inventory™ (PedsQL™). Am J Kidney Dis 2008;51:285–97.
31. Uzark K, Jones K, Burwinkle TM, et al. The Pediatric Quality of Life Inventory in children with heart disease. Progr Pediatr Cardiol 2003;18:141–8.
32. Aday LA. Designing and conducting health surveys: a comprehensive guide. 2nd edition. San Francisco (CA): Jossey-Bass; 1996.
33. Fowler FJ. Improving survey questions: design and evaluation. Thousand Oaks (CA): Sage; 1995.
34. Schwarz N, Sudman N, editors. Answering questions: methodology for determining cognitive and communicative processes in survey research. San Francisco (CA): Jossey-Bass; 1996.
35. Sudman S, Bradburn NM, Schwarz N. Thinking about answers: the application of cognitive processes to survey methodology. San Francisco (CA): Jossey-Bass; 1996.
36. Fayers PM, Hand DJ. Factor analysis, causal indicators and quality of life. Qual Life Res 1997;6:139–50.
37. Upton P, Eiser C, Cheung I, et al. Measurement properties of the UK-English version of the Pediatric Quality of Life Inventory™ 4.0 (PedsQL™) generic core scales. Health Qual Life Outcomes 2005;3(22):1–7.
38. Varni JW, Burwinkle TM, Szer IS. The PedsQL™ multidimensional fatigue scale in pediatric rheumatology: reliability and validity. J Rheumatol 2004;31:2494–500.
39. Chan KS, Mangione-Smith R, Burwinkle TM, et al. The PedsQL™: reliability and validity of the short-form generic core scales and asthma module. Med Care 2005;43:256–65.
40. Varni JW, Seid M, Knight TS, et al. The PedsQL™ 4.0 generic core scales: sensitivity, responsiveness, and impact on clinical decision-making. J Behav Med 2002;25:175–93.
41. Schwimmer JB, Burwinkle TM, Varni JW. Health-related quality of life of severely obese children and adolescents. JAMA 2003;289:1813–9.
42. Bastiaansen D, Koot HM, Bongers IL, et al. Measuring quality of life in children referred for psychiatric problems: psychometric properties of the PedsQL™ 4.0 generic core scales. Qual Life Res 2004;13:489–95.
43. Crabtree VM, Varni JW, Gozal D. Health-related quality of life and depressive symptoms in children with suspected sleep-disordered breathing. Sleep 2004; 27:1131–8.
44. Felder-Puig R, Frey E, Proksch K, et al. Validation of the German version of the Pediatric Quality of Life Inventory™ (PedsQL™) in childhood cancer patients off treatment and children with epilepsy. Qual Life Res 2004;13:223–34.
45. Williams J, Wake M, Hesketh K, et al. Health-related quality of life of overweight and obese children. JAMA 2005;293:70–6.

46. Powers SW, Patton SR, Hommel KA, et al. Quality of life in pediatric migraine: characterization of age-related effects using PedsQL 4.0. Cephalalgia 2004;24: 120–7.
47. Bastiaansen D, Koot HM, Ferdinand RF, et al. Quality of life in children with psychiatric disorders: self, parent, and clinician report. J Am Acad Child Adolesc Psychiatry 2004;43:221–30.
48. Youssef NN, Rosh JR, Loughran M, et al. Treatment of functional abdominal pain in childhood with cognitive behavioral strategies. J Pediatr Gastroenterol Nutr 2004;39:192–6.
49. Razzouk BI, Hockenberry M, Hinds PS. Influence of hemoglobin response to epoetin alfa on quality of life in anemic children with cancer receiving myelosuppressive chemotherapy. In: Program and abstracts of the 46th Annual Meeting of the American Society of Hematology; 2004 December 4–7; San Diego (CA).
50. Seid M, Sobo EJ, Gelhard LR, et al. Parents' reports of barriers to care for children with special health care needs: development and validation of the barriers to care questionnaire. Ambul Pediatr 2004;4:323–31.
51. Seid M, Varni JW, Bermudez LO, et al. Parent's perceptions of primary care: measuring parent's experiences of pediatric primary care quality. Pediatrics 2001;108:264–70.
52. Seid M, Varni JW, Segall D, et al. Health-related quality of life as a predictor of pediatric healthcare costs: a two-year prospective cohort analysis. Health Qual Life Outcomes 2004;2(48):1–10.
53. Acquadro C, Conway K, Giroudet C, et al. Linguistic validation manual for patient-reported outcomes (PRO) instruments. Lyon, France: Mapi Research Institute; 2004.
54. Uzark K, Jones K, Slusher J, et al. Quality of life in children with heart disease as perceived by children and parents. Pediatrics 2008;121:e1060–7.
55. Varni JW, Thompson KL, Hanson V. The Varni/Thompson pediatric pain questionnaire: I. Chronic musculoskeletal pain in juvenile rheumatoid arthritis. Pain 1987; 28:27–38.
56. Varni JW, Sherman SA, Burwinkle TM, et al. The PedsQL™ family impact module: preliminary reliability and validity. Health Qual Life Outcomes 2004; 2(55):1–6.
57. Varni JW, Burwinkle TM, Dickinson P, et al. Evaluation of the built environment at a children's convalescent hospital: development of the Pediatric Quality of Life Inventory™ parent and staff satisfaction measures for pediatric health care facilities. J Dev Behav Pediatr 2004;25:10–25.
58. Varni JW, Quiggins DJL, Ayala GX. Development of the pediatric hematology/oncology parent satisfaction survey. Child Health Care 2000;29:243–55.
59. Vickers AJ. Statistical considerations for use of composite health-related quality of life scores in randomized trials. Qual Life Res 2004;13:717–23.
60. Pfennings L, van der Ploeg H, Cohen L, et al. A comparison of responsiveness indices in multiple sclerosis patients. Qual Life Res 1999;8:481–9.
61. Fayers PM, Machin D. Quality of life: assessment, analysis, and interpretation. New York: Wiley; 2000.
62. Terwee CB, Dekker FW, Wiersinga WM, et al. On assessing responsiveness of health-related quality of life instruments: guidelines for instrument evaluation. Qual Life Res 2003;12:349–62.
63. Oga T, Nishimura K, Tsukino M, et al. A comparison of the responsiveness of different generic health status measures in patients with asthma. Qual Life Res 2003;12:555–63.

64. Mangione-Smith R, Schonlau M, Chan KS, et al. Measuring the effectiveness of a collaborative for quality improvement in pediatric asthma care: does implementing the chronic care model improve processes and outcomes of care? Ambul Pediatr 2005;5:75–82.
65. Seid M, Varni JW, Cummings L, et al. The impact of realized access to care on health-related quality of life: a two-year prospective cohort study of children in the California State Children's Health Insurance Program. J Pediatr 2006;149:354–61.
66. Jaeschke R, Singer J, Guyatt GH. Measurement of health status: ascertaining the minimal clinically important difference. Control Clin Trials 1989;10:407–15.
67. Wyrwich K, Tierney W, Wolinsky F. Further evidence supporting an SEM-based criterion for identifying meaningful intra-individual changes in health-related quality of life. J Clin Epidemiol 1999;52:861–73.
68. Wyrwich K, Tierney W, Wolinsky F. Using the standard error of measurement to identify important changes on the asthma quality of life questionnaire. Qual Life Res 2002;11:1–7.
69. Liang MH, Lew RA, Stucki G, et al. Measuring clinically important changes with patient-oriented questionnaires. Med Care 2002;40:II45–51.
70. Seid M, Limbers CA, Driscoll KA, et al. Reliability, validity, and responsiveness of the Pediatric Quality of Life Inventory™ (PedsQL™) generic core scales and asthma symptoms scale in vulnerable children with asthma. J Asthma, in press.
71. Varni JW, Burwinkle TM, Sherman SA, et al. Health-related quality of life of children and adolescents with cerebral palsy: hearing the voices of the children. Dev Med Child Neurol 2005;47:592–7.
72. de Wit M, de Waal HA, Alle Bokma J, et al. Monitoring and discussing health related quality of life in adolescents with type 1 diabetes improves psychosocial well-being: a randomized controlled trial. Diabetes Care 2008;31:1521–6.
73. Sallee FR, Ambrosini PJ, Lopez FA, et al. Health-related quality of life and treatment satisfaction and preference in a community assessment study of extended-release mixed amphetamine salts for children with attention-deficit/hyperactivity disorder. J Outcome Res 2004;8:27–49.
74. Schwimmer JB, Middleton MS, Deutsch R, et al. A phase 2 trial of metformin as a treatment for non-diabetic pediatric non-alcoholic steatohepatitis. Aliment Pharmacol Ther 2005;21:871–9.
75. Connelly M, Rapoff MA. Assessing health-related quality of life in children with recurrent headache: reliability and validity of the PedsQL™ 4.0 in a pediatric sample. J Pediatr Psychol 2006;31:698–702.
76. Felder-Puig R, diGallo A, Waldenmair M, et al. Health-related quality of life of pediatric patients receiving allogeneic stem cell or bone marrow transplantation: results of a longitudinal, multi-center study. Bone Marrow Transplant 2006;38:119–26.
77. Razzouk BI, Hord JD, Hockenberry M, et al. Double-blind, placebo-controlled study of quality of life, hematologic end points, and safety of weekly epoetin alfa in children with cancer receiving myelosuppressive chemotherapy. J Clin Oncol 2006;24:3583–9.
78. Cuomo AV, Gamradt SC, Kim CO, et al. Health-related quality of life outcomes improve after multilevel surgery in ambulatory children with cerebral palsy. J Pediatr Orthop 2007;27:653–7.
79. Fullerton G, Tyler C, Johnston CA, et al. Quality of life in Mexican-American children following a weight management program. Obesity 2007;15:2553–6.
80. Holterman AX, Browne A, Dillard BE, et al. Short-term outcome in the first 10 morbidly obese adolescent patients in the FDA-approved trial for laparoscopic adjustable gastric banding. J Pediatr Gastroenterol Nutr 2007;45:465–73.

81. Banks BA, Barrowman NJ, Klaassen R. Health-related quality of life: changes in children undergoing chemotherapy. J Pediatr Hematol Oncol 2008;30:292–7.
82. Cheuk DKL, Mok ASP, Lee ACW, et al. Quality of life in patients with transfusion-dependent thalassemia after hematopoietic SCT. Bone Marrow Transplant 2008;42:319–27.
83. de Vries M, van Litsenburg R, Huisman J, et al. Effect of dexamethasone on quality of life in children with acute lymphoblastic leukaemia: a prospective observational study. Health Qual Life Outcomes 2008;6:1–26.
84. Nuboer R, Borsboom G, Zoethout JA, et al. Effects of insulin pump vs. injection treatment on quality of life and impact of disease in children with type 1 diabetes mellitus in a randomized, prospective comparison. Pediatr Diabetes 2008;9:291–6.
85. Parekh AD, Thomas JC, Trusler L, et al. Prospective evaluation of health related quality of life for pediatric patients with ureteropelvic junction obstruction. J Urol 2008;180:2171–6.
86. Wade TJ, Mansour ME, Line K, et al. Improvements in health-related quality of life among school-based health center users in elementary and middle school. Ambul Pediatr 2008;8:241–9.
87. Yackobovitch-Gavan M, Nagelberg N, Demol S, et al. Influence of weight-loss diets with different macronutrient compositions on health-related quality of life in obese youth. Appetite 2008;51:697–703.

Neonatal Intensive Care Unit Collaboration to Decrease Hospital-Acquired Bloodstream Infections: From Comparative Performance Reports to Improvement Networks

Joseph Schulman, MD, MS[a,b,*], David D. Wirtschafter, MD[c],
Paul Kurtin, MD[d]

KEYWORDS

- Quality improvement
- Performance evaluation • Risk adjustment
- Central line associated bloodstream infection
- Improvement networks • High reliability organization

Left to intuition, people have trouble accurately judging their relative performance.[1] They are prone to overestimate their achievements and capabilities compared with their peers—the Lake Wobegon Effect,[2] named for the fictional town of Lake Wobegon from the radio series *A Prairie Home Companion*, where "all the children are above average." Health care workers too, are subject to this bias,[3] particularly if their notion

[a] Division of Newborn Medicine, Department of Pediatrics, Weill Cornell Medical College of Cornell University, The New York Presbyterian Hospital, 525 East 68th Street, Box 106, NY 10065, USA
[b] Division of Outcomes & Effectiveness, Department of Public Health, Weill Medical College of Cornell University, The New York Presbyterian Hospital, 525 East 68th Street, Box 106, NY 10065, USA
[c] David D Wirtschafter, MD, Inc., 5523 Voletta Pl, Valley Village, CA 91607, USA
[d] Sadler Center for Quality, Rady Children's Hospital San Diego, 3020 Children's Way, San Diego, CA 92123, USA
* Corresponding author. Division of Newborn Medicine, Department of Pediatrics, Weill Medical College of Cornell University, The New York Presbyterian Hospital, 525 East 68th Street, Box 106, NY 10065.
E-mail address: jos2039@med.cornell.edu (J. Schulman).

Pediatr Clin N Am 56 (2009) 865–892
doi:10.1016/j.pcl.2009.06.001
pediatric.theclinics.com

of quality is based largely on good intentions. Learning to provide high-quality care may be considered to derive from understanding "The degree to which health services for individuals and populations increase the likelihood of desired health outcomes and are consistent with current professional knowledge."[4] This two-part article explores several performance improvement approaches motivated by this perspective and designed to reduce hospital-acquired bloodstream infections (BSIs) in neonatal intensive care units (NICUs). Readers may be reassured that the rather specific details that follow serve to illustrate concepts with broad applicability for pediatric quality improvement.

PART 1: COMPARING INSTITUTIONAL PERFORMANCE

As suggested in the title, the critical first step in quality improvement is making providers aware of their practices and patient outcomes. Because of the paucity of evidence supporting pediatric practice, many comparative performance reports are based on provider consensus about what is important to know and measure. After describing provider performance, the critical next step is deciding what to do with that information. Because most providers are not trained in the science and practice of quality improvement, quality improvement networks/learning collaboratives/communities of practice play an essential role in disseminating the knowledge, tools, and techniques of quality improvement and in helping to actually implement improvement plans.

Comparative Neonatal ICU Hospital-Acquired Bloodstream Infection Performance Reports: How are We Doing? Do We Have a Problem?

Imagine you work at the hospital represented by the bold dot in **Fig. 1**. The display plots NICU nosocomial sepsis infection (NI) outcomes for several hundred hospitals participating in the Vermont Oxford Network.[5] Each dot represents the difference between the number of positive blood cultures in infants after day 3 of life reported by an individual hospital and the number that would be expected at that hospital after accounting for specific differences in patient characteristics—case mix—from hospital to hospital. Additionally, the dots reflect so-called "shrunken" estimates: a method that accounts for the assumption that one infant's infection is not independent of another's, and adjusts for individual hospital estimates considered relatively imprecise by moving such values closer to the mean value for all hospitals. So, how is your facility doing with these hospital-acquired infections (HAIs)? Do you have a problem with this aspect of care?

Displays as this one may appear pretty straightforward at first glance; but only at first glance. Each dot encodes the result of a complex analysis that rests upon crucial assumptions and important limitations. Tempting as it may be immediately to articulate the "answer" provided by a given dot, for several reasons, an impulsive determination is fraught with risk. First, the answer represented by each dot depends on the question posed—the hypothesis tested. Second, meaningful and fair comparison of various institutions' results depends on accounting for baseline patient characteristics that importantly influence the outcome of interest but that are independent of quality of care. Third, valid results depend on an analysis that conforms to methodological assumptions. And fourth, correctly drawn inference integrates these three considerations with explicit assessment of residual chance, bias, or confounding.[6] Let's explore some of these ideas further before we decide what the bold dot tells us about clinical performance.

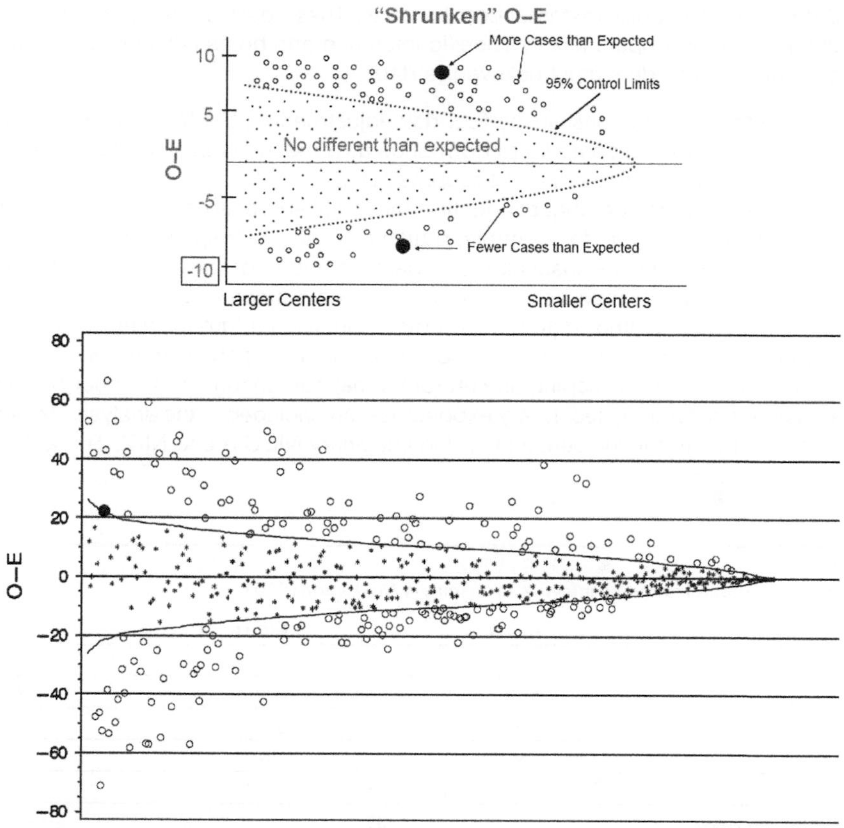

Fig.1. (*Top*) Interpretation key for lower image—observed minus expected cases adjusted for baseline characteristics and random effects. Each dot represents an individual hospital. Horizontal axis depicts absolute value of 95% control limit, considered a proxy for number of patients at a hospital (*Courtesy of* Vermont Oxford Network, Burlington, VT; with permission.) (*Lower*) Instantiates this configuration, reporting on nosocomial infection; the heavy black dot is the center of interest. The shape of the superimposed curve, marking the range of variation attributable to chance, that is, ±95% control limits—essentially 2 standard deviations for process-related data, suggests the name: funnel plot. This feature displays precision of the estimate as a function of hospital volume. Dots within the control limits are statistically indistinguishable, which means it makes no sense to rank-order those hospitals. (*From* Schulman J, Spiegelhalter DJ, Parry G. How to interpret your dot: decoding the message of clinical performance indicators. [State of the Art Article.] J Perinatol 2008;28:588–96; with permission).

Are the comparisons fair?

At the outset, it is worth discriminating at least two different and important uses for quality improvement data:

(1) Data for improvement, which do not support operationally specific inferences (concrete ideas about what to do differently) to the extent we might like, but the data nonetheless can inspire hypotheses about how to improve; and then those hypotheses must be tested.

(2) Data for accountability/external comparisons. These data are made public. They ought to support operationally specific inference and be as reliable and valid, as possible; ie, providers must believe the data.

Although the authors consider perfect risk adjustment in the NICU an impractical ideal, it is reasonable to compare performance as a means to seek opportunities for internal improvement…not external accountability.

It is crucial to appreciate that accounting for specified baseline differences among individual group members, for example, patients in various hospitals, doesn't necessarily mean that groups—hospitals—are being compared fairly. Some exposure/outcome relationships may be distorted when the outcome is also substantially affected by *un*accounted differences among individual group members. More concretely, the relationship between receiving care in a particular facility (primary exposure) and risk of developing an HAI (outcome) can change when other baseline differences—risk factors, secondary exposures—are included in the analysis. To illustrate, let's compare the incidence of HAI in imaginary NICU A and NICU B (**Table 1**).

Table 1
Incidence of hospital-acquired infection in imaginary NICU A and NICU B

All Subjects	**NICU A**		**NICU B**	**Total**
HAI	45		30	75
Infection-free	455		470	925
Total	500		500	1000
Risk	.09		.06	.075
—		Point estimate		—
Risk difference		.03		—
Risk ratio		**1.5**		—
MALES	**NICU A**		**NICU B**	**Total**
HAI	5		20	25
Infection-free	95		380	475
Total	100		400	500
Risk	.05		.05	.05
—		Point estimate		—
Risk difference		0		—
Risk ratio		**1**		—
FEMALES	**NICU A**		**NICU B**	**Total**
HAI	40		10	50
Infection-free	360		90	450
Total	400		100	500
Risk	.1		.1	.1
—		Point estimate		—
Risk difference		0		—
Risk ratio		**1**		—

The risk ratio (RR) for developing a hospital-acquired infection (HAI) in neonatal ICU (NICU) A compared with NICU B is 1.5 when all subjects are considered, but RR = 1 when stratified by gender, because gender is associated with site of care (NICU A versus NICU B) and with outcome.

The risk ratio (RR) for developing an HAI in NICU A compared with NICU B is 1.5 when all subjects are considered: ie, patients in NICU A are at 50% increased risk of developing an HAI compared with patients in NICU B. However, when only males or only females are considered, the RR is 1 (no risk difference). How can an apparently strong exposure effect disappear when we stratify by gender?

At the heart of this question is a phenomenon called Simpson's Paradox. The RR of 1.5 among all subjects disappears when analysis is stratified by gender because gender is associated with both primary exposure—the NICU in which a patient receives care, and with outcome—HAI. No real association exists between primary exposure and outcome. Rather, the association is between *secondary* exposure—*gender*—and outcome. The apparent relationship reflects unequal distribution of males and females in NICU A and NICU B. The point to underscore is that each analysis answered a different question:

- "Among the **entire** study group, what is the association between primary exposure and outcome?"
- "Among the **males** in the study group, what is the association between primary exposure and outcome?"
- "Among the **females** in the study group, what is the association between primary exposure and outcome?"

So, if apparent exposure/outcome relationships can change as additional factors are accounted for, *how does one gain confidence that an exposure/outcome relationship is real—that the important factors have indeed been accounted for?* The key idea is that patients at different hospitals may differ in various ways and some of those differences might substantially explain observed variation in outcomes among hospitals. In general, meaningful comparisons ultimately entail comparing like with like. So metaphorically speaking, the problem of comparing hospital performance centers on this question: "If asked to evaluate several bowls of fruit salad, how does one transform the diversity into a comparison of apples with apples?"

Statisticians try to achieve this via so-called risk adjustment methods. Sometimes the magic works very well and other times we are left still comparing apples with oranges, pears, and so on. Several measures exist to quantify how well a risk adjustment model has achieved the desired result.[7] Clinicians should understand at least two of these. (We emphasize that critical review is not intended to create an "excuse" for taking no action. An analytical review may be critical yet constructive by enumerating potential limitations along with speculating about the direction and magnitude of potential bias.[8] For example, in light of the identified limitations perhaps the findings represent an overestimate (or underestimate) of the effect of site of care on outcome. On the other hand, if such review suggests that the *direction* of the relationship could be different, then it may indeed be appropriate to suspend action until better data are available.)

Evaluating a risk adjustment model

One measure of model performance is discriminatory power: how well a model, on the basis of specified baseline characteristics, discriminates subjects who will experience the outcome from those who will not. Discriminatory power may be quantified as the area under a plot of model sensitivity versus 1-specificity: the receiver operating characteristic (ROC) curve (**Fig. 2**).[9] Values range from 0 to 1: 0.5 = random outcome assignment (coin toss); 1 = perfect discrimination. The *c*-statistic, using the same range of values, quantifies discriminatory power by evaluating all pairs of subjects, one of whom experienced the outcome and one of whom did not; and evaluates the

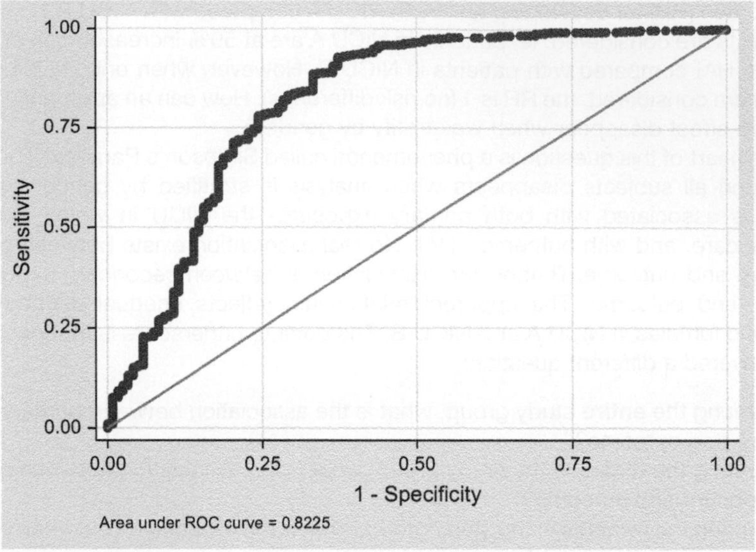

Fig. 2. Illustrative ROC curve. (*From* Schulman J. Managing your patients' data in the neonatal and pediatric ICU: an introduction to databases and statistical analysis. Oxford, UK: Blackwell; 2006; with permission.)

proportion of pairs for whom the model correctly predicts higher probability of experiencing the outcome for the subject who actually experienced the outcome.

A second model performance measure is explanatory power: the extent to which the model can explain the observed variation in outcome among subjects. Models use observed values to produce an equation summarizing the risk factor/outcome relationship. This equation predicts outcome values expected for a given profile of risk factor values; thereby describing a line. In reality, however, *observed* values don't fall precisely on the prediction line.

More specifically, models predicting a dichotomous outcome—yes/no; lived/died; infection/infection-free—assign a predicted probability of outcome occurrence to each individual subject based on that subject's risk factor values. Now, probabilities range from 0 to 1, but patients either experience the outcome or do not, so observed values are all either 0 or 1 (**Fig. 3**). Thus, observations off the line described by the predictive equation contain information that the model could not use. In general, the extent to which a model could use the observed information is measured by a quantity called R^2, or explanatory power. Theoretical R^2 values range between 0 (no association between predicted and observed values) and 1 (perfect association). The extent to which a model could *not* use information contained in the observations is measured by $1 - R^2$, also called unexplained variance. The latter represents the contribution of unmeasured factors to the observed variance. So if $R^2 = 0.16$, the model fails to explain 84% of observed variance. For dichotomous outcomes, R^2 reflects the difference between average predicted outcome probability among those who experienced the outcome and those who did not,[8] and commonly is reported as pseudo R^2. Models that account well for determinants of an infrequently occurring outcome nonetheless will have a low pseudo R^2. For example, when observed infection rate is 2% to 4%, pseudo R^2 is usually less than 0.25, because the difference between the predicted and observed values commonly is large. (Robust severity adjustment systems do

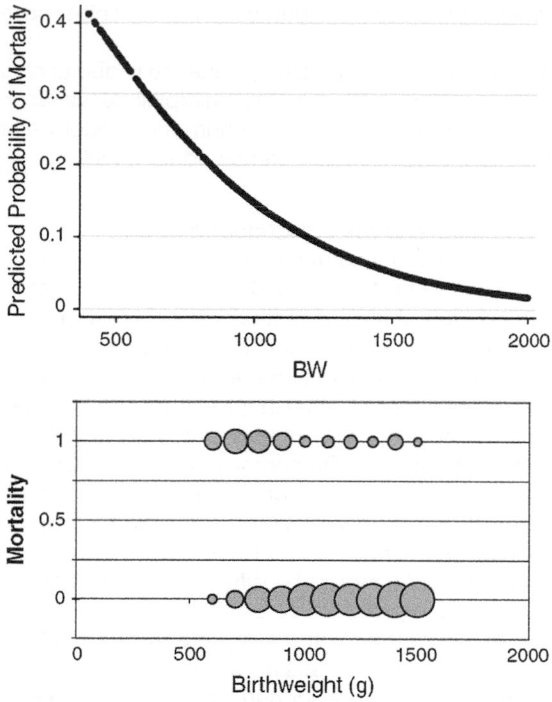

Fig. 3. Left, predicted survival probabilities as a function of birth weight (BW); right, observed outcomes by hospital, circle diameter reflects hospital volume. (*From* Schulman J, Spiegelhalter DJ, Parry G. How to interpret your dot: decoding the message of clinical performance indicators. [State of the Art Article.] J Perinatol 2008;28:588–96; with permission.)

not exist for much of pediatrics, so we need to accept imperfect risk adjustment and move forward because ultimately improvement means comparing self to self over time; if the patient population in a given NICU stays fairly similar over time then that comparison is reasonable. However, we do need agreement on operational definitions such as how to diagnose a central line associated bloodstream infection (CLABSI) or whether "clinical sepsis" is to be included in the definition. Voltaire made the essential point: "the best is the enemy of the good.")[7] One upshot of this is that detecting a change in occurrence rate for infrequent events requires both a large sample size and substantial change in risk. For example, if baseline occurrence rate is 1%, 747 subjects with the risk factor of interest and 747 subjects without that factor are needed to detect a threefold increased risk.[10]

Explained and unexplained variance are crucial ideas because some organizations consider unexplained variance a surrogate for "quality." That is, outcome differences remaining among hospitals after risk adjustment are considered to reflect care at the respective hospital. Doing so rests on two important assumptions:

1. No other factors that are independent of quality of care operate to substantially influence the relationship between site of care and outcome. That is, one is unable to think of other baseline patient characteristics that might have a substantial effect on the outcome. If otherwise, those other factors should be included in the model to

provide reassurance that exposure/outcome relationships nevertheless remain stable.

2. An unimportant proportion of the remaining variance is due to chance. The smaller the explanatory power and the larger the unexplained variance, the larger the potential contributions of irrelevant information and random error to the model; and therefore the more tenuous the inference about quality.

"Shrunken" estimates: multilevel risk adjustment models

One more type of special accounting merits further explanation to help decipher the message of the bold dot in **Fig. 1**: so-called "shrunken" estimates. Traditional risk adjustment methods assume that observations are independent of each other; for example, that a hospital-acquired infection in one patient has nothing to do with such an event in another patient in the same facility. However, what happens to one patient may not be independent of what happens to another patient in the same facility. Factors that predispose one patient to an outcome may also operate to predispose other patients to that outcome. Outcomes may be correlated: systematic differences unexplained by specified predictors may exist among hospitals. (Quality improvement is often based on understanding systemic factors as a root cause to differential performance, eg, hand hygiene rates may impact many outcomes and may be performed at very different rates by different members of the staff at different units. Other examples include presence of a PICC team; average length of time the nursing staff has worked in a given unit; having a dedicated catheter cart; who has responsibility for PICCs, housestaff versus nurse practitioners; parents' hand hygiene compliance rates.) One must therefore account for the varying roles of individual-level and group-level factors in jointly determining outcomes. This may be done via multilevel modeling, which yields "shrunken" outcome estimates. The predicted result for an individual hospital tends to "shrink," away from the hospital's observed value toward the value of the summary measure for all hospitals. How much a hospital's predicted value shrinks depends on three criteria for assessing the reliability of a particular hospital's observed result:

1. *Within-group variation*: How much do individual patients' values differ from the hospital's average outcome?
2. *Between-group variation*: To what extent does each hospital differ from the average for all hospitals?
3. *Patient volume*: Low-volume hospitals are considered a relatively less reliable data source.

Reliability here relates to the extent an observed value may have been affected by chance events and not the system of care. When an individual hospital's observations seem less reliable, the model assigns less weight to that hospital's observed outcomes and more weight to the overall experience of all hospitals.

So, how are we doing?

We are now prepared to extract the message of **Fig. 1**. The particular question the display answers—the hypothesis that was tested statistically—is not explicitly articulated in the report document provided to the institution represented by the bold dot. Instead, as is common with performance reports, one is simply provided with an implicit "answer," in this case, "observed minus expected nosocomial infections." (The model of improvement is built upon the necessity for a clearly defined AIM because from that aim will come the measures that are used to create the appropriate baseline as well as the means to assess progress.) Several questions are possible, including:[7]

1. "Which hospitals' results are not compatible with the overall average?"
2. "Which hospitals are in the top or bottom half?"
3. "Does a particular hospital come from the same distribution as all the others; is this hospital an extraordinary performer?"

The question actually posed determines the particular conformation of the funnel-shaped curve in **Fig. 1**. The report document specifies risk factors used in the risk adjustment model, but not the model's discriminatory or explanatory power; cautioning, however, that risk adjustment methods are imperfect. Nevertheless, thoughtful interpretation of risk-adjusted results depends on some factual understanding of just *how imperfect* is the comparison. "All models are wrong; the practical question is how wrong do they have to be to not be useful" (George Box, quoted in Schulman).[11]

Mindful of the foregoing caveats we can say this: lying as it does on the superimposed funnel-shaped curve, our dot in **Fig. 1** represents a borderline "outlier." The funnel curve marks the range of variation attributable to chance, ±95% control limits. Variation among dots within the control limits is more likely attributable to chance than to inherent differences in systems of care.

So, what does it mean to be an outlier? Only that if the model has done a good job transforming the evaluative task to a comparison of apples with apples, then we can be confident the dot differs from the overall average, the model expectation. However, shrunken estimates "*assume* that systematic differences exist among the hospitals; that ALL hospitals differ from the average, so confirming this in a particular case is hardly noteworthy!"[7] It is important to appreciate that larger hospitals with slightly excess risk are prone to be classified as outliers—they probably differ from the overall average, the model expectation—because the statistical method recalibrates low volume hospitals' performance so that they approximate the overall average while high volume hospitals' values change little. Thus nearly all hospitals that care for a sufficiently high patient volume will lie outside the control limits.[7]

Neonatal ICU Hospital-Acquired Bloodstream Infection Improvement Networks

The previously enumerated questions that might motivate **Fig. 1** center the focus of data-driven quality improvement efforts on individual data points describing institutional performance. Question number 3 is potentially most helpful. Outliers revealed by this hypothesis test might provide insight to structural and process-related variables whose relationships to outcomes could then be tested among the entire group.

An alternate focus with great improvement potential centers on the observed distribution of the data points: Can we favorably shift average performance of the group overall and narrow the variation among individuals? Part 2 of this article describes improvement initiatives by neonatologists in New York and California illustrating some of the possible strategies.

PART 2: COLLABORATING TO IMPROVE MANY INSTITUTIONS' PERFORMANCE

Neonatal ICU Hospital-Acquired Bloodstream Infection Improvement Networks

Part 1 of this article provided key considerations for fairly comparing individual institutional performance. Useful evaluation was shown to derive from testing a hypothesis resembling "Does a particular hospital come from the same distribution as all the others; ie, is this hospital an extraordinary performer?" In this second part, the focus shifts from individual data points (hospitals) to the observed distribution of the data points; and the corresponding hypothesis becomes "Can we favorably shift average performance of the overall group and narrow the variation among individuals?" Improvement initiatives by neonatologists in New York and California illustrate possible strategies.

New York

Background, methods

Early in 2007 all 19 regional perinatal centers (RPCs) of New York State (NYS), supported by the New York State Department of Health (NYSDOH) and the Association of Regional Perinatal Provider Networks, collaborated to decrease central line associated bloodstream infection (CLABSI) rates in their neonatal intensive care units (NICUs).[12] RPCs are State-designated to serve "...the most acutely sick or at-risk pregnant women and newborns... coordinate ... transfers of high-risk patients from their affiliate hospitals to the RPC, and are responsible for support, education, consultation and improvements in the quality of care in the affiliate hospitals within their region."[13] Representation was multidisciplinary: front-line physicians, nurse practitioners, nurses, and infection control professionals.

Despite mandated infection reporting, until this initiative began individual RPCs were unaware of how their results compared with others'. RPCs only knew their referring hospitals' performance, not other RPCs'. The extent to which centers applied best practices to prevent CLABSIs was unclear. Centers suspected that CLABSI rates and pertinent practices varied substantially among RPCs. Centers recognized that they needed an appropriate, credible standard by which to evaluate RPC performance and motivate improvement.

During the collaborative's first year, RPCs shared self-identified NICU bloodstream infection rates and agreed to set a standard of care via a bundle of practices – percutaneously inserted central catheters (PICCs) were specified because this line type accounted for the bulk of central line days. NYS Public Health Law Article 28 § 2819 required that all NYS hospitals join the National Healthcare Safety Network (NHSN),[14] which made CLABSI rate available statewide. Every individual participant had to join either a Research Panel (RP) or a Quality Improvement Panel (QIP); each established defined individual responsibilities. The RP selected performance indicators; reviewed data completeness, integrity, and analysis; and identified candidate host institutions for participants to visit and learn about potential best practices. The QIP reviewed pertinent peer-reviewed literature; coordinated the visit to a potential best performing NICU (with respect to the specified indicator; ideally, one could look for the best performance on a number of indicators, as different places often do different things well); and spearheaded creation of a care bundle. Controversy arising from collaborative activities was adjudicated by both panels. Several dozen individuals visited a NICU with low indicator rate to learn about potential best practices. Many had never before scrutinized specific care practices so carefully. Visitors observed morning rounds and hand hygiene practices; hosts described care practices for catheter insertion, maintenance, and removal; formal debriefing consolidated learning. Key "take-away" messages included the following:

- Facilitate adherence to hand hygiene practices: place hand sanitizer dispensers at each bedside.
- Use two staff members for central line placement.
- Change catheter tubing by nurse pairs using a "buddy system," according to a written policy.

- Consider line removal each day during patient rounds.
- Create a culture wherein the NICU staff, a physician "champion" and the infection control professionals consider themselves a single team working to prevent CLABSI.

Elements of the evidence-based practice bundle to prevent CLABSIs were required to derive from level-1 evidence.[15] Pertinent literature identified by the QIP was distributed to all RPCs for review.

Results

The 19 RPC NICUs shared 56,911 central line days of observation; **Fig. 4** shows birth weight (BW)-stratified and aggregate institutional performance (details available in Schulman and colleagues[12]) Each participating RPC knew which letter identified each institution.

Informed by Part 1 of this article, critical readers might now ask: "If the lower display in **Fig. 4** is the 'answer,' what's the question?" The question that indeed motivated the analysis was: "During 2007, what was the overall CLABSI rate at each NICU, and assuming no changes in circumstances—for example, stable patient demographics, stable processes of care, stable risk factor incidence—what is the underlying CLABSI risk for new patients at a particular NICU?" The lower display does not answer: "Do rates sufficiently account for differences in baseline patient characteristics among NICUs?" Nor does it answer: "How much must values differ to 'mean something'—Is variation among centers more likely due to chance than to inherent differences in their systems of care?" The actual rates depicted by each dot in **Fig. 4** are called point estimates; they are accompanied by 95% confidence intervals (CIs). Even with constant underlying risk, the proportion of neonates who will develop a CLABSI at each NICU varies every evaluation interval. CIs help to answer: "What is the true CLABSI rate for each NICU?" in the sense of establishing a *range* of underlying risk values compatible with observed outcomes. So, the overall CLABSI rate for NICU B during 2007 was approximately 12.7/1000 central line days. However, repeating the observations over a very long period, all else unchanged, the overall CLABSI rate for NICU B should lie between 4.6 and 27.6/1000 central line days. The computed interval width is an inverse function of patient volume. Larger samples will more accurately reflect the true population characteristics, ie, the individual estimate is more precise; CI narrows (compare NICU B with NICU J).[7]

Within each BW category CLABSI rates varied widely. Combining all BW strata, individual center rates ranged from 2.6 to 15.1 per 1000 central line-days, representing a nearly sixfold variation across the participating NICUs. For infants of BW less than 751 g rates ranged from 0 to 19.0 per 1000 central line days: nearly 20-fold variation across NYS's regional referral NICUs. It is unclear how much between-center variation is a result of chance (note the extensive overlap of CIs in **Fig. 4**).

The central line care bundle adopted by unanimous agreement is shown in **Box 1**.

Discussion

Health care has entered an era of mandatory statewide reporting of CLABSI rates for ICU patients.[30,31] Neonatologists at New York State's regional referral centers reframed mandated HAI reporting as an opportunity: to promote accountability and cooperation among providers and to develop a strategy to prevent CLABSIs. The strategy of a statewide collaboration is innovative for several reasons. First, because all RPCs participate, potential sampling error or bias is avoided and population-based rates can be determined. Second, because evaluated providers are directly involved in data collection, review, analysis, and interpretation, providers believe performance

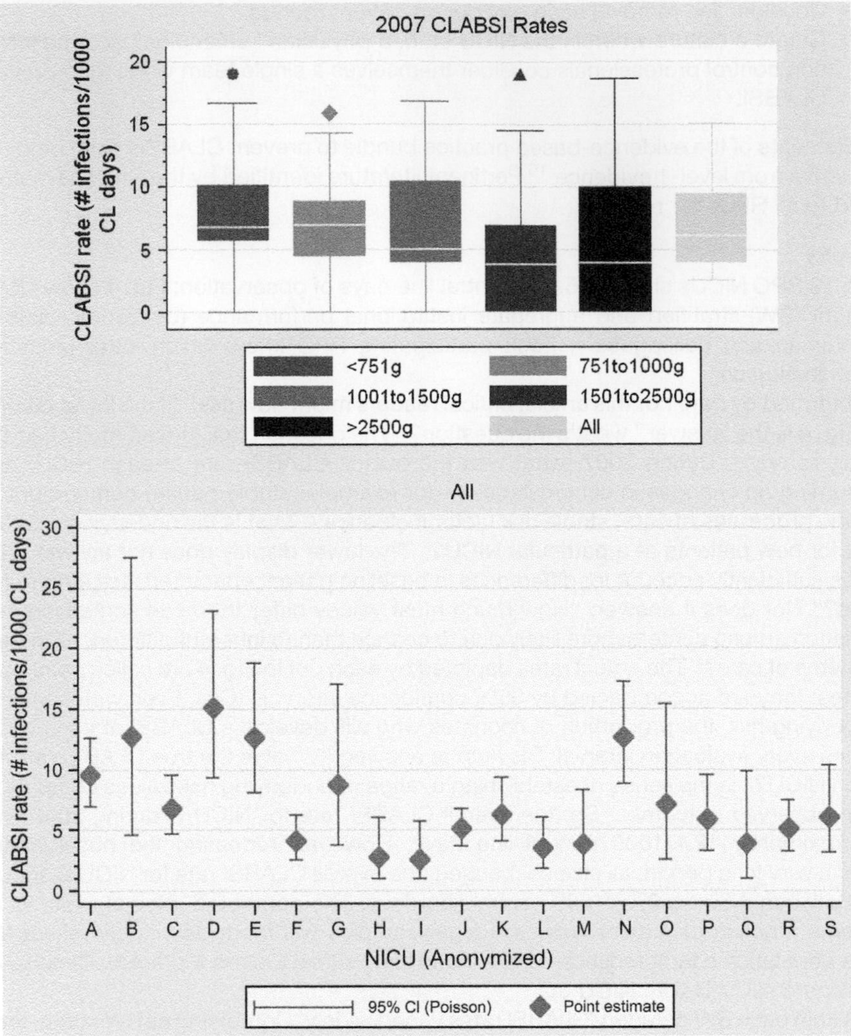

Fig. 4. (*Upper*) Range of BW-stratified CLABSI rates for participating RPCs during the calendar year 2007. Each box bounds values between the first and third quartiles, with the horizontal line within a box denoting the median value. The interquartile range (IQR) is computed by subtracting the value of the first quartile from the value of the third quartile. Values that exceed the third quartile by more than 1.5 times the IQR are identified as dots. (*Lower*) Between-RPC variation in CLABSI rate. CIs assume Poisson distribution, 95% interval. (*From* Schulman J, et al. Development of a Statewide Collaborative to decrease NICU central line associated bloodstream infections. J Perinatol, in press; with permission.)

results. If they do not, they are empowered to identify and correct their data thereby improving data accuracy. Third, the NYSDOH Office of HAI conducted site visits to assess sites' use of CLABSI case definitions and adjudicated cases.[32] Fourth, the network intends to help members improve by monitoring bundle element application and effectiveness.

Box 1
New York State Regional Perinatal Care Centers: PICC bundle

This tool specifies vital care elements to be consistently applied by credentialed practitioners

PICC Insertion

- Establish a central line kit or cart to consolidate all items necessary for the procedure (IB).[16]
- Perform hand hygiene with hospital-approved alcohol-based product or antiseptic-containing soap before and after palpating insertion sites and before and after inserting central line (IA).[17–19]
- Use maximal barrier precautions (including sterile gown, sterile gloves, surgical mask, hat, and large sterile drape) (IA).[17,20]
- Disinfect skin with appropriate antiseptic (eg, 2% chlorhexidine, 70% alcohol) before catheter insertion (IA).[17,21,22]
- Use either a sterile transparent semipermeable dressing or sterile gauze to cover the insertion site (IA).[23–25]

PICC Maintenance

- Perform hand hygiene with hospital approved alcohol-based product or antiseptic-containing soap before and after accessing a catheter or changing the dressing (IA).[17–19]
- Evaluate the catheter insertion site daily for signs of infection and to assess dressing integrity (IB).
- At a minimum, if the dressing is damp, soiled, or loose change it aseptically (IB) and disinfect the skin around the insertion site with an appropriate antiseptic (IA).[21,24,26,27]
- Develop and use standardized intravenous tubing set-up and changes (IB).[28]
- Maintain aseptic technique when changing IV tubing and when entering the catheter including "scrub the hub" (IA).[24,27,29]
- Daily review of catheter necessity with prompt removal when no longer essential (IB).[16,17]

Category IA. Strongly recommended and strongly supported by well-designed experimental, clinical, or epidemiologic studies.
Category IB. Strongly recommended and supported by some studies and strong theoretical rationale.
Centers for Disease Control and Prevention[15]

Note that *no center was without CLABSI*. Thus, the extent to which these events may be prevented, even in the best performing centers, remains uncertain.[33] Nonetheless, in adult and pediatric ICU populations, implementation of bundle strategies and checklists has been associated with substantially decreased CLABSI rates,[17,34] and the efforts of neonatologists in California, described later in this article, support the association for NICU populations. Thus, it is sensible for New York State neonatologists to try to shift average performance and narrow the variation among NICUs.

Although the bundle in **Box 1** derives from high-quality evidence, monitoring of its effectiveness is essential. The best practices collected in the bundle typically emerge by studying an individual intervention in a controlled setting (preferably a randomized controlled trial). However, in actual clinical care several best practices may be applied in combination; a procedure that assumes favorable interactions among the individual interventions. To further complicate the situation, best practices may yield varying results that depend on the myriad ways actual care settings and patients differ from the controlled circumstances operating when effectiveness was initially established.

(These are critical points because it is essential to deal with the reality of daily clinical practice – in which many changes are likely to occur simultaneously. [Unlike the randomized control trial, real-life practice is very hard to tightly control.] Organizations working to improve care will often do several interventions at once.)[35,36]

This rationale for monitoring bundle effectiveness also begs a question: Might asking whether an intervention works or not oversimplify the situation? It may be more illuminating to ask: "For *whom* might it work, and *under what circumstances*?"[35,37] Delivery of health care is a social phenomenon. As such, it may be wishful thinking to suppose that study and control groups only differ in the intervention of interest, and that no other aspects of care vary due to human factors. Local details about "how" something works and about the "what" of contexts may be crucial.[37] For example, aggregated analysis of a multicenter trial suggesting that an intervention does not "work," ie, the intervention has no effect, might obscure the reality that the intervention is beneficial for some types of patients in particular settings and harmful for other types of patients or settings. The quality improvement approach of neonatologists in California incorporates this idea.

California

Network overview

California's regional NICUs provide care to the majority of complex medical and surgical neonatal patients in the state. In 2006, California Children's Services (CCS) joined in a unique collaborative relationship with the California Children's Hospital Association (CCHA) to develop and implement a statewide initiative intended to reduce CLABSIs in these NICUs.

The project leadership team included CCS leadership (Marian Dalsey, MD, MPH, Kathy Chance, MD, and Hallie Morrow MD, MS), quality improvement expertise (Paul Kurtin, MD, Michael Seid, PhD, and Thomas Huber, M.) and neonatal medical/nursing expertise (David D. Wirtschafter, MD, and Janet S. Pettit, MSN, NNP-BC). In 2006, 13 members of CCHA joined the project (September 2006 to December 2007), and the remaining nine regional NICUs joined in January 2008. The 22 collaborating NICUs included all eight Children's Hospitals in the state, all five University of California Hospitals, and nine large regional centers, including those for three multisite hospital systems. NICU size ranged from 23 to 84 beds and patient days in 2007 ranged from 7665 to 29,565. In 2007, these 22 units provided 285,430 NICU patient care days. The original 13 NICUs had 59,182 line days in 2006 and 73,077 in 2007. The expanded cohort will report an estimated 87,500 line days in 2008.

Members worked collaboratively using three face-to face meetings to initially address project goals and methods for performing QI initiatives and later to share accomplishments, challenges and means to overcome them and form consensus around new approaches to reduce CLABSIs. Biweekly phone conferences served to update members of the collaborative on the activities of each individual site, identify potential interventions, develop consensus about data definitions and collection procedures, exchange knowledge about "best practices," and exchange ideas on "promising practices." The project's leaders provided one on-site consultation visit during 2007 to the original 13 members. These visits provided tailored consultations aimed at helping each site identify and overcome barriers to implementing necessary changes in practice. Annual project meetings included all participants and focused on lessons learned, opportunities for continued improvement, and project assessment, followed by a presentation to and celebration with the member's CEO's and CCHA's senior leadership.

Performance reports

Because we wanted to understand the performance of the collaborative as it was changing and to know whether real change was occurring, we used statistical process control (SPC) methods. Although traditional inferential statistics are commonly used to examine differences between samples from different sites or collaborative performance at different times, it requires aggregation of measures over time and thus can slow the pace of change. SPC is a branch of statistics that uses time series analysis and graphical presentation of data. Traditional inferential statistics rests on the assumption that sampled data are drawn from a stable population, whereas CLABSI rates reflect a reiterative production process whose results vary over time: ie, a NICU care system. SPC is designed to accurately characterize such variation over time—to discriminate signal from noise, how much of a change must occur for it to "mean something"; and to indicate whether the system performs predictably or not. NICU A may have the same annual infection rate as NICU B but NICU A may operate within a substantially narrower performance range than NICU B, so that one may reliably predict the coming month's results in NICU A, but not in NICU B.[38] Researchers and practitioners often find SPC data displays very useful for evaluating performance and guiding change.[39]

We created performance reports (CLABSIs per 1000 central line days) for each participating site that highlighted the large degree of variation in rates among the participating sites and compared their results with the national NHSN benchmarks.[40] The reports were primarily used to (1) create a baseline of group performance, (2) create a baseline for each site to compare itself to its own performance over time, and (3) help make the case that changes in practice are needed to both reduce variation within and between sites and to improve performance compared with national benchmarks.

CLABSI rates during the first year of the project fell 25% from 4.32 to 3.22 infections per 1000 catheter days comparing the baseline 2006 period to the whole of 2007. This represented 75 fewer infections annually in a population exposed to 73,000 line days. **Fig. 5** shows a CLABSI rate control chart for the very low birth weight (VLBW) babies. There is a downward shift in the CLABSI rate from the baseline through the intervention period. Moreover, while there is some increasing scatter during the follow-up period, this is not a strong enough shift to suggest a rising CLABSI rate. During this post-intervention period (project hiatus: July to December 2007), there were no group phone conferences and no communication regarding individual performance rates occurred.

The collaborative's CLABSI rate was 2.36/1000 line days for January to September 2008. It is not possible to directly compare this rate with the rates obtained in the previous year because of a change in the stringency of the NHSN CLABSI definition implemented on January 1, 2008.[41] The new one calls for two rather than one positive blood cultures when diagnosing a catheter-associated infection from a recognized contaminant. Since coagulase-negative staphylococci (CONS) may constitute up to one half of the organisms associated with neonatal infection,[42] this criteria change has the potential to confound neonatal HAI trend analysis. Anecdotally, the California collaborative members report that perhaps one third of their 2007 CONS infections were not diagnosed with two blood cultures, and, even though treated, they would not have been designated as CLABSI events in 2008. A similar effect was estimated in New York State (Stricof RL, December 11, 2008, personal communication).

Identifying the right ways to do the right things

The project generated many different threads of discourse and discovery, both because there exists no single vascular access "bundle" for neonates and because

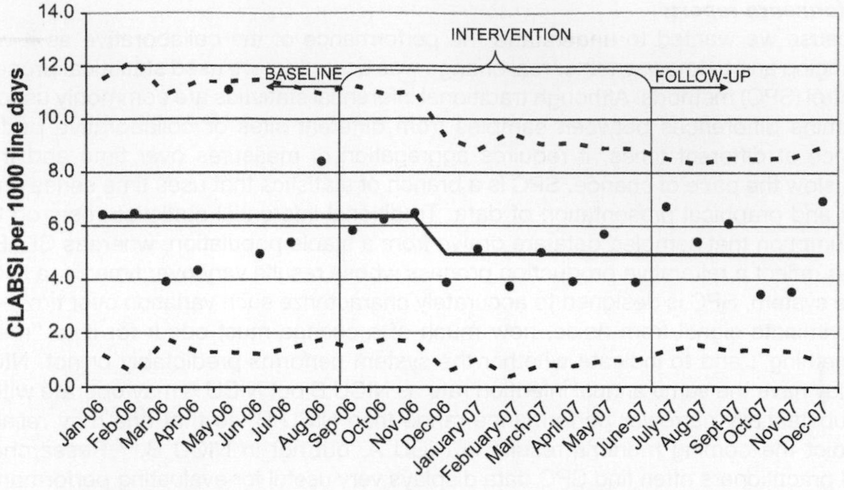

Fig. 5. CCHA-CCS NICU Collaborative: CLABSI rates among infants with birth weights <1500 g 2006–2007. Mean (*solid line*) and 99% confidence intervals (*dashed lines*) calculated using the method described by McCarty et al for binomially distributed data.

there are many technical and material challenges in meeting the needs of these patients. Thus, substantial portions of the collaborative's work consisted of developing and assessing ideas for use in the NICU. Some of the specific technical challenges considered were the following: whether, or with what restrictions, to use chlorhexidine in skin antisepsis; availability and workability of closed system vascular access devices for umbilical and peripheral vascular lines; designs of medication administration lines to lessen their exposure to bedside contaminants and to minimize the fluid load required to maintain their patency; standards on how to obtain blood cultures (considering both volume and site(s)); and revising the NSHN CLABSI criteria as they pertain to temperature assessment to reflect better the variability of neonatal temperatures and how they are measured. All of these issues, critical to the diagnosis and prevention of CLABSI, were unspecified at the beginning of the project, with no well defined and tested best practices available to be cited from the literature (**Table 2**).

Connecting upstream process steps with downstream outcomes

One of the key work products of this collaborative is a rich dataset describing the different paths taken by the individual centers in achieving their QI goals. This was possible because of our initial work to define prevention processes in greater and more practical detail than at the aggregated bundle level. The continuous real-time logging of member's work enables us to describe the progression of project activities.

The collaborative also developed a comprehensive means for assessing and recording the investigation of a positive blood culture report (**Fig. 6**). We derived its many suggested assessments from specific case reports, either published or suggested by our member's experience. Our member's anecdotal evaluation of this process indicates that a literature-based forensic approach stimulates a more far-reaching survey for both usual and unusual "suspect" practices potentially contributing to a CLABSI. Refusing to simplify explanations for unexpected events, as described above, is an example of the reflective practices of high-reliability organizations (HRO).[43]

The overarching challenge: promoting high reliability characteristics

We sought to identify and deploy feasible practices that could enhance these NICUs' adoption of "HRO characteristics." For example:

- We deployed previously available observation tools or created de novo tools for assessing the adequacy of vascular line set-ups and entry, the adequacy of hand hygiene, and the real time investigation of all CLABSIs. When our members' audits indicated performance shortfalls, for instance, hand hygiene rates falling below 90%, they responded by initiating reinforcement and re-education of desired techniques. Recently, some of our members have merged the need for on-going audit of line set-up processes with the leadership need to ensure daily contact between managers and nurses.[44] In a process they describe as "walk the line," they have asked nursing shift managers, aka "charge" nurses, to walk by each neonate's bed and review the line set-up and briefly interact with the bedside nurse. This practice also helps to enhance "situational awareness": being mindful of what is happening around oneself to understand how information, events, and one's own actions will impact one's goals and objectives; another key component of a HRO.
- We approached checklist use first by facilitating the centers' response to the mandate by the California Department of Health Care Services to comply with the Centers for Disease Control and Prevention's (CDC's) NHSN "central line insertion process."[45] We encouraged units to find other opportunities for the use of checklists; such as for line set-up, line entry, and medication administration.
- We approached "error interception," often referred to by its name: "stop the line" as originally conceived of and termed by Toyota Motor Inc.,[46] as a key characteristic of a safety culture.[47] We built on the national effort to improve the safety of line insertion, a simple instance of events that rely upon the staff's comfort level in stopping a process until their safety concerns are addressed,[48] as a first step to embracing this habit for safe care.
- We addressed the need for situational awareness by encouraging the use of huddles to identify critical issues in each unit before each shift.
- We promoted the habit of reflection and feedback about misses and near misses by transforming the "root cause analysis" process for investigating possible CLABSI events from a retrospective into a concurrent process. The concurrent process changes the analytic emphasis from intense chart review and cause documentation to bedside interview and observation. As it evolved, the positive blood culture evaluation process pulled together both the experiences of our members as well as published observations on those factors relevant to understanding the circumstances surrounding each CLABSI.
- Last, we developed auditing tools for monitoring critical processes. While this has widely been recognized and implemented for hand hygiene, we developed audit tools for line set-up and line entry with the intent that units would periodically monitor these critical performance items in the same way that they monitory hand hygiene. (Additional forms and materials at the project's Web site: http://www.dhcs.ca.gov/ProvGovPart/initiatives/nqi/Pages/default.aspx. Accessed on January 14, 2009.) (**Figs. 7** and **8**).

Accounting for the cultural dimension of neonatal ICU care

We developed a "metabundle" of recommended interventions (**Table 3**) to distinguish the adaptive or social context surrounding the implementation of the bundles'

Table 2
CCS-CCHA neonatal CLABSI prevention bundle (2008): technical aspects: http://www.dhcs.ca.gov/ProvGovPart/initiatives/nqi/Pages/default.aspx

Performance Expectations	Considerations
Insertion	
1. Maximum sterile barrier precautions used	- Cover entire infant with sterile drapes or as much as affords safe observation. - Recommend staff wear face mask when within 3 ft of sterile field
2. Skin disinfected with Chlorhexidine (CHG) or povidone iodine (PI)	- Apply over 30 seconds & allow to dry (exception aqueous CHG)
3. Dedicated team for placement & maintenance	- Insertion training course, including sterile technique, hand hygiene, use of maximum sterile barrier precautions, proper skin disinfection - Educational competencies for all aspects of care
4. All supplies required for the procedure should be available at the bedside before catheter insertion	—
5. Hand hygiene standards met	—
6. Insertion checklist used	- Standardize critical elements of line insertion - Ensure staff observers are skilled in monitoring elements of sterile technique.
7. Staff empowered to stop non-emergent procedure if sterile technique not followed	—
Maintenance	**Considerations**
Assessment & Site Care	
1. Daily assessment and documentation of catheter need included as part of multidisciplinary rounds and review of daily goals	When catheter used primarily for nutritional purposes: - Consider removal when infant reaches $\geq$120 mL/kg/day enteral nutrition - Consider discontinuing lipids when infant reaches >2.5 g/kg/day of enteral fat intake

2. Review dressing integrity and site cleanliness daily	Change PRN using sterile technique and CHG or PI for skin antisepsis
Tubing, injection ports, catheter entry	
1. Use "closed" systems for infusion, blood draws & medication administration	- May use manufactured or improvised closed system. If stopcocks are used, port(s) are capped with swabable needleless connector(s). - Define consistent practice to be used when accessing catheters
2. Assemble and connect infusion tubing using aseptic or sterile technique. Configure tubing consistently for each type of VAD.	- **Sterile** technique ideally includes sterile barrier for tubing assembly and wearing of face mask, hat, sterile gloves & 2 staff members performing connection to central catheter - **Aseptic** technique includes clean barrier for tubing assembly & wearing of clean gloves
3. Scrub needleless connector using friction with either alcohol or CHG/alcohol swab for at least 15 sec. before entry. Allow surface to dry before entry.	—
4. Clean gloves for all VAD entries & hand hygiene used before & after glove use	Standard precautions
5. Use pre-filled, flush containing syringes wherever feasible	- Higher risk of contamination when flush withdrawn from another container by a nurse
6. Staff empowered to stop non-emergent procedure if sterile technique not followed	—

Positive Blood Culture Review
Version 7: 6/30/08

Name: ___________ MR #: ___________ DOB:__/__/__ Birth WT:________ GA______wk EGA at dx:____wk
Final Dx: [ ] CABSI [ ] BSI [ ] NEC [ ] VAP [ ] Contaminant [ ]
Other:_________________

Clinical Findings at Time Blood Culture Drawn and Blood Culture Collection Data	
Risk Factors: [ ] Immunocompromised [ ] Compromised skin integrity [ ] Open body cavity [ ] Ostomy present [ ] Surgical site infection receiving Rx [ ] Other risk factors: (state)	[ ] Blood transfusion in last 72 hours [ ] NCPAP/Nasal cannula [ ] Feeding tube Enteral nutrition volume/parenteral volume ratio: ________ (approximate) [ ] Vascular Catheter [ ] Major surgery within past week [ ] or any other time Specify type of surgery:
Catheter Information: **Only relevant if line(s) present within the 48 hr prior to first blood culture**	
[ ] None [ ] PIV ____# days (if multiple site, note only longest) Estimate # IV start attempts in last 72 hrs:____ [ ] UAC_______# days [ ] UVC_______# days [ ] PICC______# days Site: ________ [ ] Other CENTRAL line ______# days Site: ________ _____Estimate total # times all lines accessed during the **last 72 hours** (including for meds/blood draws/ tubing changes, etc) Last date dressing changed: ___/___/___	[Y/N] Antibacterial patch in use [Y/N] Abnormal CL site appearance on day culture drawn [Y/N] Line-related phlebitis [Y/N] Compromised dressing [Y/N] Vomiting onto line dressing [Y/N] Stool/Urine onto line dressing [Y/N] Line repaired/exchanged in past 48 hours [Y/N] Line leaking events [ ] Care by temporary staff [ ] Care by non-NICU staff [ ] Staffing difficulties [ ] Improper line set-up [ ] Tubing/infusate NOT changed appropriately (method/time) [ ] Any other unusual event: (specify)
Infusates in Past 72 hours : [ ] TPN [ ] Lipids [ ] Blood products [ ] Steroids (3 x physiologic doses)	
Comments and Lessons Learned:	[ ] BSI (Not a CLA-BSI) after further review (e.g., meets another CDC definition and there is another clear source identified), e.g. [ ] NEC [ ] VAP [ ] Other:_____
	[ ] CLA-BSI (have data to determine that BSI fulfills CLA-BSI criteria, i.e. BSI very likely related to CL) *See page 2 for definition detail*
	[ ] Contaminant
	Adjudication Process:
	[ ] BSI Event was clearly able to be attributed/categorized into a CDC definition [ ] BSI Event required significant inferences/judgment to be attributed/categorized
	Action Plan: (Please relate to Fishbones, as applicable):

Fig. 6. Positive blood culture evaluation process (only summary page shown; remaining 3 pages available at: http://www.dhcs.ca.gov/ProvGovPart/initiatives/nqi/Pages/default.aspx. Accessed January 14, 2009).

technical features. It identifies diagnostic criteria; addresses leadership and other structural aspects of the bundle's implementation, specifies use of HRO processes including a preoccupation with failure and creating a culture of safety, the periodic and routine monitoring of processes, reflection on adverse events and feeding back of results; and encourages interdepartmental exchanges to ensure bundle compliance while the neonate is receiving care in other departments of the hospital.

This collaborative discovered the importance of context when implementing quality improvement practices. "*When you have seen one NICU…you have seen one NICU*" became a maxim of our collaborative. Although all 22 sites met the same definition of "regional NICU," there were very significant differences in staffing, the role of house staff and fellows, the mix of surgical versus VLBW neonates, other initiatives on-going in the NICU which might distract attention and resources from the CLABSI project, and

IV Tubing Change Procedure Observations

Date: ______________ Shift: __________ Observer: ______________________________

Observation #	Perform hand hygiene adequately	Gather supplies	Use disinfectant wipe to clean surface of counter	Clean or sterile barrier used for tubing assembly	Place new tubing & supplies on barrier without contamination	Perform hand hygiene adequately	Wear sterile/clean gloves during tubing assembly	Wear items required for procedure, per facility P&P H=hair covering F=face mask G=gown	Assemble tubing using all required components & without contamination	Connect IV solution to tubing & prime without contamination	Place tubing in bed without contaminating end	Place 4X4 under CVC connection site	Scrub connections 10-15 sec with alcohol/CHG before disconnecting	Perform hand hygiene & don clean/sterile gloves	Connect tubing to VAD without contamination	Perform hand hygiene after glove removal	Label tubing with date & time	Provide feedback	Comments
1	Y N	Y N	Y N	Y N	Y N	Y N	Y N NA	H F C NA	Y N	Y N	Y N	Y N	Y N	Y N	Y N	Y N	Y N	Y N	
2	Y N	Y N	Y N	Y N	Y N	Y N	Y N NA	H F C NA	Y N	Y N	Y N	Y N	Y N	Y N	Y N	Y N	Y N	Y N	
3	Y N	Y N	Y N	Y N	Y N	Y N	Y N NA	H F C NA	Y N	Y N	Y N	Y N	Y N	Y N	Y N	Y N	Y N	Y N	
4	Y N	Y N	Y N	Y N	Y N	Y N	Y N NA	H F C NA	Y N	Y N	Y N	Y N	Y N	Y N	Y N	Y N	Y N	Y N	
5	Y N	Y N	Y N	Y N	Y N	Y N	Y N NA	H F C NA	Y N	Y N	Y N	Y N	Y N	Y N	Y N	Y N	Y N	Y N	
6	Y N	Y N	Y N	Y N	Y N	Y N	Y N NA	H F C NA	Y N	Y N	Y N	Y N	Y N	Y N	Y N	Y N	Y N	Y N	
7	Y N	Y N	Y N	Y N	Y N	Y N	Y N NA	H F C NA	Y N	Y N	Y N	Y N	Y N	Y N	Y N	Y N	Y N	Y N	
8	Y N	Y N	Y N	Y N	Y N	Y N	Y N NA	H F C NA	Y N	Y N	Y N	Y N	Y N	Y N	Y N	Y N	Y N	Y N	
9	Y N	Y N	Y N	Y N	Y N	Y N	Y N NA	H F C NA	Y N	Y N	Y N	Y N	Y N	Y N	Y N	Y N	Y N	Y N	
10	Y N	Y N	Y N	Y N	Y N	Y N	Y N NA	H F C NA	Y N	Y N	Y N	Y N	Y N	Y N	Y N	Y N	Y N	Y N	

Fig. 7. Intravenous tubing change procedure audit tool.

Catheter Entry Observations

Date: ____________ Shift: ____________ Observer: ______________________

Observation #	Reason for entry: B=blood draw T=tubing change M=med administration	Type of catheter P=PIV, UA=UAC; UV=UVC; PI=PICC O=Other	Perform hand hygiene	Apply clean gloves	Place clean/sterile barrier under port	Scrub port for 10-15 sec using friction	Port scrubbed using: A = Alcohol C = Chlorhexidine	Allow anti-microbial to dry	Enter port without contamination	Flush obtained from vial without contamination	Single use prefilled flush syringe used only 1 time	All blood/residue flushed clear from injection port	Wipe blood from port surface following blood draw	Remove gloves	Perform hand hygiene	Provide feedback	Comments
1	B T M	P UA UV PI O	Y N	Y N	Y N NA	Y N	A C	Y N	Y N	Y N NA	Y N NA	Y N NA	Y N NA	Y N	Y N	Y N	
2	B T M	P UA UV PI O	Y N	Y N	Y N NA	Y N	A C	Y N	Y N	Y N NA	Y N NA	Y N NA	Y N NA	Y N	Y N	Y N	
3	B T M	P UA UV PI O	Y N	Y N	Y N NA	Y N	A C	Y N	Y N	Y N NA	Y N NA	Y N NA	Y N NA	Y N	Y N	Y N	
4	B T M	P UA UV PI O	Y N	Y N	Y N NA	Y N	A C	Y N	Y N	Y N NA	Y N NA	Y N NA	Y N NA	Y N	Y N	Y N	
5	B T M	P UA UV PI O	Y N	Y N	Y N NA	Y N	A C	Y N	Y N	Y N NA	Y N NA	Y N NA	Y N NA	Y N	Y N	Y N	

Fig. 8. Catheter entry audit tool.

the staff and technical resources available to undertake such an effort. The project team rigorously maintained focus on the intent of the project, to reduce CLABSIs, but permitted significant freedom in how individual sites tried to achieve that goal. Also emphasized was the critical role played by the unit's culture of safety and how that is manifested in the interpersonal, interdisciplinary relationships within the unit.

Implementation issues included: whether, and how, to implement feedback to the staff about days without an infection; whether or not to allow parents to become aware of these data; how to involve the parents in the hand hygiene campaigns, even to the extent of empowering them to "stop the line" if they had concerns; and how to approach nonconforming colleagues.

We addressed communication problems and the possibility of infections attributable to line manipulation outside of the NICU by encouraging dialog with non-NICU departments such as Anesthesiology and Radiology, who also need access to these lines but are variably educated and trained to the same standards for their set up and entry. We proactively sought improved communication with Infection Control Departments, whose focus is on ensuring each report's completeness and accuracy and whose routine reporting lag can delay the timely assessment of the clinical situation surrounding an event and its feedback to the NICU. We encouraged NICU leaders to interact with their Hospital's leadership about their efforts and results to reduce CLABSIs, as these leaders were now being addressed externally by the Joint Commission, the Centers for Medicare and Medicaid Services and state initiatives to publicly release adverse event rates.[49,50] We encouraged the NICU teams to address staff communication challenges within their units by adopting techniques such as "huddles" at shift change; immediate bedside consultation with and by the staff as soon as any positive blood culture report was received; and "rounding for outcomes."

Summary, Part 2

In our experience, improvement collaboratives must have two closely linked goals. The first is to improve current performance such as reducing the rate of CLABSIs by 50% over 6 months. The second goal must be to sustain those improvements over time even in the face of competing priorities and the never-ending distractions of everyday clinical care. To achieve the first goal, the California collaborative emphasized the technical aspects of care such as proper line set up and medication administration supported by appropriate bundles, checklists, and audits to encourage clinicians to do the right thing. To help sustain the gains, which is often much harder than making the initial improvements, we focused on the adaptive changes[51] the social and cultural aspects of interdisciplinary care within the NICU including the need for open communication with staff (and families); open questioning by any staff member of the usual way of doing things; continuous learning; appropriate modeling of behavior by leaders; and a focus on failures and ways to prevent, identify and mitigate them.

Our experience highlights the notion that productive improvement collaboratives entail fundamental and transformative change in the way providers deliver and evaluate their care. Far from mere platitude, the point is that "every system is perfectly designed to achieve the results that it gets" (attributed to Deming, by Pauker and colleagues[52]) so to get better results requires changing the system. California and New York neonatologists have learned that achieving and sustaining such change is a monumental undertaking; demanding affirmation that the current reality is unacceptable, a clear and shared vision of the desired future, and dogged determination – over many years.

Table 3
CCS-CCHA neonatal central line associated bloodstream infection prevention bundle (2008): adaptive aspects

Administrative Leadership	Considerations
1. Demonstrable administrative involvement in and support for achieving Zero Health care–Associated Infections	—
2. Engage Staff with feedback: Posting days since last CABSI Posting CABSI rates	- Annotate CABSI rates with descriptions and dates of practice changes - Celebrations of successes
3. Perform investigation and analysis of each CABSI	- Begin process ASAP & within 24 hours of CABSI notification. Review opportunities for system improvements after each event.
4. Surveillance activities of critical processes related to sustaining the gains: a. Hand Hygiene b. Adherence to unit catheter management and entry standards c. Monitor patient processes off unit for bundle compliance d. Unit personnel support for the "Stop the Line" safety culture	a. Capture 50 HH observations/month/activity using consistent observers b. As above initially, then smaller volume less frequently. c. Prospectively establish and maintain bundle compliance with off unit service departments, eg, operating rooms (Anesthesiology and Pediatric Surgery), radiology suite (Radiology). d. Empower staff to stop intervention at any time when technique is being breached.
5. Competent trained personnel to perform specialized maintenance activities	- Consider specialized team for dressing changes, catheter repair, catheter clearance of blockage
CABSI Diagnosis and Classification	
1. Two blood cultures drawn from separate sites, following skin disinfection with PI or CHG, within 48 hours of each other.	- One culture may be from a central line site if a second peripheral site is not feasible, taking into account circumstances such as vessel accessibility, pain and the infant's clinical status. - The recommended neonatal culture volume is $\geq$1 mL

2. The diagnosis of a laboratory confirmed (LC) catheter-associated BSI (CABSI) can only be made in the absence of another clinically appreciated infectious focus, the presence of one or more positive blood cultures, and one of the following three criteria being met: Criteria 1: at least one blood culture growing a recognized pathogen (see Considerations); or Criteria 2: at least two blood cultures growing a recognized contaminant (see Considerations) and the presence of one (or more) clinical signs of generalized infection (either Fever >38°C (see Considerations) or Hypotension; or Criteria 3: Age <1y AND one of the following: Fever (see Considerations), Hypothermia (<37°C rectal), apnea, or bradycardia. See: http://www.cdc.gov/ncidod/dhqp/pdf/nhsn/NHSN_Manual_PatientSafetyProtocol_CURRENT.pdf	- Recognized pathogens are those not named as common skin contaminants. - Common skin contaminants: diphtheroids, Bacillus species, Propionibacterium species, coagulase-negative staphylococci including *S epidermidis*, viridans group streptococci, Aerococcus or Micrococci - Fever: per the CDC's NHSN, the neonatal equivalents of >38°C rectal are: (38°C rectal/tympanic/temporal art 37°C oral = 36°C axillary) - Hypotension is not defined further. - Hypothermia: per the CDC's NHSN, the neonatal equivalents of <37°C are: (37°C rectal/tympanic/temporal artery = 36°C oral = 35°C axillary) However this collaborative does not believe the temperature equivalences specified by NHSN realistically reflect their neonatal populations' temperature data. Instead the collaborative recommends that **axillary temperatures should be considered as a screening method; axillary temperatures** < 36.0°C (<96.8°**F) should be tentatively labeled as "hypothermia" and axillary temperatures › 38.0°C (>100.4°F) should be tentatively labeled as fever.** *Because of the variability in axillary temperature readings, the presence of an elevated or hypothermic temperature will only be termed* ***confirmed*** if there have been ***at least two consecutive abnormal axillary measurements or one abnormal axillary and one abnormal rectal (or other core) measurement.***

Available at: http://www.dhcs.ca.gov/ProvGovPart/initiatives/nqi/Pages/default.aspx.

REFERENCES

1. Kruger J, Dunning D. Unskilled and unaware of it: how difficulties in recognizing one's own incompetence lead to inflated self-assessments. J Pers Soc Psychol 1999;77(6):1121–34.
2. Wikipedia. Lake Wobegon effect. Available at: http://en.wikipedia.org/wiki/Lake_Wobegon_effect; August 9, 2006. Accessed August 10, 2008.
3. Davis DA, Mazmanian PE, Fordis M, et al. Accuracy of physician self-assessment compared with observed measures of competence. JAMA 2006;296(9):1094–102.
4. Chassin MR, Galvin RW. National Roundtable on Health Care Quality. The urgent need to improve health care quality. JAMA 1998;280(11):1000–5.
5. Vermont Oxford Network. The Vermont Oxford Network. Available at: http://www.vtoxford.org/. 2008. Accessed July 24, 2008.
6. Hennekens CH, Buring JE. Epidemiology in medicine. Boston: Little, Brown and Company; 1987.
7. Schulman J, Spiegelhalter DJ, Parry G. How to interpret your dot: decoding the message of clinical performance indicators. [State of the Art Article]. J Perinatol 2008;28:588–96.
8. Ash AS, Schwartz M. Evaluating the performance of risk-adjustment methods: dichotomous outcomes. In: Iezzoni LI, editor. Risk adjustment for measuring healthcare outcomes. Chicago: Health Administration Press; 1997. p. 427–70.
9. Schulman J. Managing your patients' data in the neonatal and pediatric ICU: an introduction to databases and statistical analysis. Oxford, UK: Blackwell; 2006.
10. van Belle G. Statistical rules of thumb. In: Balding DJ, Bloomfield P, Cressie NA, editors. Wiley series in probability and statistics. New York: Wiley-Interscience; 2002. p. 221.
11. Schulman J. Transforming risk factors into an unbiased mortality model. J Perinatol 2008;28:243–6.
12. Schulman J, Stricof RL, Stevens TP, et al. Development of a Statewide Collaborative to decrease NICU central line associated bloodstream infections. J Perinatol, in press.
13. Bureau of Women's Health. N.Y.S.D.O.H. NYS Hospitals and perinatal designation level. Available at: http://www.health.state.ny.us/community/pregnancy/health_care/perinatal/hospital_designations.htm. September, 2005. Accessed June 30, 2008.
14. Division of Healthcare Quality Promotion and National Center for Infectious Diseases. The National Healthcare Safety Network (NHSN) user manual. Department of Health and Human Services, Centers for Disease Control and Prevention; 2006.
15. Centers for Disease Control and Prevention. Guidelines for the prevention of intravascular catheter-related infections. MMWR Recomm Rep 2002;51(RR-10):1–29.
16. Berenholtz SM, Pronovost PJ, Lipsett PA, et al. Eliminating catheter-related bloodstream infections in the intensive care unit. Crit Care Med 2004;32:2014–20.
17. Provonost P, Needham D, Bernholtz S, et al. An intervention to decrease catheter-related bloodstream infections in the ICU. N Engl J Med 2006;355(26):2725–32.
18. Centers for Disease Control and Prevention. Guideline for hand hygiene in health-care settings: recommendations of the Healthcare Infection Control Practices Advisory Committee and the HICPAC/SHEA/APIC/IDSA Hand Hygiene Task Force. MMWR Recomm Rep 2002;51(RR-16):1–45.

19. Boyce JM, Pittet D. Guideline for hand hygiene in health-care settings: recommendations of the Healthcare Infection Control Practices Advisory Committee and the HICPAC/SHEA/APIC/IDSA Hand Hygiene Task Force. Infect Control Hosp Epidemiol 2002;23(Suppl 12):S3–40.
20. Raad II, Hohn DC, Gilbreath BJ, et al. Prevention of central venous catheter-related infections by using maximal sterile barrier precautions during insertion. Infect Control Hosp Epidemiol 1994;15(4 Pt 1):231–8.
21. Mimoz O, Villeminey S, Ragot S, et al. Chlorhexidine-based antiseptic solution vs alcohol-based povidone-iodine for central venous catheter care. Arch Intern Med 2007;167(19):2066–72.
22. Chaiyakunapruk N, Veenstra VL, Lipsky BA, et al. Chlorhexidine compared with povidone-iodine solution for vascular catheter–site care: a meta-analysis. Ann Intern Med 2002;136:792–801.
23. McGee DC, Gould MK. Preventing complications of central venous catheterization. N Engl J Med 2003;348:1123–33.
24. Maki DG. A prospective, randomized trial of gauze and two polyurethane dressings for site care of pulmonary artery catheters: implications for catheter management. Crit Care Med 1994;22:1729–37.
25. Gillies D, O'Riordan L, Carr D, et al. Gauze and tape and transparent polyurethane dressings for central venous catheters. Cochrane Database Syst Rev 2003;(3):1–19.
26. Crnich CJ, Maki DG. The promise of novel technology for the prevention of intravascular device–related bloodstream infection. I. Pathogenesis and short-term devices. Clin Infect Dis 2002;34:1232–42.
27. Salzman MB, Isenberg HD, Shapiro JF, et al. A prospective study of the catheter hub as the portal of entry for microorganisms causing catheter-related sepsis in neonates. J Infect Dis 1993;167(2):487–90.
28. Aly H, Herson V, Duncan A, et al. Is bloodstream infection preventable among premature infants? A tale of two cities. Pediatrics 2005;115:1513–8.
29. Garland JS, Alex CP, Sevallius JM, et al. Cohort study of the pathogenesis and molecular epidemiology of catheter-related bloodstream infection in neonates with peripherally inserted central venous catheters. Infect Control Hosp Epidemiol 2008;29:243–9.
30. Association for Professionals in Infection Control and Epidemiology, I., Healthcare-Associated Reporting Laws and Regulations. 2008.
31. McGiffert L. Summary of state activity on hospital-acquired infections. Austin, Texas: Consumers Union; 2007. Available at: http://www.consumersunion.org/campaigns/CU%20Summ%20HAI%20state%20rpting%20laws%20as%20of%201-08.pdf.
32. Department of Health. N.Y.S., New York state hospital-acquired infection reporting system: pilot year–2007 2008. Available at: http://www.nyhealth.gov/nysdoh/hospital/reports/hospital_acquired_infections/2007/docs/hospital-acquired_infection-full_report.pdf. Albany (NY).
33. Pronovost PJ, Goeschel CA, Wachter RM. The wisdom and justice of not paying for "preventable complications". JAMA 2008;299(18):2197–9.
34. Costello JM, Morrow DF, Graham DA, et al. Systematic intervention to reduce central line-associated bloodstream infection rates in a pediatric cardiac intensive care unit. Pediatrics 2008;121(5):915–23.
35. Pawson R, Tilley N. Realistic evaluation. London: Sage Publications, Ltd; 1997.
36. Horn SD. Performance measures and clinical outcomes. JAMA 2006;296(22):2731–2.
37. Berwick DM. The Science of improvement. JAMA 2008;299(10):1182–4.

38. Schulman J. Evaluating the processes of neonatal intensive care. London: BMJ Books; 2004.
39. Benneyan J, Lloyd R, Plsek P. Statistical process control as a tool for research and healthcare improvement. Qual Saf Health Care 2003;12:458–64.
40. Edwards JR, Peterson KD, Andrus ML, et al. National Healthcare Safety Network (NHSN) report, data summary for 2006, issued June 2007. Am J Infect Control 2007;35:290–301.
41. Division of Healthcare Quality Promotion. The National Healthcare Safety Network (NHSN) manual: patient safety component protocol. Atlanta (GA): National Center for Infectious Diseases; 2008.
42. Bizzarro M, Raskind C, Baltimore RS, et al. Seventy-five years of neonatal sepsis at Yale: 1928–2003. Pediatrics 2005;116:595–602.
43. Luria JW, Schoettker PJ. Reliability science and patient safety. Pediatr Clin North Am 2006;53:1121–33.
44. Studer Q. Hardwiring excellence. Gulf Breeze (FL): Fire Starter Publishing; 2003.
45. National Healthcare Safety Network (NHSN). Central Line Insertion Practices (CLIP) adherence monitoring. Available at: http://www.cdc.gov/ncidod/dhqp/nhsn_CLIP_AdherenceMonitoring.html. Accessed December 22, 2008.
46. Glauser E. The Toyota phenomenon, 2005.
47. ECRI Institute (2005) Health Care Risk Control-Culture of Safety. Risk Management Reporter Volume.
48. Pronovost P, Berenholtz SM, Goeschel CA, et al. Creating high reliability in health care organizations. Health Serv Res 2006;41:1599–617.
49. HAI prevention emphasized in 2009 National Patient Safety Goals. Healthcare Benchmarks Qual Improv 2008;85–8.
50. Jarvis W. The Lowbury lecture. The United States approach to strategies in the battle against healthcare-associated infections, 2006: transitioning from benchmarking to zero tolerance and clinician accountability. J Hosp Infect 2007; 65(Suppl 2):3–9.
51. Goeschel C, Pronovost P. Harnessing the Potential of Health Care Collaboratives: lessons from the keystone ICU project, in Advances in patient safety: new directions and alternative approaches. Volumes 1–4, AHRQ Publication Nos. 08-0034 (1–4). July 2008. Rockville (MD): Agency for Healthcare Research and Quality; 2005.
52. Pauker S, Zane E, Salem D. Creating a safer health care system: finding the constraint. JAMA 2005;294(22):2906–8.

Standardize to Excellence: Improving the Quality and Safety of Care with Clinical Pathways

Paul Kurtin, MD[a,*], Erin Stucky, MD[a,b]

KEYWORDS

• Quality • Safety • Clinical pathways • House staff • Hospitalist

Clinical pathways, also known as clinical practice guidelines, have a fundamental role in the delivery of high quality, safe care. Far from being "cookbook medicine" or interfering with physician autonomy in directing their patients' care, clinical pathways improve care by reducing or eliminating many barriers to the delivery of safe, effective, and efficient care.

High quality care can be defined as care that is safe, timely, effective, efficient, equitable, and patient and family centered.[1] The first of five barriers or challenges to high quality care addressed by clinical pathways is the widespread unnecessary variation in care.[2] Unnecessary variation in care can be defined as diagnostic or therapeutic interventions performed at the discretion of the ordering physician and not required by the patient's condition. Whether looked for at the national, regional, or local level, unnecessary variation can be found. Similar patients should be treated similarly based upon the best available evidence or expert consensus while patients with important differences in their condition should be treated differently. Unnecessary variation in any process, including clinical care, leads to two important and unwanted outcomes—increased cost and decreased quality. Clinical pathways, when based upon the best available evidence or consensus of experts, combined with significant input from local practitioners standardize care processes and have the potential to reduce unnecessary variation in care, improve clinical outcomes, and reduce the costs of care. At Rady Children's Hospital, we have more than a decade of experience with clinical pathways and have repeatedly documented improved clinical outcomes and reduced costs of care via the use of clinical pathways.[3] We call this approach

[a] Rady Children's Hospital San Diego, 3020 Children's Way, MC 5064, San Diego, CA 92123, USA
[b] Department of Pediatrics, University of California San Diego, La Jolla, CA 92093, USA
* Corresponding author.
E-mail address: pkurtin@rchsd.org (P. Kurtin).

Pediatr Clin N Am 56 (2009) 893–904
doi:10.1016/j.pcl.2009.05.005
pediatric.theclinics.com

"standardize to excellence." Standardizing care processes for all eligible children also helps reduce and avoid disparities in care delivery. If there is a best way to manage a specific condition, all children with that condition should be, and are, treated that way. With significant financial pressures on all providers of health care, if two practices yield similar clinical outcomes yet one approach is consistently less expensive, all patients should be managed using the less expensive approach.

A second barrier to high quality care that is addressed by clinical pathways is the gap between knowledge and practice. This gap, which can be as large as 17 years, is the time it takes a proven new practice to go from the medical literature into routine clinical care. In our approach to developing clinical pathways, the pathways are living documents that must be reviewed and updated on a regular basis. Our current approach to updating pathways, including the involvement of house staff, is described herein. By updating pathways on a predetermined schedule and modifying pathways in real time when an important new medication or treatment approach is reported in the literature, clinical pathways help physicians provide the most up to date care possible. Each pathway has designated "content" experts who evaluate the importance and relevance of new information before it is considered to be included in a pathway for general use. With this approach, the gap between knowledge and practice can be reduced from years to months or even weeks.

The third barrier to high quality care addressed by clinical pathways is the failure of many physicians to appreciate, understand, and work within the complex systems of care that exist within hospitals today. Inpatient care is multi- and interdisciplinary and involves a large number and variety of patient-provider interactions and therapeutic interventions. Much more is involved in the care of most inpatients than simply the primary physician-patient relationship. The process to develop clinical pathways includes all providers who will take part in caring for the patient, including nurses, social workers, dieticians, pharmacists, and respiratory therapists. By including all involved disciplines in the development of clinical pathways, we can explicitly address issues of care coordination by examining the many interacting systems needed to provide safe, high quality care to a child with a given condition. When designed and used in this way, clinical pathways also help physicians meet the American Board of Pediatrics certification requirement of system-based learning.[4]

A fourth challenge to high quality care that is addressed by clinical pathways and currently attracting a great deal of national attention is the need to improve patient safety. Beginning with the Institute of Medicine's publication of "To Err is Human,"[5] the focus of patients and their families, payers, regulators, and providers is on ways to reduce or eliminate harm and improve patient safety. Any given care process that varies and is implemented differently from provider to provider and from patient to patient presents a greater risk for error and potential harm. Standardizing via clinical pathways the way in which clinical interventions and processes are chosen and performed improves the safety of those interventions.

The fifth challenge to high quality care addressed by clinical pathways is the slow adoption and routine use of practices by providers that can improve clinical outcomes and patient safety. One root cause of this slow adoption of proven practices is the lack of a "business case" for quality. In brief, providers spend considerable resources (eg, people, technology, training) to improve care while the financial benefits of these quality improvement efforts often go to the payers. In our experience,[6] as we improved care processes and patient outcomes, including shortening lengths of stay for many common conditions, our reimbursement for this improved care actually fell. Because we are paid on a per diem basis, as days in the hospital decreased, reimbursement also decreased. This decreased revenue has been at least partially offset by our widespread use of clinical pathways and our ability to actually document improved clinical outcomes that has helped us gain significant market share. Clinical pathway development and routine use are also potentially helpful in pay for performance programs in which providers are rewarded for reliably and routinely delivering well-specified, evidence-based processes of care. When firmly embedded into routine care processes and the organization's clinical culture, pathways can make it easy for providers to "do the right thing" and deliver the expected care.

A component of our pathway process that supports widespread use is the explicit statement that nothing interferes with physician autonomy when it comes to the care of a specific child. Physicians are free to deviate from the pathway if they feel such a course would improve the care of their patient. These deviations from expected practices are reviewed to determine if the pathway needs to be altered to include the care required by that one patient. In addition, physicians routinely receive feedback information on their adherence to specific components of pathways and on their patients' outcomes, such as their length of stay, readmission rate, or transfer to a higher level of care. No physician should be expected to change their practices without knowing on a regular and timely basis the impact of those changes on their patients' outcomes. Transparency with pathway results helps to build physician confidence and comfort with the pathway process.

The potential benefits of pathway use as described previously provided enough information and motivation for early adopter physicians to at least try clinical pathways;[7] however, it was a vote by the medical staff making pathways the default mechanism of care that lifted the pathway adherence rate from 30% to 40% to greater than 90% for the past decade (**Table 1**). Early results of pathway outcomes comparing patients on a pathway with patients with the same condition but not on a pathway showed that pathway patients consistently did much better. Rigorously analyzing clinical care processes and outcomes and then widely sharing that information forms the foundation of our clinical pathway efforts.

Until the full potential of the electronic health record is realized, obtaining actionable information from clinical practice involves a trade-off between the clinical robustness and expense of chart review versus the relatively easy yet less detailed search through administrative databases. We use a hybrid approach in which analysis of administrative databases is supplemented with chart reviews when more clinical detail is needed.

Sharing valid, risk-adjusted data on practice patterns and outcomes with physicians provides motivation for change to improve patients' outcomes. The perceived need for change arises when physicians see that their patients' outcomes are not as good as they might like when compared with the outcomes reported by other local providers or national databases. Most physicians do not routinely receive or review data on the outcomes of their patients other than for poor outcomes reviewed at clinical morbidity and mortality meetings. Even less frequently are those results compared with the results of other providers caring for similar patients. Once physicians become comfortable with the reliability and validity of their own data and with the comparisons in performance being made, they will actively seek ways to improve their performance. In addition to identifying differences in outcomes, this approach to assessing physician practices always, in our experience, reveals wide variation in the care of similar patients. Reducing this variation in care when not clinically necessary provides the opportunity to improve clinical outcomes by standardizing processes of care with evidence-based, consensus-driven, locally adapted clinical pathways.

The creation of pathways takes time and resources; therefore, there must be an approach to prioritize pathway development. Our approach to prioritization includes

Table 1
Pathway report example: rates for use and select key pathway measures

Parameter	Baseline	April–June 2006	July–September 2008	PHIS 2007 Average	RCHSD Target
Asthma					
Eligible patients (number)	105	112	97	—	—
Preprinted order set use	77%	86%	99%	—	90%
Chest radiography	62%	59%	58%	67%	<45%
Systemic steroids	98%	99%	100%	96%	98%
Relievers	—	100%	100%	95%	100%
Average length of stay (days)	1.70	1.46	1.30	2.34	—
Readmits within 7 days	—	—	1.0%	0.6%	0

Parameter	Baseline December 2005	April–June 2006	July–September 2008	PHIS 2007 Average	RCHSD Target
Appendicitis					
Eligible patients (number)	49	141	191	—	—
Preprinted order set use	—	64%	100%	—	90%
CT at RCHSD	51%	49%	62%	39%	—
Perforation rate	—	36%	38%	35%	—
12-Month rolling average perforation rate	39%	39%	33%	—	—
Appropriate use of antibiotics	71%	95%	99%		90%
Average length of stay (days)	4.50	3.12	3.36	3.4	—
Readmits within 30 days	—	4.2%	3.1%	5.2%	0

Percentages noted equal use/eligible patients.
Abbreviation: RCHSD, Rady Children's Hospital San Diego.

the following variables: (1) the number of patients potentially impacted by a pathway (the more patients, the higher the priority); (2) the cost of caring for children with a specific condition (the higher the cost, the higher the priority); (3) the need for high-risk procedures when patient safety might be a concern; and (4) the physician's interest and requests for pathways to be developed to help them care for their patients. Because the use of pathways is a foundation of our clinical care, even if the number of patients to be managed with a pathway is small, we develop a pathway when requested by a physician.

Over time, pathway use in our organization has spread to create a consistent continuum of care (inpatient, emergency department, specialty clinics, primary care office, and home care) for common chronic conditions such as asthma. Pathways specific for caring for patients in the emergency department and in various specialty clinics have also been developed.

When creating multidisciplinary pathways, a representative from each included discipline is a member of the pathway team. In addition to providing discipline-specific content to the pathway, each representative is also expected to be a "champion" for pathway dissemination and use by their peers. The quality management department of the hospital is responsible for tracking pathway process and outcome metrics and routinely reporting them back to the pathway users. These results are also shared with the medical staff executive committee and with the hospital board. Visible board and chief executive officer support as well as strong support from the organized medical staff are critical in gaining and maintaining staff interest and involvement in the pathway process.

The Joint Commission recognized our work in clinical pathways by awarding its Ernest A. Codman Award in 2002 to Rady Children's Hospital San Diego. Our approach to the development and implementation of clinical pathways is well described in a recent book entitled "Organizing for Quality: The Improvement Journeys of Leading Hospitals in Europe and the United States."[8]

THE ROLE OF HOSPITALISTS IN CREATING, IMPLEMENTING, AND SUSTAINING CLINICAL PATHWAYS

Hospitalists, physicians whose primary professional focus is the general medical care of hospitalized patients, gained attention in 1996 when Dr. Robert Wachter coined the term in the *New England Journal*.[9] Hospitalist activities may include patient care, teaching, research, advocacy, and leadership related to hospital care. Hospital medicine is a "geographic" specialty organized around a site of care rather than a body system, age, or disease state. Hospitalists practice beyond the traditional ward setting, often providing care, consultation, and special services (such as sedation) throughout the hospital system. Pediatric hospitalists have been rendering care in this manner for over 3 decades, with the oldest division of hospital medicine having started in at Rady Children's Hospital San Diego in 1978.[10] The culture of hospital medicine, and in particular of pediatrics, is one of advocacy for the patient and the system that is centered around excellence in clinical care. Pediatric hospitalists are board certified or eligible pediatricians working in varied settings and numbered over 600 as of 2008 (personal communication, N. Alexander, MPP, American Academy of Pediatrics Section on Hospital Medicine, February 2008). A 2007 Pediatric Research in the Inpatient Setting survey of 208 pediatric hospitalists at over 40 sites in the United States and Canada reported that 92% spend some time in administration, with 53% spending 20% or more.[11] Most (85%) are on hospital committees and lead initiatives in practice guidelines (61%) or quality improvement (52%).

Although only 7% reported time spent in research, of these, 57% focused on quality improvement or health services delivery.

Pediatric hospitalists are uniquely positioned to engage in quality and safety efforts at the bedside, in units, in the hospital, and within hospital network systems; however, most have not had formal training beyond residency, with 13% having completed a chief residency and 19% a nonhospitalist fellowship.[11] Only about a dozen have completed pediatric hospitalist fellowship training, which includes dedicated quality improvement education and projects. Most pediatric hospitalists cite a need for more formal training in quality improvement and safety (>70%), preferring residency tracks or fellowship to attain these skills.[11] Despite the lack of formal training, pediatric hospitalists have accepted and developed quality improvement roles from the level of participation in Joint Commission preparations to more objectively clarified and broad positions such as Director of Quality or Clinical Effectiveness. Involvement in quality improvement is rapidly being accepted as part of the hospitalists' job description.[12] The role in development, implementation, and maintenance of clinical pathways, that is, evidence-based algorithms and associated standardized order sets, fits well with pediatric hospitalists who are clinically focused, close to the "sharp end" of patient care, and have experience working with teams. This role at community hospitals is particularly valuable and pairs well with advocacy for the pediatric patient within larger predominantly adult health care systems.

Creation of Pathways

The pediatric hospitalists at Rady Children's Hospital participate in all general pediatric pathway processes. The Medical Director for Quality, a pediatric hospitalist, is responsible for oversight of the entire pathway program in partnership with the Chief Quality and Safety Officer and a quality management department data analyst. Pediatric hospitalists serve in a variety of roles on clinical pathway teams, including the following:

- Team leader
  - Schedules and chairs team meetings
  - Sets the agenda
  - Records team activities
  - Reports to management
- Team facilitator
  - Owns the process
  - Oversees the dynamics of the team and helps to ensure each team member has a voice
  - Clarifies decision-making processes
- Team member
  - Brings fundamental knowledge about a topic
  - Helps with implementation of proposed interventions
  - Should evolve into future team leaders
  - Represents all of the key process owners, stakeholders

Review of baseline internal data displayed by the group, unit, or physician can result in long and often unproductive discussions regarding the reliability and validity of the data. Pediatric hospitalists at our institution are expected to understand the methods used to obtain the data, assist in its interpretation, and help the group objectively use the information to select specific measures for tracking processes and outcomes of care. Pediatric hospitalists are expected to be system early adopters and to model features of good teamwork such as inclusiveness, openness, and consensus-seeking behavior. For example, in developing a pathway for complicated pneumonia, divergent discussions involving competing literature on the timing and best method of imaging can often be best resolved by the pediatric hospitalist. Assessment of issues such as the availability of a procedure, sedation risk, radiation exposure, and the likelihood of change in clinical management based on the results requires a view of the whole child and the whole system, which are the realm of the pediatric hospitalist. Final clinical, process, safety, financial, and balancing measures chosen to track the outcomes of the pathway should reflect the interdisciplinary nature of care, internal data capabilities, and the literature.

Implementation of Pathways

Pathway implementation, following the Plan Do Study Act (PDSA) process, often reveals systemic operational and cultural barriers not anticipated during the development process. Pediatric hospitalist programs at nonacademic centers and those established to offset house staff patient load have been created with, among other things, an explicit responsibility for efficiency, adherence to hospital policies, and the flow of patients through the hospital. Pediatric hospitalists' responsibilities at academic centers have grown to include, or have had from inception, an additional responsibility to educate students and house staff. Pediatric hospitalists are constantly involved in team care with respiratory therapists, registered nurses, child life specialists, and others, allowing for real-time observation of "what works." At the authors' center, pediatric hospitalists respond to pathway concerns at the bedside, making the process real and patient oriented rather than separate and didactic. Feedback is given to the pathway team leader for quick incorporation as appropriate, often with same day reimplementation. Examples include adding "stat" to medication orders on a fever without source pathway to ensure timely medication administration or addressing the inability to obtain a routine renal sonogram on a Sunday afternoon for an infant with pyelonephritis.

In addition to writing and overseeing the writing of orders, pediatric hospitalists are physician champions for pathways and influence the culture surrounding their use. Pediatric hospitalists are visible to nonhospitalist general pediatricians, family practitioners, midlevel providers, and house staff who may work with or in parallel to the pediatric hospitalist. In environments in which pediatric hospitalist services are relatively new or in which these services have overlapped with subspecialty services, this interaction can be a challenge. Because key practitioners should always be part of the pathway development team, the pediatric hospitalist can assist in their recruitment with targeted personal e-mail and phone calls before formal implementation and can offer to answer any concerns. Inherent in this collaborative relationship is trust in and an understanding of the evidence-based, consensus-driven pathway process. Depending on the issue raised regarding the use of a pathway, the specific pathway team facilitator, leader, or a content expert can be called upon to speak directly with the concerned physician or midlevel provider. At the authors' center, pediatric hospitalists have been practicing in a collaborative manner for over 30 years, caring for almost 80% of general pediatric admissions. Long-standing relationships have been built, in part, due to turnover of only seven physicians since inception. Solid partnerships with primary care and subspecialty colleagues are a cornerstone of successful pathway implementation. Similar to their physician colleagues, pediatric hospitalists can assist with engagement of key leaders/early adopters from nursing, respiratory therapy, and other disciplines. Our pediatric hospitalists have a presence on many hospital committees and serve as liaisons to or medical directors for multiple clinical units and nonphysician clinical groups. Through these relationships, pediatric hospitalists can listen to ideas and support changes to pathways suggested by these nonphysician groups.

Maintenance of Pathways

Sustained use pathways are the result of embedded processes, default systems, belief in the pathway process, consistent periodic analysis of outcomes, and new evidence-based information using PDSA cycles and timely action. Pediatric hospitalists can influence each of these components to varying degrees. Variability in practices has been reported to be less for pediatric hospitalists than for community-based pediatricians,[13] although variation in reported use of unproven therapies by pediatric hospitalists exists.[14] Although this observation suggests that pediatric hospitalists may integrate validated practices with more consistency than generalists whose practice is not hospital based, it also highlights an important point—the need to assess what should not be done as well as what should be done. A pathway may appear to be followed as designed if administrative dataset review excludes, for example, a new therapy being used which is not part of the planned pathway order set. Pediatric hospitalists provide a window into daily operations, often catching small variations in expected practice soon after they surface. These discrepancies in planned care can often be rapidly resolved through e-mail exchange with pathway members. Examples may include the use of acyclovir for all neonates admitted with fever, daily chest radiographs for patients with pneumonia, or placement of a peripherally inserted central catheter for home intravenous antibiotics for a patient with uncomplicated pyelonephritis. Pediatric hospitals should support integration of positive system changes commonly recommended by hospital colleagues from nursing, respiratory, pharmacy, social work, nutrition, and child life. These changes often result in enhancements to the processes, safety, and parent/child satisfaction with care. Pediatric hospitalists are viewed as avid supporters of the entire care team, sharing a common goal of safe, efficient, effective, patient-centered, timely, and equitable care. Pediatric hospitalists are also expected to help expedite agreed upon changes and to educate and hold their physician colleagues accountable for implementing these changes. The PDSA cycle alone, although embedded in the pathway process, will not be successful in sustaining the use of pathways. Pediatric hospitalists are a critical integrated part of the hospital framework necessary to sustain pathways. They possess the teamwork, leadership, and clinical skills necessary to nurture the culture of quality and ensure ongoing pathway development, use, evaluation, and improvement.

Future Directions

Pediatric hospitalist engagement in local, state, and national clinical quality efforts is growing. Hospitalist competencies for internists have been published,[15] with those for pediatric hospitalists anticipated in 2009, which include active participation and leadership in quality improvement. Sharing of pathways is occurring on Web sites and at pediatric hospitalist national meetings and is defining areas for clinical research.[14] Integration of pediatric hospitalists into informal and formal quality improvement roles in a consistent manner should be viewed as a "best or at least promising practice" for institutions. These partnerships between pediatric hospitalists and their local hospitals and between pediatric hospitalists and larger hospitalist networks are a means by which to sustain robust and relevant clinical pathways within and between institutions.

PATHWAYS AND STANDARD ORDER SETS AS TEACHING TOOLS: THE ROLE OF HOUSE STAFF

The Institute of Medicine and American Board of Pediatrics' expectations for rendering care that adheres to principles of quality and for continuing education and activity in quality improvement send a strong message to all in graduate medical education. The obvious prequel to meaningful quality improvement activities in practice is the learning and application of the theories of quality improvement within residency. The Accreditation Council for Graduate Medical Education (ACGME) Pediatric Residency Review Committee expects residents to "participate in a quality improvement project," "participate in identifying system errors and implementing potential system solutions," and be educated in "systems approach to examining health care delivery practices."[16] Looking more carefully at the ACGME six core competencies, involvement in the pathway process can address medical knowledge, communication skills, practice-based learning, professionalism, and systems-based practice quite readily. In addition, patient care, best evaluated at the bedside, is at least influenced by discussions surrounding the patient/family education included in pathways. Building a continuum of training in the science and practice of quality improvement in the medical profession allows for development of habits for professional success in the twenty-first century; however, a long-term commitment to quality improvement as a daily habit is not merely a reflexive response to external agency mandates and societal pressures. It is a return to basic tenets of medicine which require physicians to "do no harm or injustice" to patients.[17] Harm or injustice can be found in many areas of medical practice, ranging from inappropriate medication ordering to failure to educate families in a culturally competent manner. Although many residency programs address such issues independently, a comprehensive program addressing quality and safety is currently lacking in most US programs and is evident in only a few.[18] In addition, validation of the importance of quality improvement in improving clinical processes and outcomes by the academic sector is leading to evolution of quality improvement as a science and, with it, more research focused on improving health care delivery.

Resident involvement in the pathway process is an effective method for teaching skills such as literature search and evidence-based medicine critical review. At the authors' center, the Innovative Quality Improvement Research in Residency (INQUIRY) program was begun in spring 2006 to better address the need for focused quality improvement didactic and hands-on learning. Quality improvement theory, tools, data analysis, and data presentation are topics covered in core didactic sessions. Residents are taught the basics of statistics, including common and special cause variation and control charts. As part of the pathway team, they work in triplets, choosing an algorithm branch point or other specific question of interest to address (**Fig. 1**). Working in groups of three allows for attendance of at least one member at all face-to-face meetings and accommodates the need to balance pathway work with resident schedules. House staff collaborate with content experts to review their work and draft recommendations that are sent to the pathway team. Residents are critical to the annotation of the entire algorithm under review and receive recognition for their work, with names posted on the hospital intranet pathways page.

Engagement of house staff in pathway work presents both challenges and opportunities. The INQUIRY program is a longitudinal process, which is a more realistic method by which to embed lifelong learning habits, yet is difficult to maintain in the current resident block schedule structure. It is also hospital focused, although discussions and algorithms often extend from emergency department to outpatient care. Participation in the INQUIRY program is elective; therefore, it attracts early adopters

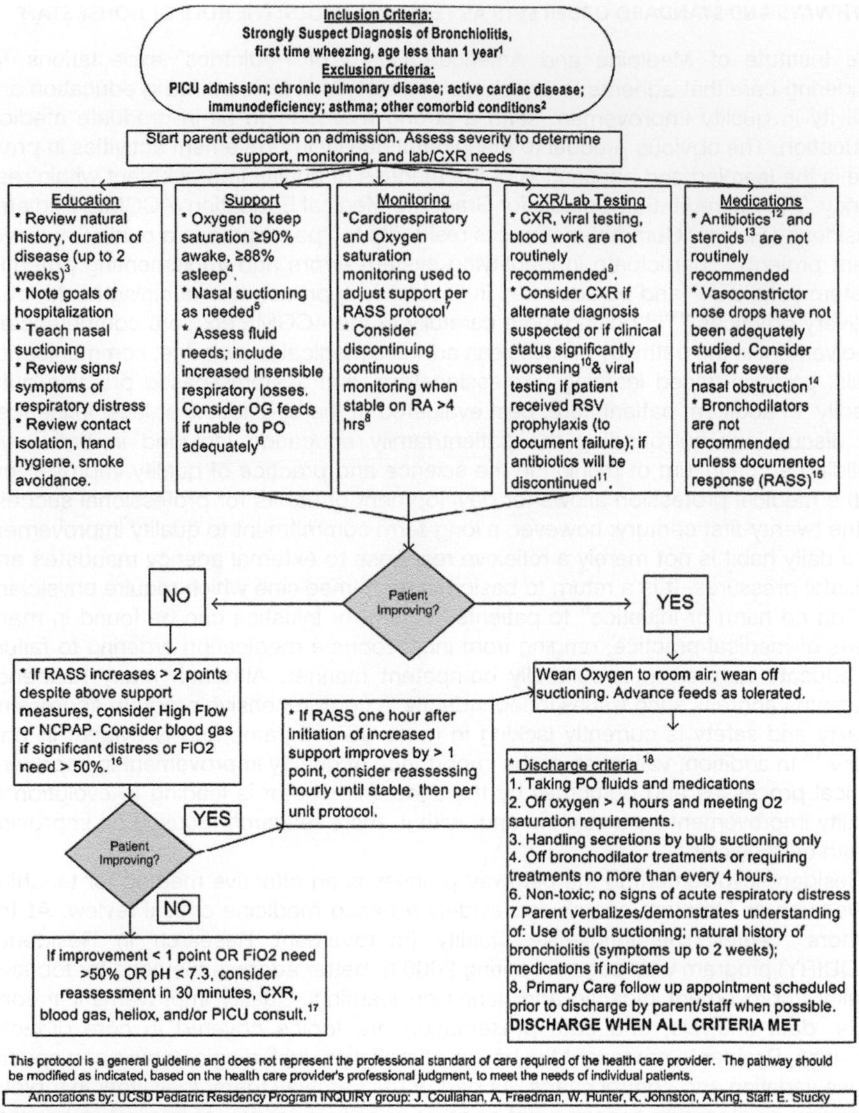

Fig. 1. Example of Rady Children's Hospital San Diego algorithm with annotations for bronchiolitis. (*Courtesy of* Rady's Children's Hospital, San Diego, CA; with permission.)

and change leaders. The obvious benefit is the ability for residents to educate their peers on the use and relevance of quality improvement and specific pathways. Working with hospital staff outside of the typical ward environment has lead to more awareness of teamwork and collaboration when on the wards. Focus on specific algorithm branch point questions has lead to a "pride of ownership" and interest in follow-up on outcomes of instituted interventions. Understanding of basic statistics and recognition of the clinical impact of measurable change has lead to formal research projects. Hospital staff, residents, and physician faculty agree that residents offer unique and important contributions to pathway processes, and residents, in return, gain valuable skills to lead future institutional initiatives.[19]

Future Directions

Resident education in quality improvement should emphasize exposure to and collaboration with hospital and outpatient administrative structures and staff, offer experience using basic quality improvement tools, and allow ample time for active involvement in specific clinical projects. To best allow for true education in and assessment of the six core competencies, current block-based electives will need to be restructured to allow quality and safety rotations, integrate quality improvement into continuity clinic curriculum, and foster quality improvement as research. Ideally, these resident quality improvement projects could extend into fellowship and clinical practice and could be part of initial board certification as well as recertification.

SUMMARY

Providing practitioners with locally developed, consensus-driven, evidence-based clinical pathways can improve the quality of care by (1) incorporating national guidelines and recommendations into routine care practices, increasing the use of validated practice; (2) reducing unnecessary variation in care by a single physician or group of physicians, improving efficiency, timeliness, and reducing disparities; and (3) standardizing care processes and improving safety. Pathways make it easier to identify opportunities for future improvements in care processes while simultaneously making those improvements easier to enact. In the authors' experience, pediatric hospitalists have a vital role in all aspects of creating, implementing, evaluating, and improving clinical pathways. Involving house staff in the pathway process enriches the scholarly components of pathway development while also actively engaging them in the science and practice of quality improvement.

REFERENCES

1. Hurtado MP, Swift EK, Corrigan JM, editors. Crossing the quality chasm: a new health system for the 21st century. Washington (DC): National Academies Press; 2001.
2. AHRQon variation. Improving health care quality. Available at: www.AHRQ.gov/news/qualfact.hm. Accessed January 2, 2009.
3. Applied child health services research. In: Sobo EJ, Kurtin PS, editors. Child Health Services Research: application, innovations, and insights. San Francisco: Jossey-Bass; 2003.
4. ABP citation. Maintenance of certification/core competencies. Available at: www.ABP.org/ABPwebsite. Accessed January 2, 2009.
5. Kohn LT, Corrigan JM, Donaldson MS, editors. To err is human: building a safer health system. Washington (DC): National Academies Press; 1999.
6. Homer C, Iles D, Dougherty D, et al. Exploring the business case for improving the quality of health care for children. Health Aff 2004;23(4):159–66.
7. Rogers EM. The diffusion of innovation. 4th edition. New York: Free Press; 1995.
8. Bate P, Mendel P, Robert G. Organizing for quality: the improvement journeys of leading hospitals in Europe and the United States. London: Radcliffe Publishing; 2007.
9. Wachter R, Goldman L. The emerging role of "hospitalists" in the American health care system. N Engl J Med 1996;335(7):514–7.
10. Stucky E, Evolution of a new specialty: a twenty year pediatric hospitalist experience [abstract]. In: Proceedings of the National Association of Inpatient Physicians Conference, New Orleans, Louisiana, April 21, 1999.

11. Ottolini M, Stucky E, Dhepyasuwan N, et al, Current roles and training needs of pediatric hospitalists: a study from the Pediatric Research in Inpatient Settings (PRIS) Network [abstract 754348]. In: Proceedings of the Pediatric Academic Society Annual Meeting, Honolulu, Hawaii, May 6, 2008.
12. Halasyamani L, Stucky ER. Quality improvement for the hospitalist. In: McKean SC, Bennett AL, Halasyamani LK, editors. Hospital medicine: just the facts. McGraw Hill Publishing; 2008. p. 41–5.
13. Conway PH, Edwards S, Stucky ER, et al. Variations in management of common inpatient pediatric illnesses: hospitalists and community pediatricians. Pediatrics 2006;118:441–7.
14. Landrigan CP, Conway PH, Stucky ER, et al. Variation in pediatric hospitalists' use of proven and unproven therapies: a study from the Pediatric Research in Inpatient Settings (PRIS) Network. J Hosp Med 2008;3(4):292–8.
15. Pistoria M, Amin A, Dressler D, et al. The core competencies in hospital medicine: a framework for curriculum development by the Society of Hospital Medicine. J Hosp Med 2006;1(S1):2–95.
16. Program requirements for graduate medical education in pediatrics. Available at: http://www.acgme.org/acWebsite/RRC_320/320_prIndex.asp. Accessed December 30, 2008.
17. The hippocratic oath. Available at: http://www.nlm.nih.gov/hmd/greek/greek_oath.html. Accessed December 30, 2008.
18. Voss JD, May NB, Schorling JB, et al. Changing conversations: teaching safety and quality in residency training. Acad Med 2008;83(11):1080–7.
19. Swanson C, Stucky E Quality improvement: the ultimate in systems-based teaching for residents [abstract 753225]. In: Proceedings of the Pediatric Academic Society Meeting. Toronto (ON, Canada), May 5, 2007.

Transforming Safety and Effectiveness in Pediatric Hospital Care Locally and Nationally

Keith E. Mandel, MD[a,*], Stephen E. Muething, MD[b],
Pamela J. Schoettker, MS[c], Uma R. Kotagal, MBBS, MSc[d]

KEYWORDS

- Quality improvement • Transformation • Safety
- Reliability • Measurement • Leadership

Although most pediatric care is provided in the community-based primary care setting, much of the care required by children who have complex and chronic conditions is provided by hospitals,[1] making them a high-priority focus for assessing and improving the safety and effectiveness of pediatric care delivery. Yet, despite significant efforts, national measures of the quality of hospital-based pediatric health care reveal that gaps persist in each of the quality dimensions defined by the Institute of Medicine (ie, safety, effectiveness, timeliness, patient-centeredness, equity, and efficiency).[2]

Achieving dramatic, sustainable improvements in the safety and effectiveness of care for children requires a transformational approach to how hospitals individually focus on improvement and how they learn from each other to achieve national goals. On the basis of the authors' journey at Cincinnati Children's Hospital Medical Center, knowledge acquired from other sites, and national transformation initiatives, this article describes how the following theoretic framework can locally and nationally transform the safety and effectiveness of hospital-based pediatric care.

[a] Physician–Hospital Organization, Division of Health Policy and Clinical Effectiveness, Cincinnati Children's Hospital Medical Center, 3333 Burnet Avenue, Mail Location 7023, Cincinnati, OH 45229, USA
[b] Division of General and Community Pediatrics, Cincinnati Children's Hospital Medical Center, 3333 Burnet Avenue, Mail Location 2011, Cincinnati, OH 45229, USA
[c] Division of Health Policy and Clinical Effectiveness, Cincinnati Children's Hospital Medical Center, 3333 Burnet Avenue, Mail Location 7014, Cincinnati, OH 45229, USA
[d] Division of Health Policy and Clinical Effectiveness, Cincinnati Children's Hospital Medical Center, 3333 Burnet Avenue, Mail Location 3025, Cincinnati, OH 45229, USA
* Corresponding author.
E-mail address: keith.mandel@cchmc.org (K.E. Mandel).

Pediatr Clin N Am 56 (2009) 905–918
doi:10.1016/j.pcl.2009.05.002 pediatric.theclinics.com

STRATEGIC APPROACH TO QUALITY AND SAFETY

Through a strategic planning effort based on clear direction from the board of directors, hospitals can achieve transformational change in their delivery system. Five steps are recommended: (1) set system-level priorities, (2) match a single measure or family of measures to each system-level priority, (3) identify breakthrough targets for each priority, (4) pilot test interventions to get results, and (5) spread successful interventions throughout the organization.

A strong strategic plan confirms quality as a core business strategy and commits the institution to achieving sustainable breakthroughs in improving clinical outcomes, reducing medical errors, delivering cost-effective care, improving care coordination, and enhancing access to care and timeliness of services delivered.[3] A plan that emphasizes the importance of integrating research with delivery system design to accelerate transfer of new knowledge to the bedside achieves the best medical and quality-of-life outcomes.

Establishing system-level improvement priorities with broad-based input from providers and patients and families is essential; these priorities could be modeled on the Institute of Medicine's six quality dimensions.[2] Examples include access to care, delays in the system, safe care, clinical excellence (including evidence-based care), reduced hassles, team well-being, and family-centered care (**Fig. 1**). Whatever the choice, system-level priorities should be clearly defined and consistently communicated to the entire staff.

A set of system-level measures is linked to each strategic improvement priority. System-level measures reflect performance across the entire organization or system of care, as opposed to measures of project- or condition-specific performance. A parsimonious set of system-level measures is preferable to a large set of highly-specific measures that reflects discrete aspects of hospital performance.[4] Monthly review of system-level measures by senior leadership and the board of directors keeps teams focused and moving forward (**Table 1**).

Underlying the system-level priorities is a horizontal integrating improvement structure that promotes integration across traditional boundaries (**Fig. 2**). System-level improvement priorities are aligned with quality improvement efforts within the academically organized clinical units, with measures and progress toward goals reported to senior leadership on a quarterly basis. Within clinical divisions, performance measures at the individual provider level[5,6] are vertically aligned with the strategic improvement priorities.

Perfection (100% performance and 0 defects) and breakthrough improvement goals reinforce the focus on transformation, as opposed to incremental improvement. Senior leadership designates specific initiatives underlying the strategic improvement priorities and works closely with improvement team leaders to establish annual and quarterly milestone goals linked to aim statements that are specific, measurable, achievable, realistic, and timely.[7] Improvement teams organize their work around 90-day improvement cycles (M. Pugh, unpublished data, 2003) and produce monthly reports that document progress toward goals and describe tests of change.[8]

Beyond transforming care within the local delivery system, there also needs to be a focus on impacting pediatric populations at the regional, state, national, and international levels through strategic partnerships (**Fig. 3**). A few examples from Cincinnati Children's Hospital Medical Center are reviewed in a later section.

On the basis of this general framework, the authors believe the following key drivers of transformation are essential (**Table 2**).

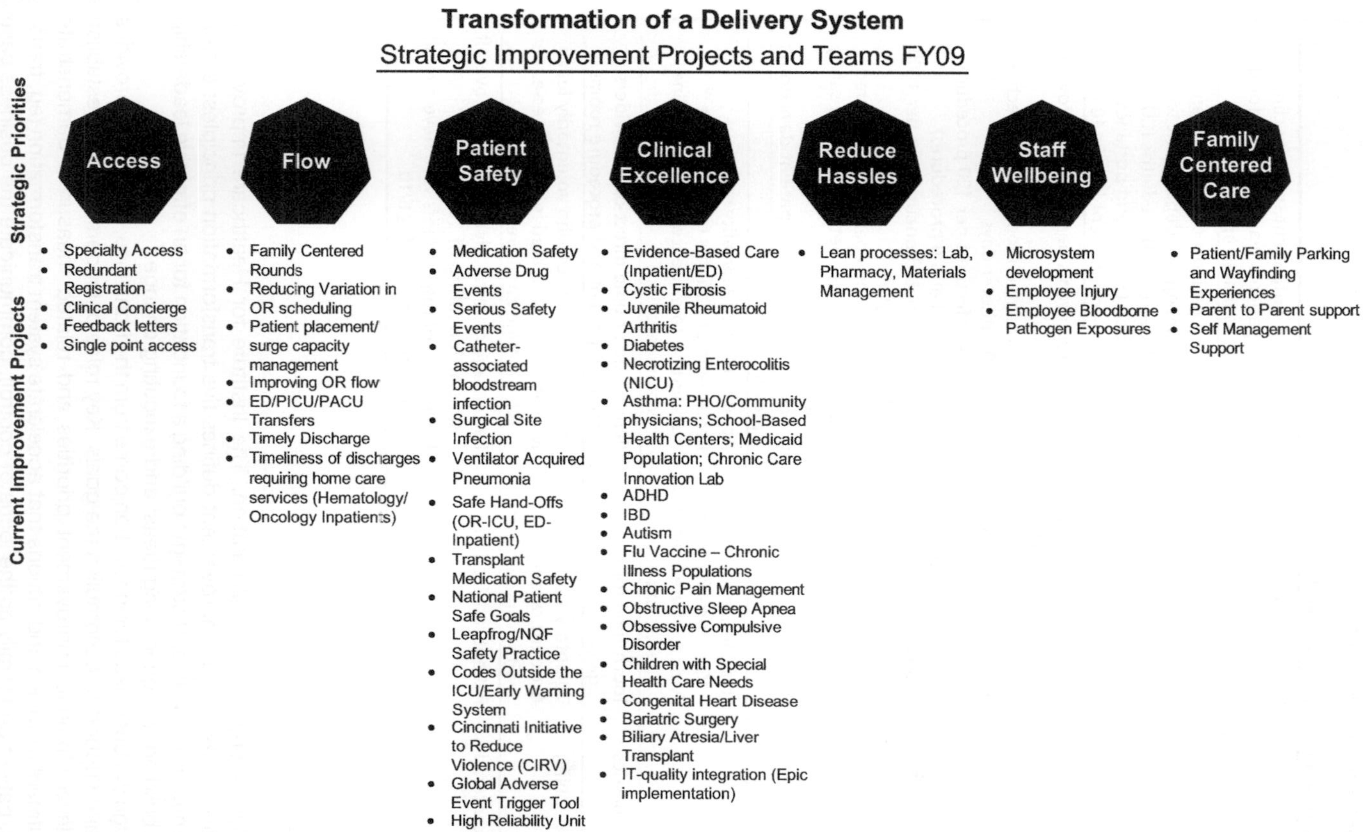

Fig. 1. An example of strategic priorities and portfolio of improvement projects at Cincinnati Children's Hospital Medical Center. ADHD, attention-deficit/hyperactivity disorder; ED, emergency department; IBD, inflammatory bowel disease; IT, information technology; NICU, neonatal ICU; NQF, National Quality Forum; OR, operating room; PHO, physician-hospital organization; PICU, pediatric ICU; PACU, postanesthesia care unit.

Table 1
Examples of system-level measures linked to strategic improvement priorities at Cincinnati Children's Hospital Medical Center

Strategic Priorities	System-level Measures	Definitions
Access	Third next available appointment	Percentage of outpatient specialty clinics with new patients waiting ≤10 d for the third next available appointment
Flow	Patients who have delays	Percentage of patients delayed in transfers from the emergency department to an inpatient bed (≤1 h), pediatric ICU to an inpatient bed (≤1 h), and postanesthesia care unit to an inpatient bed (≤10 min)
Patient safety	Adverse drug events Bloodstream infection rate Surgical site infection rate Ventilator-associated pneumonia rate Serious safety events Codes outside the ICU	Adverse drug events per 1000 doses (overall; preventable) Catheter-associated bloodstream infections per 1000 catheter days Surgical site infections per 100 procedure days (Classes I and II procedures) Ventilator-associated pneumonias per 1000 ventilator days Serious safety events per 10,000 adjusted patient days; days between serious safety events Codes per 1000 non-ICU patient days (total; preventable)
Clinical excellence	Standardized pediatric ICU mortality ratio Evidence-based care for eligible patients	Actual/expected mortality rate Percentage of patients receiving care according to evidence-based guideline recommendations
Reduced hassles	Touch time for care givers	Percentage of time direct-care providers spend in patient and procedure rooms
Staff well-being	Voluntary staff turnover Accident rate for staff with workdays lost	Percentage of nurses who voluntarily leave Number of work-related injuries/illnesses per 100 full-time employees
Family-centered care	Patient satisfaction	Percentage of respondents who have overall satisfaction rating of 10/10 Percentage of respondents who have overall satisfaction rating of ≤6/10

LEADERSHIP

Leadership is critical to transformation. The Institute for Healthcare Improvement framework for leadership improvement defines five transformation principles: establishing a mission, vision, and strategy; building a foundation for an effective leadership system; building will; generating ideas; and executing change.[9]

Although the best ideas for innovation come from the front lines, leadership provides the will and support to accomplish the goals. Key roles of leadership are to establish system-level strategic improvement priorities and related measures; demonstrate a commitment to values and actions that accelerate system transformation (eg, transparency, patient and family as the locus of control); communicate the business case for quality; understand and manage the inherent risks (eg, transparency); and maintain a high level of accountability for results.

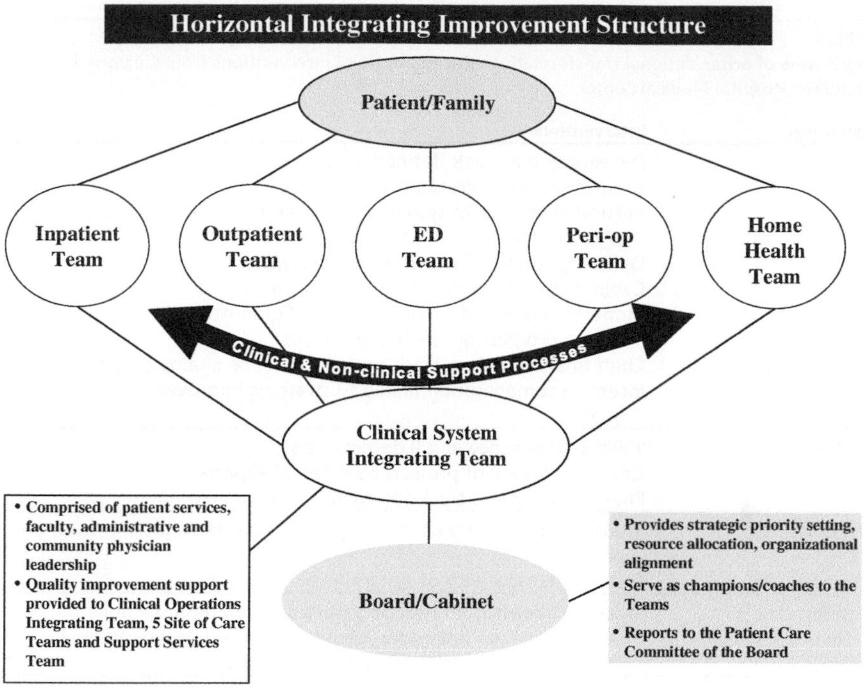

Fig. 2. An example of a clinical system improvement integrating structure at Cincinnati Children's Hospital Medical Center. ED, emergency department; Peri-op, perioperative.

Transformation can be accelerated by the board of directors' full commitment to transparency, by establishing improvement as the core business strategy, by requiring progress updates relative to annual safety and quality goals, and by ensuring the availability of resources to achieve goals. The board chair and senior leadership team make rounds on inpatient units to learn first-hand about issues and challenges; each board meeting begins with an update on safety issues and sentinel events, including a review of root cause analyses and actions taken; and a portion of the chief executive officer/management's compensation is tied to achieving goals for strategic improvement priorities.

BUILDING WILL

Relative to building will for transformation, a sense of urgency shared among providers, patients and families, and policymakers is essential.[10] This sense of

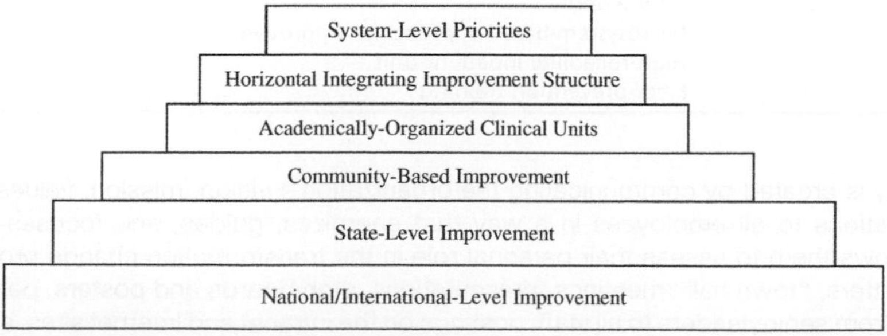

Fig. 3. Organizing for quality and transformation.

Table 2
Key drivers of organizational transformation with examples of interventions from Cincinnati Children's Hospital Medical Center

Key Driver	Interventions
Leadership	Delivery system goals defined in strategic plan Annual review of strategic improvement priorities Vertical alignment of system-level measures throughout the organization Quarterly review of system-level measures Cabinet champions on improvement teams Monthly meeting of the Patient Care Committee of the board to review progress on quality initiatives Chief financial officer leads business case for quality efforts Incentive compensation linked to strategic improvement priorities/goals
Building will	100% performance and 0 defect goals Quarterly review of projects by external experts Physician academic track for quality improvement
Transparency	Internal transparency of monthly reports for strategic improvement projects External transparency of system-level measures
Business case for quality	Financial impact from reducing hospital-acquired infections (eg, surgical site infections, ventilator-associated pneumonia, catheter-associated blood stream infections)
Patient/family engagement	Family Advisory Council Parents on improvement teams Family faculty: parents working full-time on quality and transformation Parents on board committees
Infrastructure: quality improvement and data analysis	Centralized and department-based quality improvement experts Use of statistical process control methods Clinical system improvement infrastructure to address horizontal integration across boundaries Evidence-based practice teams
Improvement capability	Intermediate improvement science training program Advanced improvement methods training program Quality improvement training program for residents Quality improvement fellowship program
Reliability and standardization	Learning from other industries (eg, industrial engineering principles, human factors science) Learning from innovators (eg, Agency for Healthcare Research and Quality; Institute for Healthcare Improvement high-reliability network) Microsystem-based approach to improvement High-reliability inpatient unit Error-prevention training

urgency is created by communicating the organization's vision, mission, values, and expectations to all employees in a way that energizes, guides, and focuses them and allows them to assess their personal role in the transformation change process. Newsletters, "town hall" meetings, presentations, storyboards and posters, personal letters from senior leaders to all staff, postings on the intranet and internet sites, annual reports, and special brochures are used to accomplish this goal.

TRANSPARENCY

Internal transparency has a powerful effect in raising the level of collective accountability for quality and transformation. Improvement data, including organizational scorecards, graphic displays of process and outcome measures, and monthly reports for strategic improvement initiatives, are made available to all employees by way of an intranet site. For example, at Cincinnati Children's Hospital Medical Center, the intranet home page features a patient safety tracker that is updated daily and indicates the number of days since the last serious safety event. Extensive information on safety initiatives is posted, including details of actual safety events and lessons learned through root cause analyses. The patient safety officer also communicates with all employees on a weekly basis through a journal posted on the intranet.

Regarding external transparency, system-level measures, measure specifications, and links to other sites where data are publicly reported (eg, the Leapfrog Group, the Joint Commission) are available on a hospital's public Web site.

BUSINESS CASE FOR QUALITY

Lack of a "business case for quality" (ie, improved financial outcomes as a result of investing in quality improvement[11,12]) is often cited as a major barrier to committing to transformational change.[13] Documenting the internal business case for quality is important to inspiring and sustaining improvement efforts from an individual hospital perspective, whereas articulating the external business case for quality is essential to recruiting support for improvement from purchasers and commercial and governmental payors. Independent validation of the financial impact of quality improvement efforts by the hospital finance team is important.

The board of directors must truly believe that quality improvement is essential to long-term success and viability, with board decisions regarding budgeting and capital allocation linked to providing demonstrably better, safer care for patients and families. At the same time, there must be a firm belief that better care also makes good business sense. Improvement initiatives have been shown to reduce costs, increase demand, promote more efficient use of scarce hospital resources, generate higher margins, and offer families improved overall value. For example, the authors found that, on average, the length of stay for each patient who had a preventable surgical site infection is increased by 10.6 days (15.0 days versus 4.4 days for children who do not develop a surgical site infection);[14] avoiding these infections would have resulted in an additional 1 million dollars per year in revenue through increased bed capacity for other patients.

ENGAGING PATIENTS AND FAMILIES

The patient and family as the locus of control is key to transformation. Patients and families help drive priorities and refocus the system on what matters most. Full commitment to the following areas is essential to successful transformation: (1) having patients and families involved on all improvement teams to ensure their values and perspectives are incorporated into the design of the care delivery system, to keep teams focused on priorities important to patients, and to promote the role of families as active advocates and partners; (2) full transparency of outcomes data for populations; and (3) allowing patients and parents to access the medical record. Parents participate on board committees and serve as advisors to improvement teams. With patients and families as equal partners, even the most reluctant participants can be persuaded to change and resistance can be overcome.

INFRASTRUCTURE

Responsibility for quality should be embedded into line management, rather than a separate quality structure or council. Improvement teams are accountable for achieving goals and are co-led by a physician and a nonphysician, with patient or parent involvement or a combination of the two. There is a persistent, intense focus on improving outcomes. Monthly reports document progress and include annotated run and control charts;[15] descriptions of Plan-Do-Study-Act (PDSA) cycles[8] accelerate the pace of change. Monthly meetings with the senior leader champion keep teams focused on data, PDSA cycles, and achieving 90-day goals. The senior leader champion also helps teams overcome organizational barriers, obtain resources, foster energy for change, and plan for spread to other parts of the organization. Improvement teams must be supported by a robust infrastructure that includes highly skilled and experienced quality improvement consultants and decision support analysts (who have at least a master's degree) who can effectively mine data and develop predictive models to drive improvement.

IMPROVEMENT CAPABILITY

To transform care delivery, a hospital needs leaders and staff who have improvement capability. Advanced improvement training programs (eg, Intermountain Healthcare[16]) help build a strong critical mass of improvement leaders. To sustain progress and accelerate the pace of cultural change, however, it is important to rapidly increase the number of individuals who have expertise in leading and executing improvement initiatives. To accomplish this, hospitals need to develop their own intermediate and advanced improvement programs to prepare staff to execute and teach improvement science and to lead improvement teams. For academic institutions, the use of improvement science methods, including planned experimentation, factorial designs, and control charts to understand common and special-cause variation, is critical.[17] When quality improvement is not fully embraced as a science, discipline and will can be lost and coalitions can degrade. Integrating improvement science with pediatric residency programs and establishing a quality improvement fellowship program are vital to ensuring that the next generation of clinicians has the quality improvement knowledge and skills to improve care delivery and patient outcomes.

RELIABILITY AND STANDARDIZATION

In health care, reliability is defined as the measurable capability of a process, procedure, or health service to perform its intended function in the required time, under commonly occurring conditions.[12] Weick and colleagues[18] identified five characteristics common to organizations that practice high reliability. Leaders are *preoccupied with failure* and extract the maximum learning from each failure, flaw, and near miss. There is a *reluctance to simplify interpretations*; instead, diverse opinions and experiences are embraced. High-reliability organizations are *sensitive to operations*; with a high level of situational awareness, they recognize that successful frontline operations are key to failure prevention. High-reliability organizations are *committed to resiliency*, with an increased ability to predict and respond to potential errors; they also believe that issues should be addressed as close to the front line as possible, with deference to local expertise in times of crisis (*underspecification of structures*). The principles of reliability science can be used to prevent failures, to identify and mitigate the impact of failures that inevitably occur, and to redesign the system to prevent future failures.[17,19]

RELIABILITY EXAMPLES FROM CINCINNATI CHILDREN'S HOSPITAL MEDICAL CENTER

The following examples demonstrate how this framework for transformation can be used to improve safety (such as reducing surgical site infections and ventilator-associated pneumonias [VAPs]) and to achieve highly reliable delivery of evidence-based care for common, important conditions. These examples were selected to emphasize the alignment of improvement initiatives with system-level priorities and measures.

Application of Evidence for Common Conditions

The system-level priority target in this instance is clinical excellence: providing evidence-based care. The system-level measure is a composite measure of the percentage of patients receiving care according to evidence-based guideline recommendations for five common conditions (bronchiolitis, acute gastroenteritis, fever of uncertain source, acute exacerbation of asthma, and community-acquired pneumonia). The leadership champion for two teams (one in the emergency department and one for inpatient care) is the chief of staff, a practicing physician. A quality improvement consultant and a data analyst provide 1 to 1.5 days of support each week. The goal is to improve the reliability of care delivery and to achieve 95% compliance with guideline recommendations.

The most fundamental step toward high reliability is standardizing key processes and decision making. Through education forums (eg, presentations at medical and nursing grand rounds and resident teaching conferences), educational materials (eg, posters and pocket cards with guideline summaries), and companion documents and tools (eg, electronic order sets, clinical pathways, parent versions of the guidelines, discharge goals, discharge instruction sheets, and education records)[20], the authors' institution achieved 82% adherence to key guideline recommendations.[21] To increase adherence, the authors used a quasi-experimental approach to examine the separate and combined effect of two interventions—a clinical protocol and a method to identify and mitigate failures. The clinical protocol gave nurses and respiratory therapists permission to administer appropriate evidence-based recommendations for guideline-eligible patients. No physician order was required to initiate the protocol; of note, a physician order was necessary if the protocol was not followed. Thus, the desired action was the default. The second intervention designated a charge nurse to identify guideline-eligible patients each shift. When a guideline-eligible patient did not receive care according to the guideline recommendations, the nurse identified the cause and attempted to remedy or mitigate the situation by speaking with the staff or physician assigned to the patient, thus identifying and preventing a potential error. The composite measure of compliance increased to 92% with the "identify and mitigate" strategy, with sustained results.

Reducing Ventilator-associated Pneumonias

The system-level priority is improving patient safety. Reliable application of evidence is the key to decreasing VAPs. The improvement team was co-led by the medical director of the pediatric ICU, an intensivist. The project was modeled as an internal learning collaborative between all the hospital ICUs, led by respiratory therapists on each unit and supported by a quality improvement consultant and a data analyst. Ambitious targets were set.[22] A key driver diagram (**Fig. 4**) was created to clarify and prioritize improvement interventions. Interventions were designed using reliability principles, with the goal to achieve 95% for the composite measure of the care bundle. The VAP rate dropped from a baseline average of 5.6 infections per 1000 ventilator days to 0.3 infections per 1000 ventilator days over a 9-month period.[22]

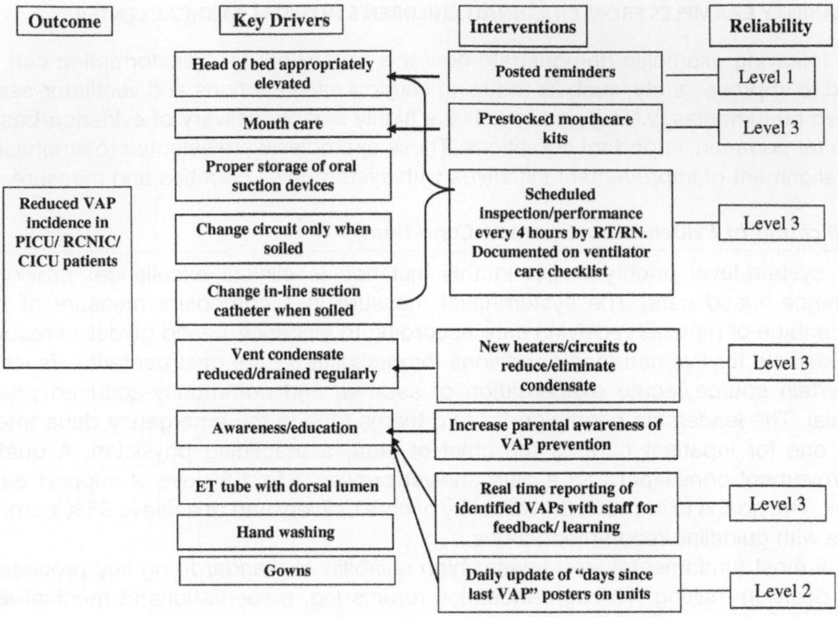

Fig. 4. Key driver diagram for reducing VAPs at Cincinnati Children's Hospital Medical Center. CICU, cardiac ICU; ET, endotracheal tube; PICU, pediatric ICU; RCNIC, Regional Center for Newborn Intensive Care; RT/RN, respiratory therapist/registered nurse.

Linking system transformation, ambitious goals, and the use of reliability and improvement science, and executing with a robust improvement infrastructure and the laser-like focus of leadership, can lead to dramatic improvements in safety and evidence-based care. All of the components described earlier must be executed with a sense of urgency and a relentless pursuit of perfection to dramatically improve quality and safety.

TRANSFORMING CARE AT THE NATIONAL LEVEL

Transformation at individual sites is important; however, national evidence of poor performance requires us to work across hospitals to make care safer and more effective at all locations.

Hospitals providing pediatric care have a strong history of participating in multihospital improvement collaboratives, of supporting development of national quality measures (eg, asthma measures endorsed by the Joint Commission[23] and pediatric patient safety indicators developed by the Agency for Healthcare Research and Quality[24]), and of advocating for public policy changes at the state and national levels that promote efforts to measure and improve care to children.

Although these efforts are impressive in terms of scope and results achieved, moving national, system-level measures toward near-perfection goals will require more than hospital participation in a series of project-specific improvement collaboratives. Improving national system-level measures will require each hospital to pursue its own transformation journey and, at the same time, collaborate across hospitals and other organizations. To maximize success, the following issues need to be addressed: (1) creating a sense of urgency for improvement and raising the level of collective accountability for improving quality measures at the national level,[25] (2) providing leadership for improvement at the board, senior-leadership, and management levels, (3) enhancing improvement capability and capacity, (4) increasing the level of patient and parent engagement, (5) documenting the business case for quality, and (6) pursuing a supportive policy environment.

Aligning efforts across organizations committed to quality and transformation is essential. An example of an integrating force in this regard at the national level is the Alliance for Pediatric Quality[26], a collaboration among the American Academy of Pediatrics, the American Board of Pediatrics, the Child Health Corporation of America, and the National Association of Children's Hospitals and Related Institutions. A high-priority focus for the Alliance for Pediatric Quality is to raise the level of collective accountability for achieving near-perfection, transformational goals by defining a core set of national quality measures for pediatric care. Recognizing the complexity involved with establishing national system-level measures and near-perfection goals, the Alliance for Pediatric Quality can build on other national quality measurement development efforts (eg, the National Initiative for Children's Healthcare Quality, the Child and Adolescent Health Measurement Initiative, the National Quality Forum, the Agency for Healthcare Research and Quality, the Joint Commission, the Ambulatory Quality Alliance, the Hospital Quality Alliance, and the American Medical Association Physician Consortium for Performance Improvement). Potential system-level measures for assessing the quality of hospital-based care for children across the United States are shown in **Table 3**.[4]

CREATING URGENCY: THE NEED TO GO PUBLIC

A sense of urgency that is shared among providers, patients and families, and policy-makers is essential to successful transformation at the national level.[10] This sense of urgency can be created by establishing a core set of measures that document the current state of quality of care within and across hospitals caring for children. Hospitals can proactively embrace this opportunity to take the lead in establishing the "national scorecard" and can communicate progress achieved in improving the system-level measures to various stakeholder groups, including the public-at-large, purchasers, payors, and government entities. Strong leadership from the Alliance for Pediatric Quality and each hospital is essential to documenting the current state of quality and will entail at least the following steps: (1) supporting standardized reporting among hospitals, (2) establishing a centralized data source to support comparative performance reporting and to meet private- and public-sector reporting requirements, and (3) committing to internal and external transparency of aggregate and comparative hospital data. Transparency will have a powerful effect in elevating the level of collective accountability for quality of care at the national level; in addition, the variation in comparative performance will fundamentally change the nature of how hospitals learn from each other and interact at all levels (eg, board, senior management, frontline care givers, parents/patients).

SUPPORTIVE PUBLIC POLICY ENVIRONMENT

Hospitals providing pediatric care are dramatically improving quality and safety, but these efforts would be greatly enhanced by a far more supportive policy environment. Although this is true for improvement initiatives for all populations, it is particularly salient for children due to the heavy reliance on publicly financed care (eg, Medicaid and the State Child Health Insurance Program [SCHIP]). The necessary federal and state authority and the attendant improvement capacity in terms of staff, expertise, and resources within

Table 3
Potential system-level measures for assessing the quality of hospital-based care for children across the United States (based in part on the Institute of Healthcare Improvement's Whole System Measures)

Institute of Medicine Quality Dimension	National System-level Measure
Safe	Adverse events: overall, drug-related, inpatient, outpatient
Effective	Standardized mortality ratio: overall, ICU
Effective	Composite measure of functional outcomes for populations that have chronic conditions
Effective	Composite measure of reliability of evidence-based care delivery: inpatient, emergency department, ICU
Effective, Safe	Nosocomial infection rates: catheter-associated bloodstream infections, surgical site infections, VAPs
Effective, Safe	Codes outside the ICU
Effective	Readmission rate
Effective	Admission rates for ambulatory-sensitive conditions
Patient/family centered	Satisfaction: inpatient and outpatient
Timely	Days to third next available appointment: primary care, specialty care
Efficient	Bed turnover rate
Efficient	Health care costs per capita
Efficient	Risk-adjusted cost per discharge
Efficient	Care giver time with patient/family
Efficient	Composite measure of delay in patient transfers: emergency department, postanesthesia care unit, ICU
Equitable	Above measures stratified by payor and race/ethnicity

Data from Institute of Medicine, Committee on Quality Health Care in America. Crossing quality chasm—new health system for the 21st century. Washington, DC: National Academy Press; 2001; and Martin L, Nelson E, Lloyd R, et al. Whole system measures. IHI innovation series white paper. Available at: http://www.ihi.org/IHI/Results/WhitePapers/WholeSystemMeasuresWhitePaper.htm. Accessed January 20, 2009.

Medicaid and SCHIP are insufficient compared to Medicare.[27] Although some progress can be made under current rules, congressional action is needed to provide these authorities and resources to Medicaid and SCHIP. The time for action is now because both of these programs are undergoing significant scrutiny and changes.

SUMMARY

Hospitals providing pediatric care are uniquely positioned to accelerate improvement and achieve transformational goals for populations within and beyond their walls. The strong history of collaboration among hospitals providing pediatric care, especially children's hospitals, sets the stage for successfully transforming care at a national level; however, a parsimonious set of system-level measures, a collective commitment to ambitious goals, a clear business case for quality, and transparent comparative data are essential to create a sense of urgency and to drive change. A strong leadership commitment to accelerate the transformation journey within and across hospitals delivering pediatric care is crucial.

REFERENCES

1. All children need children's hospitals. Alexandria (VA): National Association of Children's Hospitals and Related Institutions; 2007.
2. Institute of Medicine, Committee on Quality Health Care in America. Crossing the quality chasm—a new health system for the 21st century. Washington, DC: National Academy Press; 2001.
3. Britto M, Anderson J, Kent W, et al. Cincinnati Children's Hospital Medical Center: transforming care for children and families. Jt Comm J Qual Patient Saf 2006; 32(10):541–8.
4. Martin L, Nelson E, Lloyd R, et al. Whole system measures. IHI innovation series white paper. Available at: http://www.ihi.org/IHI/Results/WhitePapers/WholeSystemMeasuresWhitePaper.htm. Accessed January 20, 2009.
5. Blacklidge M, Kotagal U, Lazaron L, et al. Challenges to performance-based assessment for community physicians. J Healthc Qual 2005;27(5):20–7.
6. Myers S, Clark M, Russell J, et al. Focusing measures for performance-based privileging of physicians on improvement. Jt Comm J Qual Patient Saf 2008; 34(12):724–33.
7. Monaghan J, Channell K, McDowell D, et al. Improving patient and carer communication, multidisciplinary team working and goal-setting in stroke rehabilitation. Clin Rehabil 2005;19(2):194–9.
8. Langley GJ, Nolan KM, Nolan TW, et al. The improvement guide. A practical approach to enhancing organizational performance. San Francisco CA: Jossey-Bass; 1996.
9. Provost L, Miller D, Reinertsen J. A framework for leadership improvement. Available at: http://www.ihi.org/NR/rdonlyres/E0B13EEA-71FE-41A9-9616-3977A0EB14FD/2813/IHILeadershipFramework_FEB2006versionFINAL.pdf. Accessed January 20, 2009.
10. Kotter J. Leading change: why transformation efforts fail. Harv Bus Rev 1995;73: 59–67.
11. Homer C, Child Health Business Case Working Group. Exploring the business case for improving the quality of health care for children. Health Aff (Millwood) 2004;23(4):159–66.
12. Leatherman S, Berwick D, Iles D, et al. The business case for quality: case studies and an analysis. Health Aff (Millwood) 2003;22(2):17–30.
13. Reiter K, Kilpatrick K, Greene S, et al. How to develop a business case for quality. Int J Qual Health Care 2007;19(1):50–5.
14. Sparling K, Ryckman F, Schoettker P, et al. Financial impact of failing to prevent surgical site infections. Qual Manag Health Care 2007;16(3):219–25.
15. Amin S. Control charts 101: a guide to health care applications. Qual Manag Health Care 2001;9:1–27.
16. Institute of Health Care Delivery Research. Advanced training program. Available at: http://intermountainhealthcare.org/about/quality/institute/courses/atp/Pages/home.aspx. Accessed January 22, 2009.
17. Moen RD, Nolan TW, Provost LP. Quality improvement through planned experimentation. 2nd edition. New York: McGraw-Hill; 1999.
18. Weick K, Sutcliffe K, Obstfeld D. Organizing for high reliability: processes of collective mindfulness. Res Organ Behav 1999;21:81–123.
19. Luria J, Muething S, Schoettker P, et al. Reliability science and patient safety. Pediatr Clin North Am 2006;53(6):1121–33.

20. Gerhardt W, Schoettker P, Donovan E, et al. Putting evidence-based clinical practice guidelines into practice: an academic pediatric center's experience. Jt Comm J Qual Patient Saf 2007;33(4):226–35.
21. Muething S, Schoettker P, Gerhardt W, et al. Decreasing overuse of therapies in the treatment of bronchiolitis by incorporating evidence at the point of care. J Pediatr 2004;144(6):703–10.
22. Bigham M, Amato R, Bondurrant P, et al. Ventilator-associated pneumonia in the pediatric intensive care unit: characterizing the problem and implementing a sustainable solution. J Pediatr 2009;154:528–7.
23. The Joint Commission. Performance measurement initiatives. Children's Asthma Care (CAC) performance measure set. Available at: http://www.jointcommission.org/PerformanceMeasurement/PerformanceMeasurement/Childrens+Asthma+Care+(CAC)+Performance+Measure+Set.htm. Accessed January 28, 2009.
24. Agency for Healthcare Research and Quality. AHRQ quality indicators. Pediatric quality indicators overview. Available at: http://www.qualityindicators.ahrq.gov/pdi_overview.htm. Accessed January 29, 2009.
25. American Academy of Pediatrics Steering Committee on Quality Improvement and Management, American Academy of Pediatrics Committee on Practice and Ambulatory Medicine, Hodgson E, et al. Principles for the development and use of quality measures. Pediatrics 2008;121(2):411–8.
26. Alliance for Pediatric Quality. Measurably improving the quality of health care for America's children. Available at: http://www.kidsquality.org/. Accessed January 29, 2009.
27. National Association of Children's Hospitals and Related Institutions. A summary of N.A.C.H. recommendations to improve quality performance measurement in Medicaid and SCHIP. Available at: http://www.childrenshospitals.net/AM/Template.cfm?Section=Publications_Media&;Template=/CM/HTMLDisplay.cfm&ContentID=22422. Accessed January 29, 2009.

Implementing a Pediatric Rapid Response System to Improve Quality and Patient Safety

Kerry T. Van Voorhis, MD[a,*], Tina Schade Willis, MD[b,c]

KEYWORDS

- Rapid response team • Medical emergency team • Pediatrics
- Cardiac arrest • Emergency • Patient safety

Hospitals today are complex environments serving sicker patients than ever before. Patients who are not acutely ill are often managed as outpatients, leaving inpatient units to care for those with more severe conditions. According to the World Health Organization, the proportion of emergency admissions continues to rise in most countries,[1] while pressures to contain health care costs have resulted in shorter inpatient length of stay.[2] At the same time, recruiting and retaining trained nurses is increasingly difficult,[3] and physician work hours are trending downward.[4] The result is a more intricate inpatient milieu with proportionally fewer staff equipped to care for sicker patients who are more likely to experience life-threatening events, including cardiopulmonary arrest and unplanned admission to the intensive care unit (ICU).

Life-threatening events frequently arise in the hospital setting. Recent estimates suggest that 370,000 to 750,000 in-hospital resuscitation attempts are made every year in the United States.[5] The incidence of adult in-hospital cardiac arrest ranges from 1 to 5 events per 1000 hospital admissions,[5] while the incidence in children's hospitals is significantly lower at 0.19 to 2.45 events per 1000 admissions.[6] These events often result from preventable medical errors. Given the dismal survival rate of in-hospital cardiac arrest, it is critical to develop systems that recognize predictable clinical warning signs and intervene before patients reach the point of arrest.

[a] Division of General Pediatrics, Levine Children's Hospital at Carolinas Medical Center, P.O. Box 32861, Charlotte, NC 28232-2861, USA
[b] Division of Pediatric Critical Care Medicine, University of North Carolina at Chapel Hill, Suite 20160 Women's Hospital, 101 Manning Drive, Chapel Hill, NC 27599-7221, USA
[c] North Carolina Children's Center for Clinical Excellence, NC, USA
* Corresponding author. Division of General Pediatrics, Levine Children's Hospital, Carolinas Medical Center, P.O. Box 32861, Charlotte, NC 28232-2861.
E-mail address: kerry.vanvoorhis@carolinashealthcare.org (K.T. Van Voorhis).

Pediatr Clin N Am 56 (2009) 919–933
doi:10.1016/j.pcl.2009.05.017
pediatric.theclinics.com

MEDICAL ERROR AND ADVERSE EVENTS

A problem closely linked to the rising complexity of hospitals, and a factor in a significant proportion of life-threatening events, is medical error. In its 2000 report, *To Err is Human*, The Institute of Medicine concluded that between 44,000 and 98,000 patients die each year in US hospitals as a result of preventable clinical errors.[7] There are many terms used to describe inappropriate care and adverse outcomes experienced by patients. A list compiled by Andrews and colleagues[8] includes "adverse or untoward events, maloccurrences, complications, medical injuries, therapeutic misadventures, substandard care, unexpected outcomes, preventable deaths, iatrogenic injuries, mishaps, errors, negligence, and malpractice." Resar and colleagues[9] have defined medical error as "the failure of a planned action to be completed as intended or the use of a wrong plan to achieve an aim."

Estimates of the incidence of harm caused by medical error vary widely, depending on the research methodology and population studied. The Harvard Medical Practice Study, a retrospective chart review published in 1990, showed that 3.7% of more than 30,000 patient records from New York hospitals revealed an incident that two physicians agreed was adverse and caused serious harm.[10] Investigators in this study defined adverse events according to a legal-policy model, as their goal in measuring the event rate was to determine the feasibility of a no-fault system of compensation for medical malpractice.[8] Given the nature of the study, the authors only included errors that were clearly documented in the medical record. However, evidence from other studies suggests that fewer than 10% of adverse events are revealed in the medical record because documentation by hospital staff is often voluntary, time intensive, and perceived as potentially punitive.[11]

Other studies have demonstrated much higher rates of harm from medical error. For example, Steel and colleagues[12] found that an alarming 36% of 815 consecutive patients admitted to a general medical service at a university hospital had an iatrogenic illness, and 9% had an iatrogenic event that was life threatening or resulted in subsequent disability. This 1981 study reached the following conclusion: "Given the increasing number and complexity of diagnostic procedures and therapeutic agents, monitoring of untoward events is essential, and attention should be paid to educational efforts to reduce the risks of iatrogenic illness."

Rather than relying on medical records alone, Andrews and colleagues[8] searched for medical errors associated with 1047 adult surgical patients during inpatient rounds and case conferences. They reported that adverse events as a result of medical error occurred in 480 (46%) of the patients. Eighteen percent of patients experienced serious injury caused by medical error, with outcomes ranging from temporary physical disability to death. Patients who experienced adverse events stayed longer in the hospital (24 days versus 9 days for those without medical errors), and longer stays were associated with more medical errors. Adverse events were more likely to occur in patients with severe illness. Fifty-five percent of patients who required ICU care during their hospital stay experienced harm from medical error, compared with 38% of patients who did not spend time in the ICU.[8]

One or more causes of error were identified for just over half of the adverse events. Errors by an individual, such as poor technical performance, poor judgment, or failure to obtain or act on information contributed to 38% of the adverse events. Flawed interactions between individuals, such as failure of a consultant team to communicate adequately with the requesting team, were found to be responsible for 16% of the errors. About 10% of the errors were related generally to administrative decisions or protocols, such as inadequate staffing or defective equipment.[8]

Compared with adults, published estimates of adverse events in pediatric patients are few. Three studies using the "first-generation" methodology of the Harvard Medical Practice Study (nontargeted retrospective chart review) revealed similar low rates of adverse events in pediatric inpatients (2.3%, 2.9%, and 3.7%).[11] Studies using trigger tools, methods for increasing the efficiency of detection, have revealed higher rates of error. For example, in a 12-site children's hospital quality and safety collaborative study, Takata and Currier[13] reported a rate of 11.1 adverse drug events per 100 pediatric inpatients. Twenty-two percent of these errors were deemed preventable.

While post hoc analysis often links adverse events in the medical setting to "human error," many can be traced to a systems problem, defined by Bright and colleagues[2] as a sequence of events in the macro- and micro-environment that involve deficiencies in the structure and organization of health care. Cook and colleagues[14] point out that gaps in the continuity of care, such as the loss of information that occur at change of shift and transfer to a different facility, makes it more difficult to appreciate trends in a deteriorating patient's condition. Resolving systems problems and eliminating preventable medical errors is an important means of reducing adverse events, including cardiac arrest.

OUTCOMES FOR CARDIAC ARREST

Research over the past several decades has led to improved understanding of the epidemiology and pathophysiology of cardiac arrest in both adults and children. Corresponding advances in resuscitation, particularly coordinated strategies to strengthen the community chain of survival, have resulted in a marked improvement in outcomes for arrests that occur outside of the hospital setting.[15] Efforts by the American Heart Association and other groups have brought these advances to the public in effective ways. As a result, an increasing segment of the general public is equipped to react quickly to an unresponsive person outside the hospital setting. Peberdy and colleagues[15] point out that today one can find automated external defibrillators in schools, theaters, grocery stores, restaurants, shopping malls, airports, and many other public places. In addition to police and firefighters, many security officers, airline flight attendants, and trained laypersons are trained to use them while waiting for paramedics to arrive. In an effort to make the technical aspects of resuscitation easier to remember, elements of popular culture have been incorporated into education. The 1970s song "Staying Alive" by the Bee Gees is now immortalized as the proper tempo for chest compressions (100/minute). "Another One Bites the Dust" by Queen is a less hopeful but acceptable alternative. As a result of these developments, resuscitation in the prehospital setting is gradually moving closer to that in the hospital setting.

In contrast, procedures and outcomes for in-hospital resuscitation have remained relatively unchanged over the past 30 years.[5,16] In most hospitals, a "code team" responds to cardiac arrest in a general ward area. However, this approach has not been associated with a significant improvement in the mortality rate.[17] According to prospective data from 14,720 in-hospital cardiac arrests recorded by National Registry of Cardiopulmonary Resuscitation (NRCPR), fewer than half (44%) of adult in-hospital arrest victims had return of spontaneous circulation, and only 17% survived to hospital discharge. Pediatric patients (<18 years of age) in the study had a higher survival rate of 27%. Thirty-four percent of pediatric survivors had a poor neurologic function postarrest.[15,18] A 1999 meta-analysis of 554 in-hospital pediatric cardiac arrests demonstrated a similar survival rate of 24%. Twenty-two percent of survivors had poor neurologic function postarrest.[19]

For both children and adults in the NRCPR study, survival rates were higher when arrests occurred in monitored units and when the resuscitation team arrived quickly. Ninety-five percent of the pediatric arrests in the NRCPR study were either monitored or directly witnessed by a member of the health care team at the time of the event. In 86% of the 207 hospitals submitting data for the study, an organized emergency team responds 24 hours per day.[15]

Berg and colleagues[20] carefully analyzed the 880 pediatric arrests reported in the NRCPR study. Pediatric cardiac arrests occurred in the intensive care unit (ICU; 65%), emergency department (ED; 13%), general pediatric ward (14%), operating room (OR) or postanesthesia care unit (3%), diagnostic area (2%), and other/unknown location (2%). Immediate causes of pediatric cardiac arrests included acute respiratory insufficiency (57%), hypotension (61%), arrhythmia (49%), metabolic/electrolyte disturbance (12%), airway obstruction (5%), and acute pulmonary edema (4%). Many patients had more than one immediate cause.

WARNING SIGNS AND SYMPTOMS

Observations over the past two decades have changed the belief that most incidents of cardiopulmonary arrest are sudden and unpredictable. In fact, cardiopulmonary arrest is often preceded by up to several hours of warning signs and symptoms that predict subsequent deterioration. This pattern has been demonstrated repeatedly and reliably in a series of prospective studies of adult patients who experience cardiac arrest on a general inpatient ward. In each of the studies listed in **Table 1**, patients who arrested in other locations (ED, OR, ICU) and those who had "do not resuscitate"

Table 1
Landmark adult studies demonstrating clinical antecedents to cardiac arrest

Publication	Major Findings
Sax 1987	95% (19 of 20) had acute clinical instability and/or high burden of baseline comorbidities
Schein 1990	84% (54 of 64) had new complaints or clinical deterioration within 8 hours of arrest 70% had abnormal respiratory or neurologic function; 25% had both No consistent laboratory findings were found before arrest 77% had underlying diseases not expected to cause death during hospitalization
Franklin 1994	66% (99 of 150) had documented clinical deterioration within 6 hours of arrest Former ICU patients had significantly higher risk of arrest compared with patients never in the ICU (14.7 versus 6.8 per 1000 admissions) Failures: notifying physician, obtaining/interpreting labs, ICU triage, stabilization on floor
Hodgetts 2002	68% (80 of 118) had documented clinical deterioration before arrest 100% of patients with potentially avoidable arrests received inadequate pre-arrest treatment Avoidable arrests five times more likely for patients on general wards than in ICU
Hillman 2002	70% (386 of 551) had serious antecedents within 8 hours of urgent transfer to ICU Most commonly: tachycardia, hypotension, tachypnea, sudden change in mental status

(DNR) orders were excluded. Each study builds on the findings of its predecessors, resulting in a clear pattern of events that typically precede in-hospital cardiac arrest.

Franklin and Mathew[21] investigated nurse and physician responses to the pre-arrest decline of 150 adult inpatients. In 99 (66%) of 150 patients, a nurse or physician documented deterioration in the patient's condition within 6 hours of arrest. Of the 51 arrests that could not be anticipated, 2 were in-hospital suicides and 4 occurred in association with medical procedures. Several pitfalls were appreciated in the 99 potentially predictable arrests. In 25 cases, a nurse documented deterioration but failed to notify a physician. In 42 cases, the ward physician was notified but failed to alert the ICU physician. With another group of patients, the ward physician failed to obtain (30 cases) or respond to an abnormal arterial blood gas (8 cases) in the setting of respiratory distress and/or altered mental status. ICU triage error was noted in 32 cases, most of which involved failure of the ICU physician to stabilize the patient before transfer to the ICU. The authors concluded that strategies to prevent cardiac arrest should include training for nurses and physicians that concentrates on cardiopulmonary stabilization and how to respond to neurologic and respiratory deterioration.[21]

Hodgetts and colleagues[22] reviewed records from 32,348 consecutive adult admissions over a 1-year period and found 118 in-hospital cardiac arrests that prompted code team involvement. An expert panel reviewed each case and unanimously agreed that 68% of in-hospital arrests were potentially avoidable. Cardiac arrests were more likely to occur on weekends than weekdays. The odds of potentially avoidable cardiac arrest were five times greater for patients on general wards than critical care areas, and patients who arrested in critical care areas were more likely to survive. The odds of a potentially avoidable cardiac arrest was 12.6 times greater for patients in a clinical area judged "inappropriate" for their main complaint, compared with those in "appropriate" areas. The panel agreed that 100% of potentially avoidable arrests were judged to have received inadequate treatment before arrest. The authors noted several common errors including delays and errors in diagnosis, inadequate interpretation of test results, incomplete treatment, inexperienced physicians, and management in inappropriate clinical areas.

Hillman and colleagues[23] studied the characteristics and incidence of serious abnormalities in 551 adult patients before unplanned ICU admission. They found that patients transferred urgently to ICU from the general ward were more severely ill, had longer ICU stays, and higher mortality (47.6% mortality) than those admitted from the ED (31.5%) and OR (19%). Seventy percent of ward patients had serious documented antecedents during the 8 hours before transfer, most commonly including hypotension, tachycardia, tachypnea, and/or sudden change in level of consciousness.

A prospective study of 6300 hospitalized adults by Buist et al.[17] further clarified a set of abnormal antecedent clinical parameters with a high predictive value for subsequent cardiac arrest. These included a decrease in Glasgow Coma Score by two points, onset of coma, hypotension (<90 mm Hg), respiratory rate less than 6/minute, hypoxia (oxygen saturation <90%, on or off oxygen therapy), and bradycardia higher than 30/minute. The presence of any of these six factors was associated with a 6.8-fold increase in the risk of in-hospital mortality. Risk of mortality was higher for patients with multiple abnormalities (88% risk with four) compared with a single factor (16% risk). The authors recommended that these criteria be used for activating a rescue response before further deterioration.

These and other studies[24,25] clearly demonstrate that most adult patients who suffer cardiac arrest on the general inpatient floor exhibit antecedent abnormal signs and symptoms. Prospective studies documenting the reliable presence of similar patterns in children are lacking. While some hospitalized children may suffer sudden and unexpected cardiac arrests from acute arrhythmia, airway obstruction, seizure, or other events, the more common pattern is thought to be a gradual progression of hypoxemia and hemodynamic instability.[6] "Vital signs" have earned that distinction for good reason.

The limitation of these studies, and resulting challenge for hospital personnel, is the absence of a reliable denominator (ie, how many patients exhibiting abnormal signs and symptoms did *not* suffer cardiac arrest). No doubt, the denominator is very large. For example, Buist and colleagues[17] found that serious clinical abnormalities resolved spontaneously in 67% of patients. However, given universally poor outcomes for in-hospital cardiac arrest, the need to respond urgently to patients with serious abnormalities is compelling, prompting the Institute for Healthcare Improvement and others to call for the implementation of rapid response systems to recognize and respond to deteriorating hospitalized patients of all ages to prevent cardiac arrest.

There are multiple single institution studies in adult populations showing statistically significant decreases in cardiac arrest and mortality rates after the development of a rapid response system.[26] However, the only multicenter cluster randomized control study examining the effects of a rapid response system on cardiac arrests and mortality in adult populations showed no significant differences between groups, although both control and intervention institutions experienced significant improvements in cardiac arrest rates at the end of the study period.[27] There are few published studies examining rapid response systems in single pediatric institutions and no multicenter studies in a pediatric population. Despite the paucity of published studies, several pediatric studies report significant decreases in cardiac and/or respiratory arrest rates[28–32] and one study reports a significant decrease in hospital-wide mortality rates.[31]

OUTCOME MEASURES OF PEDIATRIC RAPID RESPONSE SYSTEMS

As rapid response systems are implemented and sustained with specific outcomes in mind, process and outcome measures must be followed to detect changes at the institution level as well as provide a framework for benchmarking. In 2007, the International Liaison Committee on Resuscitation (ILCOR) published "recommended guidelines for monitoring, reporting, and conducting research on medical emergency team, outreach, and rapid response systems: an Utstein-style scientific statement."[33] In addition to patient and hospital demographics, peri-event data, and universal nomenclature, there are specific recommendations for patient and hospital outcomes data reporting. According to their recommendations, hospital outcomes should include total acute care discharges whether alive or dead, hospital deaths, DNR deaths, number of emergency team activations, total number of in-hospital cardiac arrests, and cardiac arrests occurring in non-ICU, operating room, or emergency departments.

Although most of the adult literature has used similar outcomes in published studies, there remain many differences in the definitions of reported outcomes in published studies of pediatric rapid response systems (**Table 2**). These differences make it difficult to assess and compare the small number of pediatric rapid response system studies in the literature. For example, Tibballs and colleagues[28] and Hanson and colleagues,[32] like in adult studies, report cardiac arrests as one of their main outcome variables. Brilli and colleagues[29] and Sharek and colleagues[31] use the term "code" to include respiratory and cardiac arrests and Hunt and colleagues[30] report both "cardiopulmonary" and "respiratory" arrests. In addition, these outcomes are indexed differently in pediatric

Table 2
Clinical outcomes for pediatric rapid response systems

Publication	Institution	Statistically Significant Outcomes
Tibballs 2005	Royal Children's Hosp. Melbourne, Australia	No significant decrease in total cardiac arrest or mortality rates except in those deaths and cardiac arrests the transgressed MET criteria: Decrease in mortality 0.11 → 0 per 1000 admissions Decrease in Cardiac Arrests 0.16 → 0 per 1000 admissions
Brilli 2007	Cincinnati Children's Hospital; Cincinnati	Decrease in Non-ICU codes 1.54 → 0.62 per 1000 admissions 0.27 → 0.11 per 1000 patient days
Sharek 2007	Lucile Packard Children's Hospital; Stanford University	Decrease in non-ICU codes: 2.45 → 0.69 per 1000 discharges 0.52 → 0.15 per 1000 patient days
Hunt 2008	Johns Hopkins Hospital Baltimore, Maryland	No significant change in cardiopulmonary arrests Decrease in respiratory arrest: 1.46 → 0.40 per 1000 discharges 0.23 → 0.06 per 1000 patient days
Hanson 2008 (*In press*)	North Carolina Children's Hospital, Chapel Hill	Increase in mean time interval between non-ICU cardiac arrests: 2512 → 9418 patient days between cardiac arrests Decrease in median duration of clinical instability before ICU assessment: 9 h 55 m → 4 h 15 m

studies with many reporting arrest events per 1000 patient days instead of or in addition to 1000 admissions/discharges. Although patient days likely offer a more accurate measure of effect on the patient population, it is not standardized for reporting in the literature. Effects on wards mortality before and after rapid response system development were reported by Brilli and colleagues,[29] Hunt and colleagues,[30] and Tibballs and colleagues,[28] whereas Sharek and colleagues[31] and Hanson and colleagues[32] focused on hospital-wide mortality rates. It is clear that pediatric institutions need further recommendations for standardized measures of rapid response systems. One immediate solution would be to follow the ILCOR recommendations for data reporting for all rapid response systems including those in pediatric populations.

IMPLEMENTATION OF A SUCCESSFUL RAPID RESPONSE SYSTEM

According to the Medical Emergency Team Consensus Conference, successful rapid response systems include four necessary components: (1) an afferent limb, (2) an efferent limb, (3) an evaluative/process improvement limb, and (4) an administrative limb.[34] The afferent limb is defined as the component of the emergency response system that is able to detect an event and trigger a response. The efferent limb provides a crisis response including resources such as a medical emergency team (MET) or rapid response team (RRT) and equipment. The evaluative/process improvement component exists to improve patient care and safety. Finally, the administrative limb exists to implement and sustain the service. To highlight the process of developing a pediatric rapid response system and measuring its effects on patient safety, we share case examples that describe our experiences at the North Carolina Children's Hospital at the University of North Carolina-Chapel Hill and Levine Children's Hospital in Charlotte, North Carolina.

CASE EXAMPLE: UNIVERSITY OF NORTH CAROLINA-CHAPEL HILL

An institution-wide pediatric rapid response system (PRRS) has been active at North Carolina Children's Hospital since August 2005. Antecedents described in the adult literature along with pattern antecedents identified in detailed institution-specific chart reviews were used to establish the criteria for activation of the RRT. Calling criteria were designed without numeric vital sign parameters to be highly sensitive for pre–cardiac arrest states. The criteria for activation are displayed in poster format throughout the hospital. The PRRS includes all four consensus conference components.

The afferent limb relies on human assessment and interpretation of monitoring to detect an event and activate the RRT. The primary system change is the empowerment of any member of the hospital staff or family member to activate the RRT. The RRT is activated though both a pager call to team members and a public announcement. A public announcement is used not only to notify the RRT members but also the primary team to assist in the decision-making process and foster acceptance of the team to other hospital staff.

The efferent limb, or RRT, includes a pediatric critical care fellow or attending, a senior resident, a critical care charge nurse, and a pediatric respiratory therapist. The primary team for the patient is also expected to be present and participate as members of the RRT. The RRT has all of the following competencies: (1) ability to prescribe therapy; (2) advanced airway management; (3) capability to establish central venous access; and (4) ability to begin ICU level of care at the bedside.[34] The team responds to all areas excluding the neonatal and pediatric intensive care units. This includes clinics within the hospital building, adult patient areas where pediatric visitors may be present, inpatient wards, burn unit, bone marrow transplant unit, radiology, or any other physical space within the institution walls.

On arrival to the patient's bedside, the RRT provides immediate medical evaluation and treatment as required. The team then communicates further treatment plans to the patient's primary medical team and family. The team is trained to perform a debriefing with immediate feedback to the resident physicians and nurses regarding recognition of clinical deterioration and strategies for improvement. The RRT members are instructed to adopt a supportive attitude and not to make negative comments. An RRT activation form is completed by the pediatric critical care physician and then collected for performance improvement.

The administrative and process improvement limbs are necessary for implementing and sustaining the system. Before implementation, a 4-month period of educational sessions for all medical staff including physicians, nurses, respiratory therapists, chaplains, security, and communications staff was completed. During these sessions, criteria for activation of the RRT were reviewed, illustrative cases discussed, and concerns and questions addressed.

Once education was complete, the system changes were initiated without a run-in period. From that time onward the rapid response system has been evaluated by prospectively collected data recorded on RRT activation forms and existing performance improvement database information. The administrative committee meets monthly to review the data collected and discuss individual cases that prompted additional safety concerns. Further root cause analyses are performed as needed to address these safety concerns. As a result, several changes to the system have been made to further decrease variation in response and improve safety. For example, a new policy preventing the cancellation of a "code blue" or RRT call was implemented to reinforce the concept that there are no false alarms. In addition, the pediatric ICU staff began activating the RRT for urgent consults when it was identified that the team was not being used fully. Individual cases are discussed formally at a monthly resident conference to reinforce management and resuscitation of the critically ill pediatric patient.

As a result of the PRRS, the mean time interval between cardiac arrests increased significantly from a baseline of 2512 to 9418 days, indicating a significant decrease in non-ICU cardiac arrests. In addition, median duration of predefined clinical instability before assessment by ICU personnel decreased from 9 hours 55 minutes to 4 hours 15 minutes postintervention ($P = .028$).[32] The duration of clinical instability significantly decreased for unplanned ICU admissions whether assessed by the RRT or not, indicating that implementation of a PRRS resulted in a hospital-wide culture change favoring early assessment by critical care personnel. This culture change is likely the most important aspect of rapid response systems leading to early recognition and treatment of clinical deterioration. One recent study similarly found that DNR orders and delayed MET activation are the strongest independent predictors of mortality in patients receiving a Medical Emergency Team review. The investigators stressed that avoidance of delayed MET activation should be a priority for hospitals operating rapid response systems.[35]

CASE EXAMPLE: LEVINE CHILDREN'S HOSPITAL

An institution-wide Pediatric Early Response Team (PERT) was initiated at Levine Children's Hospital (LCH) in 2004, and has evolved considerably since then. The initial afferent system for identifying a deteriorating patient used evidence-based criteria for airway, breathing, circulatory, and neurologic concerns, but activating the efferent response was inefficient and cumbersome. The nurse typically paged the inpatient physician and charge nurse and waited for recommendations or "permission" to have the ICU team evaluate the patient. In spring 2007, a multidisciplinary task force including representatives from critical care, inpatient general pediatrics, nursing, respiratory care, and risk management began a collaboration to enhance the system by adopting the latest evidence-based strategies. LCH adopted the simple age-neutral activation criteria listed in **Box 1**.

The revised system empowers concerned staff members to activate PERT by calling the hospital paging operator. A group text page immediately informs PERT members, including a pediatric hospitalist, supervising resident physician, critical care charge nurse, and pediatric respiratory therapist. Each PERT member has authority to implement a wide range of standing orders shown in **Box 2**, including transfer to a higher level of care. After the patient has been stabilized, a brief record is completed to document which staff member initiated the call, reason for the call, assessment and intervention measures, and outcomes. In addition, the patient's bedside nurse completes a feedback tool to record response time; quality of communication between the PERT members, primary inpatient team, nursing staff, and patient/family; and suggestions for improvement. Staff members initiate PERT are acknowledged for their commitment to patient safety by a personalized letter from the chief nursing officer and chief medical officer. There are no "false alarms."

Box 1
Pediatric Early ResponseTeam activation criteria at Levine Children's Hospital

Acute change in HR, BP, RR, O2 Sat

Acute change in mental status

Pain or agitation that is difficult to control

New or prolonged seizure

Staff member is worried about a patient

PERT calls at LCH increased significantly since implementation of the direct activation mechanism in May 2007. The average number of PERT events per 1000 discharges was 1.37 during the 12 months before implementation, compared with 8.42 during the 18 months after implementation. There were 80 PERT events between July 1, 2006, and December 31, 2008. PERT was predominantly activated by the patient's bedside nurse (84%), and occasionally by the physician (9%), charge nurse (5%), or respiratory therapist (2.5%). Activation triggers included acute changes in heart rate (22%), blood pressure (7.5%), respiratory rate (41%), hypoxia (35%), mental status (25%), and other/staff concern (68%). More than one reason for calling PERT was frequently documented. PERT arrival occurred within 5 minutes of the call in 95% of cases, and within 10 minutes in all remaining cases. Assessments and interventions provided by PERT are documented in **Table 3**.

PERT intervention was typically brief, lasting less than 30 minutes in 86% (69/80) of cases. Nine cases lasted 30 to 60 minutes, and two cases lasted 60 to 90 minutes.

Box 2
Standing orders for Pediatric Early ResponseTeam at Levine Children's Hospital

Patient weight: —— kg

Obtain HR, BP, RR, O2 saturation and continue to monitor

Assess Airway Breathing status

Assess Circulatory status

Obtain situation and background information from bedside nurse

—— Oxygen to keep saturations above 92% or for respiratory distress

—— Albuterol 2.5 mg neb (or 2 puffs MDI), repeat × 3 doses PRN wheezing/respiratory distress

—— Epinephrine 2.25% (Racemic Epi) 0.5 mL dilutes to 3 mL nebulized × 1 dose PRN stridor

—— Obtain blood glucose. If below 40, give D25% 2 mL/kg IV × 1 dose.

—— Initiate IV access based on patient condition

—— Normal Saline 20 mL/kg IV × 1 dose based on patient condition

—— Narcan 0.1 mg/kg IV for known narcotic administration with altered mental status/resp depression. May repeat × 1 dose (max dose 2 mg)

—— Transfer to PICU based on patient condition; PICU attending notified: Dr. ——————

—— Notify primary attending/service of patient's condition: Dr. ——————

Table 3
Assessment and intervention by Pediatric Emergency ResponseTeam at Levine Children's Hospital (n = 80)

Intervention	Number of Cases (%)
Airway suctioning	23 (29%)
Supplemental oxygen	47 (59%)
Bag-valve mask ventilation	15 (19%)
Oral/nasal airway	5 (6%)
Beta-agonist inhalation	2 (2.5%)
Racemic epinephrine inhalation	5 (6%)
Chest x-ray	8 (10%)
IV placement	11 (14%)
IV fluid bolus	17 (21%)
Naloxone (Narcan)	2 (2.5%)
Blood glucose measurement	16 (20%)
Dextrose administration (D25 IV)	3 (4%)
Other medications given	17 (21%)
No intervention necessary	6 (7.5%)

Education to initiate ICU transfer for interventions lasting more than 30 minutes was subsequently provided. Following PERT intervention, 56% (45/80) of patients remained on the general or progressive floor, whereas 39% (31/80) were transferred to the ICU, including three cases where the patient required resuscitation for cardiac arrest on the general ward. Four patients requiring PERT intervention were admitted to the hospital from an outpatient area such as radiology or dialysis following the event.

Levine Children's Hospital opened in December 2007, 6 months after implementation of the revised PERT system. Despite a 10% increase in inpatient volume in 2008 compared with 2007, the mean rate of non-ICU codes (defined at LCH as either cardiac or respiratory arrest) decreased to 1.5 per 1000 discharges. The rate of codes outside the ICU had previously been approximately four cases per 1000 discharges. Interestingly, there were zero non-ICU codes during the period of intense education about upcoming changes to PERT. Since the PERT revision, the rate of non-ICU codes has remained below 2.25 per 1000 discharges, even during periods when total pediatric codes (ICU + non-ICU) exceeded 10 per 1000 discharges.

IMPLEMENTATION OF FAMILY ACTIVATION

At Levine Children's Hospital, family members are encouraged to immediately notify a staff member when they are concerned about their child. The NC Children's Hospital used a similar approach initially. During the first year after implementation of the PRRS at NC Children's Hospital, "family concern" was one of the reasons for activation in 8% of the calls. More than half of those patients required transfer to the ICU, demonstrating that the calls were appropriate and necessary. In the spring of 2007, after piloting the system in two units, family activation was introduced throughout the institution, allowing families to directly activate the RRT using the same system as the hospital staff without a triage step.[36] Researchers at the University of Pittsburgh Medical Center recently described their patient and family activation system. At their institution, a call by a family member results in the activation of a special Condition HELP team (a physician, a nursing supervisor, and a patient advocate) who evaluates whether to elevate the situation and activate a rapid response emergency team, called Condition A (cardiopulmonary arrest) or Condition C (a crisis that might result in imminent arrest).[37]

The 2009 National Patient Safety Goals have identified partnership with patients and families as "an important characteristic of a culture of safety" and according to the Institute for Family-Centered Care, the core concepts of patient- and family-centered care are dignity and respect, information sharing, participation, and collaboration.[38,39] These goals are even more important in pediatrics, where patients are reliant on parents and caregivers for most of their needs.

At NC Children's Hospital, members of the medical staff feared that family activation would result in numerous calls for nonemergent situations as well as calls that would be better routed to patient relations representatives. Focus groups, open communication, and finally a pilot of family activation on two units of the institution reassured the medical staff and families that the introduction of family activation would not disrupt or overwhelm the existing rapid response system. The rule of "no false alarms" helps all staff understand that any serious concern of a family member or a member of the child's medical team is valid cause for activating the system.

At the time of admission, all patients and families are educated about the RRT by their nurse. If families are not educated at the time of admission, several educational tools are available to ensure that families are fully equipped to activate the RRT. The key elements of the family activation and education include staff education and mock scripts, bilingual flyers in visitor areas and waiting rooms, electronic chart education reminders for nurses, and large colorful bilingual posters in each patient room. The posters serve as a both a reminder of the number to call and a prompt for nurses to provide education at the time of admission. A tear-off card mechanism for activation by non–English-speaking families is available next to the poster in every room.

Audits and interviews with families to assess their understanding of the RRT in their own words are conducted routinely, with feedback provided to the unit staff. Through audits, it has been discovered that the poster alone is not sufficient education for families. In fact, many families have never read the information unless their nurse mentioned it at the time of admission. Without the poster, however, it may be difficult to remember the phone number to call to activate the team. In addition to the other tools, information about the RRT is included in the hospital guide that is provided to families at the time of admission.

Since the introduction of family activation, the mean number of RRT calls has increased significantly from 16 to 24 calls per 1000 discharges (Willis, unpublished data, 2009). The number of rapid response calls made directly by a family member is very low—only two calls during the first year of implementation. Many staff members have indicated that families prefer to have a medical professional call on their behalf. Despite this fact, family concern continues to be recorded as a reason for activation in 6% of all calls. Efforts to provide education to patients and families about rapid response systems serve not only to help them summon care in a time of need, but also to move toward a hospital-wide culture of recognizing families as critical members of the medical team.

USE OF RAPID RESPONSE SYSTEM FOR QUALITY IMPROVEMENT

There are many reported benefits of rapid response systems beyond a reduction in cardiac arrest and mortality rates. These include improved staff satisfaction and safety culture, improved nursing documentation, earlier palliative care, and improved education for physician trainees.[26,40–43] In addition, rapid response and medical emergency team activations can be used for detection of medical errors and system safety issues. In fact, at one institution, more than 30% of RRT activation reviews detected a medical error, and a focus on standardization of hospital processes was completed to improve hospital-wide safety.[44] These processes included standardized protocols for hypoglycemia and transfer of patients. Standardized protocols can also be used by RRTs to improve care of sepsis patients.[45] RRT activations can easily be incorporated into existing morbidity and mortality reviews and used as a trigger tool for system reviews and further improvement in hospital processes.

SUMMARY

Life-threatening events are common in today's complex hospital environment, where an increasing proportion of patients with urgent admission for severe illness are cared for by understaffed, often inexperienced personnel. Medical errors play a key role in causing adverse events and failure to rescue deteriorating patients. Outcomes for in-hospital cardiac arrest in both adults and children are generally poor, but these events are often preceded by a pattern of deterioration with abnormal vital signs and mental status. Fortunately, when hospital staff or a family member observes warning signs and triggers timely intervention by a rapid response team, rates of cardiac arrest and mortality can be reduced. Moreover, rapid response team involvement can be used to trigger careful review of preceding events to help uncover important systems issues and allow for further improvements in patient safety.

REFERENCES

1. World Health Organization report: emergency medical services. 2008.
2. Bright D, Walker W, Bion J. Clinical review: outreach—a strategy for improving the care of the acutely ill hospitalized patient. Crit Care 2004;8(1):33–40.
3. Buchan J. Global nursing shortages. BMJ 2002;324(7340):751–2.
4. Philibert I, Friedmann P, Williams WT, et al. New requirements for resident duty hours. JAMA 2002;288(9):1112–4.
5. Sandroni C, Nolan J, Cavallaro F, et al. In-hospital cardiac arrest: incidence, prognosis and possible measures to improve survival. Intensive Care Med 2007;33(2): 237–45.
6. Tibballs J, van der Jagt EW. Medical emergency and rapid response teams. Pediatr Clin North Am 2008;55(4):989–1010.
7. Kohn LT, Corrigan JM, Donaldson MS. To err is human: building a safer health system. 1999.
8. Andrews LB, Stocking C, Krizek T, et al. An alternative strategy for studying adverse events in medical care. Lancet 1997;349(9048):309–13.
9. Resar RK, Rozich JD, Classen D. Methodology and rationale for the measurement of harm with trigger tools. Qual Saf Health Care 2003;12(Suppl 2):ii39–45.
10. Harvard Medical Practice Study. Patients, doctors and lawyers and medical injury, malpractice litigation, and patient compensation in New York. 1990.
11. Sharek PJ, Classen D. The incidence of adverse events and medical error in pediatrics. Pediatr Clin North Am 2006;53(6):1067–77.
12. Steel K, Gertman PM, Crescenzi C, et al. Iatrogenic illness on a general medical service at a university hospital. N Engl J Med 1981;304(11):638–42.

13. Takata G, Currier K. Enhancing patient safety through improved detection of adverse drug events.
14. Cook RI, Render M, Woods DD. Gaps in the continuity of care and progress on patient safety. BMJ 2000;320(7237):791–4.
15. Peberdy MA, Kaye W, Ornato JP, et al. Cardiopulmonary resuscitation of adults in the hospital: a report of 14720 cardiac arrests from the National Registry of Cardiopulmonary Resuscitation. Resuscitation 2003;58(3):297–308.
16. Ballew K, Philbrick J. Causes of variation in reported in-hospital CPR survival: a critical review. Resuscitation 1995;30:203–15.
17. Buist M, Bernard S, Nguyen TV, et al. Association between clinically abnormal observations and subsequent in-hospital mortality: a prospective study. Resuscitation 2004;62(2):137–41.
18. Nadkarni VM, Larkin GL, Peberdy MA, et al. First documented rhythm and clinical outcome from in-hospital cardiac arrest among children and adults. JAMA 2006; 295(1):50–7.
19. Young KD, Seidel JS. Pediatric cardiopulmonary resuscitation: a collective review. Ann Emerg Med 1999;33(2):195–205.
20. Berg MD, Nadkarni VM, Zuercher M, et al. In-hospital pediatric cardiac arrest. Pediatr Clin North Am 2008;55(3):589–604, x.
21. Franklin C, Mathew J. Developing strategies to prevent inhospital cardiac arrest: analyzing responses of physicians and nurses in the hours before the event. Crit Care Med 1994;22(2):244–7.
22. Hodgetts TJ, Kenward G, Vlackonikolis I, et al. Incidence, location and reasons for avoidable in-hospital cardiac arrest in a district general hospital. Resuscitation 2002;54(2):115–23.
23. Hillman KM, Bristow PJ, Chey T, et al. Duration of life-threatening antecedents prior to intensive care admission. Intensive Care Med 2002;28(11):1629–34.
24. Kause J, Smith G, Prytherch D, et al. A comparison of antecedents to cardiac arrests, deaths and emergency intensive care admissions in Australia and New Zealand, and the United Kingdom–the ACADEMIA study antecedents to hospital deaths clinical antecedents to in-hospital cardiopulmonary arrest. Resuscitation 2004;62(3):275–82.
25. Nurmi J, Harjola VP, Nolan J, et al. Observations and warning signs prior to cardiac arrest. Should a medical emergency team intervene earlier? Acta Anaesthesiol Scand 2005;49(5):702–6.
26. Barbetti J, Lee G. Medical emergency team: a review of the literature. Nurs Crit Care 2008;13(2):80–5.
27. Hillman K, Chen J, Cretikos M, et al. Introduction of the medical emergency team (MET) system: a cluster-randomised controlled trial. Lancet 2005;365(9477): 2091–7.
28. Tibballs J, Kinney S, Duke T, et al. Reduction of paediatric in-patient cardiac arrest and death with a medical emergency team: preliminary results. Arch Dis Child 2005;90(11):1148–52.
29. Brilli RJ, Gibson R, Luria JW, et al. Implementation of a medical emergency team in a large pediatric teaching hospital prevents respiratory and cardiopulmonary arrests outside the intensive care unit. Pediatr Crit Care Med 2007;8(3):236–46 [quiz: 247].
30. Hunt EA, Zimmer KP, Rinke ML, et al. Transition from a traditional code team to a medical emergency team and categorization of cardiopulmonary arrests in a children's center. Arch Pediatr Adolesc Med 2008;162(2):117–22.

31. Sharek PJ, Parast LM, Leong K, et al. Effect of a rapid response team on hospital-wide mortality and code rates outside the ICU in a children's hospital. JAMA 2007;298(19):2267–74.
32. Hanson C, Randolph GD, Erickson J, et al. A reduction in cardiac arrests and duration of clinical instability after implementation of a pediatric rapid response system. Qual Saf Health Care, in press.
33. Peberdy MA, Cretikos M, Abella BS, et al. Recommended guidelines for monitoring, reporting, and conducting research on medical emergency team, outreach, and rapid response systems: an Utstein-style scientific statement: a scientific statement from the International Liaison Committee on Resuscitation (American Heart Association, Australian Resuscitation Council, European Resuscitation Council, Heart and Stroke Foundation of Canada, InterAmerican Heart Foundation, Resuscitation Council of Southern Africa, and the New Zealand Resuscitation Council); the American Heart Association Emergency Cardiovascular Care Committee; the Council on Cardiopulmonary, Perioperative, and Critical Care; and the Interdisciplinary Working Group on Quality of Care and Outcomes Research. Circulation 2007;116(21):2481–500.
34. Devita MA, Bellomo R, Hillman K, et al. Findings of the first consensus conference on medical emergency teams. Crit Care Med 2006;34(9):2463–78.
35. Calzavacca P, Licari E, Tee A, et al. A prospective study of factors influencing the outcome of patients after a Medical Emergency Team review. Intensive Care Med 2008;34(11):2112–6.
36. Patient safety alert. Initiative gives families access to rapid response team. Healthcare Benchmarks Qual Improv 2008;15(1 Suppl):1–2.
37. Dean BS, Decker MJ, Hupp D, et al. Condition HELP: a pediatric rapid response team triggered by patients and parents. J Healthc Qual 2008;30(3):28–31.
38. The Joint Commission. 2009 National Patient Safety Goals.
39. FAQ. 2008; 2008 August, 21.
40. Santiano N, Young L, Hillman K, et al. Analysis of Medical Emergency Team calls comparing subjective to "objective" call criteria. Resuscitation 2009;80(1):44–9.
41. Chen J, Flabouris A, Bellomo R, et al. The Medical Emergency Team System and not-for-resuscitation orders: results from the MERIT study. Resuscitation 2008; 79(3):391–7.
42. Chen J, Hillman K, Bellomo R, et al. The impact of introducing medical emergency team system on the documentations of vital signs. Resuscitation 2009;80(1):35–43.
43. Jacques T, Harrison GA, McLaws ML. Attitudes towards and evaluation of medical emergency teams: a survey of trainees in intensive care medicine. Anaesth Intensive Care 2008;36(1):90–5.
44. Braithwaite RS, DeVita MA, Mahidhara R, et al. Use of medical emergency team (MET) responses to detect medical errors. Qual Saf Health Care 2004;13(4): 255–9.
45. Sarani B, Brenner SR, Gabel B, et al. Improving sepsis care through systems change: the impact of a medical emergency team. Jt Comm J Qual Patient Saf 2008;34(3):179–82, 125.

Quality Improvement and Patient Safety in the Pediatric Ambulatory Setting: Current Knowledge and Implications for ResidencyTraining

Daniel R. Neuspiel, MD, MPH[a,*], Daniel Hyman, MD, MMM[b], Mariellen Lane, MD[c]

KEYWORDS

• Quality • Safety • Ambulatory • Residency training • Pediatrics

The pediatric outpatient environment varies greatly in setting, population served, the presence of trainees, and the types of providers caring for patients. There is also great variability in the quality and effectiveness of care across and within various pediatric ambulatory settings. The knowledge of the extent of this variability is fairly limited, although it is increasing coincident with more attention to quality and the expanded number of measures used by various agencies and entities. The outpatient environment has been the leading edge of improvement work in pediatrics and it has similarly served as an effective locale for the training of pediatric residents in the science of improvement.

This review summarizes what is known about the measurement of quality and patient safety in pediatric ambulatory settings. The current Accreditation Council for Graduate Medical Education (ACGME) requirements for resident training in improvement and their application in these settings are discussed. Some approaches and challenges to meeting these requirements are reviewed. Finally, some future directions that this work may follow are presented; the goal is to strengthen the effectiveness of improvement methods and their linkage to professional education.

[a] Division of General Pediatrics, Levine Children's Hospital of Carolinas Medical Center, PO BOX 32861, Charlotte, NC 28232-2861, USA
[b] The Children's Hospital, Denver, 13123 East 16th Avenue Box 080, Aurora, CO 80045, USA
[c] Morgan Stanley Children's Hospital of New York-Presbyterian, New York, NY, USA
* Corresponding author.
E-mail address: Daniel.neuspeil@carolinashealthcare.org (D.R. Neuspiel).

Pediatr Clin N Am 56 (2009) 935–951
doi:10.1016/j.pcl.2009.05.011
0031-3955/09/$ – see front matter

QUALITY IN THE AMBULATORY ENVIRONMENT: WHAT IS KNOWN?

Measurement of quality in ambulatory environments has evolved over the past 15 years since the introduction of the Healthcare Effectiveness Data and Information Set (HEDIS) (see http://www.ncqa.org/tabid/29/Default.aspx) by the National Committee for Quality Assurance in 1993.[1] HEDIS provides measurement of the quality of care, primarily in ambulatory settings, and offers comparative performance data between different health plans. Since the introduction of HEDIS, quality measurement has been promoted and implemented by numerous other stakeholders and national organizations to provide information about health providers, ostensibly to inform decision-making by consumers. Although profiling with HEDIS may not be valid for comparison between providers,[2] these measures are frequently of great benefit for the purpose of quality improvement across ambulatory practices.

The American Academy of Pediatrics (AAP) recently published a review of measurement of quality in pediatric settings.[3] The AAP defines appropriate measures by the following criteria:

1. Measures should address issues that are significant for children's health, by severity, prevalence or functional status, and should have the potential to influence improvement.
2. Measures should be scientifically valid and must be found to be reliable after a period of "field testing."
3. Measures should be feasible to collect.

The AAP has endorsed similar recommendations for the "measure" definition outlined by the American Academy of Family Physicians, particularly with respect to measures for use in pay for performance programs. These recommendations reflect support for the patient–physician relationship, and seek to link all measures to clinical guidelines or other evidence-based medicine principles.[4]

The child health field has not received the degree of attention and focus on measurement or pay for performance from government, payers, and other health care stakeholders as adult medicine. While Medicare has, in recent years, introduced an incentive payment system for outpatient providers called "Physician Quality Reporting Initiative" (PQRI) (see http://www.cms.hhs.gov/pqri/), Medicaid has no such national program, although some states have implemented local programs to provide incentives for quality performance. In 2003, a study found that children covered by Medicaid were less likely to be fully immunized (69% versus 54%); less likely to have received recommended well-child visits in the first 15 months of life, (53% versus 31%); and far more likely to undergo myringotomy tubes (35 versus two per 1000 members), compared with children on commercial health insurance.[5]

In contrast with adult care, most pediatric quality measurement has focused on the ambulatory environment. Pediatric HEDIS measures (**Box 1**) include such elements of outpatient pediatric care quality as childhood immunization rates and appropriate care of pediatric asthma. Over the past twenty years, other managed care measures have been used by various health plans (eg, rates of lead screening, use of antibiotics for respiratory infections, and adherence to various preventive services like dental care). Some of these measures (**Table 1**) have been included in various national data sets and endorsed by the National Quality Forum and the Ambulatory Quality Alliance.

The seminal study by Mangione-Smith and colleagues[6] assessing the quality of ambulatory pediatric care was a follow-up to an earlier RAND Corporation study of the quality of adult outpatient care in the United States. Similar to the adult study,[7] Mangione-Smith and colleagues reported that children received only 46.5% of

Box 1
2009 HEDIS measures pertaining to children's health

Weight assessment counseling for nutrition and physical activity for children and adolescents
Childhood immunization status
Lead screening in children
Appropriate testing for children with pharyngitis
Appropriate treatment for children with upper respiratory infection
Use of appropriate medications for asthma
Follow-up care for children prescribed ADHD medications
Access to care (# of visits) as measured at various age ranges
Annual dental visit
Cost of care measures/relative resource use
Guidelines for effectiveness of care measures

recommended care for preventive services, acute illness management, and ongoing care of chronic conditions. The measures considered in the pediatric study included care for: acne, asthma, attention deficit hyperactivity disorder, adolescent preventive health, allergic rhinitis, depression, diarrhea, fever, immunizations, urinary tract infections, vaginitis/sexually transmitted diseases, and routine health care maintenance.

Other landmark studies of quality of care for children were the National Healthcare Quality Report and the National Healthcare Disparities Report issued by the Agency for Healthcare Research and Quality in 2005.[8] These reports demonstrated both general gaps in care, as well as inequity of care in such critical factors as: infant mortality (4.6 per 1000 live births in Massachusetts as compared with 12.1/1000 in Washington D.C.); overuse of antibiotics (twice as frequent in children as compared with adults); incomplete immunizations (67% of black children fully immunized, compared with a 73% average rate and 75% for white children); and hospitalization for asthma (29.5/10,000 children overall but 59.6 hospitalizations per 10,000 black children).

Many of these gaps had been documented previously in studies examining the quality of pediatric care for asthma, immunizations, and well-child care. Unfortunately, documenting gaps and disparities is easier than demonstrating effective strategies for narrowing them. For example, the National Cooperative Inner City Asthma Study reported that its Inner City Asthma Intervention toolkit was implemented in more than 20 sites. The program was felt to be effective but did not include an evaluative component that could objectively demonstrate the program's impact.[9] Similarly, Homer and colleagues[10] reported in 2005 that a rigorous assessment of a commonly used quality improvement intervention had not demonstrated significant impact on either process or outcome measures of care for asthma.

Quality in pediatrics has more often been measured in processes rather than outcomes. A "process measure" assesses the performance of the health system itself, as contrasted with an "outcome measure" that illustrates patient health results. For example, asthma measures are often focused on whether children are prescribed appropriate therapy, not whether the child required hospitalization or missed school days. Immunization measures are typically reported as adherence to recommended vaccination schedules and do not necessarily address the outcome measure of effective prevention of vaccine-preventable diseases.

Table 1
National Quality Forum voluntary consensus measures

Category of Measures	Measures Pertinent for Children
Ambulatory surgery center measures	Prophylactic antibiotics for surgical cases (timing, choice, discontinuation) Falls Never events (Wrong site, side, procedure)
Asthma and respiratory illness	Asthma assessment Management plan Appropriate asthma meds Appropriate treatment for upper respiratory infection Appropriate testing for pharyngitis
Bone and joint disease	(None; osteoporosis, low back pain)
Diabetes	Adult inclusion criteria only (age 18–75 years old)
Eye care	(All adult measures)
Geriatrics	None
Heart disease	None
Hypertension	None
Medication management	Med lists Allergies documented Annual monitoring for selected drugs Drug avoidance in elderly
Mental health and substance use	ADHD diagnosis based on DSM-IV criteria Follow up care for ADHD
Obesity	BMI documented in children 2–18 years
Patient experience with care	None (CAHPS survey-based Medicare pts only)
Prenatal care	
Prevention immunization and screening	Tobacco use or exposure documentation and prevention Childhood immunization status

Data from National Quality Forum, Washington, DC. Available at: http://www.qualityforum.org.

Several pediatric subspecialty societies are developing common measure sets, although none have been endorsed to date by NQF or other national entities. The Cystic Fibrosis (CF) Foundation has published clinical quality measures for CF programs across the country (see http://www.cff.org/LivingWithCF/QualityImprovement/). These process measures include benchmarked outcome measures for pulmonary status, nutritional status, and adherence to clinical care guidelines. Although other specialty societies have issued outcome-oriented measures (eg, clinical oncology group), most have been research-focused and not publicly available or usable for quality improvement efforts. Recently, a network of pediatric gastroenterologists has initiated an improvement collaborative ("Trailblazer Collaborative") that aims to improve care and outcomes for children with inflammatory bowel disease.[11]

Although the principle of equity is one of the six central domains of the definition of quality,[12] there is no national definition for measurement of equity and no NQF-endorsed measure that is specifically evaluated by race and/or ethnicity. Conditions, such as sickle cell disease, which differentially impact children from minority racial and ethnic backgrounds, have been underrepresented in emerging quality efforts and will require systematic advocacy and support for these efforts.[13]

Measurement efforts can be either for comparative reporting and benchmarking, or primarily for improvement.[3] Scrutiny of measures used for comparative reporting is essential to ensure validity, risk adjustment, and assurance that differences in performance are caused by differences in care. Studies regarding adults who have diabetes have demonstrated that less than 5% of differences in measured outcomes were attributable to provider decision-making and behavior.[2] Caution is desirable in the rush to develop and disseminate national measures to assess and compare quality across providers.

PATIENT SAFETY IN THE AMBULATORY ENVIRONMENT: WHAT IS KNOWN?

There is a small but growing body of information available on the types of errors that occur in ambulatory care,[14–22] Studies on pediatric ambulatory medical errors are also limited.[23–26] Research suggests that adverse events and near misses are frequent occurrences, but little is known about types of errors, risk factors, or effective interventions.

Most reports of errors in ambulatory pediatric care have centered on medication safety. In one study,[27] 21 percent of outpatient prescriptions in a family medicine practice had at least one error. Other investigators found that medication samples were dispensed with inadequate documentation.[28] High rates of medication documentation errors were found in another family medicine practice.[29] In a pediatric emergency department in Canada, 100 prescribing errors and 39 medication administration errors occurred per 1000 patients.[30] In a sample of new prescriptions for 22 common medications in outpatient pediatric clinics, approximately 15% were dispensed with potential dosing errors.[24]

Several studies have examined antipyretic-dosing errors in children seen in pediatric emergency departments. Li and coworkers[31] found that over half of surveyed caregivers gave inaccurate doses of acetaminophen or ibuprofen, especially to infants. Another study[32] determined that 53% of children received an improper antipyretic dose at home. Goldman (2004)[33] noted that most parents under-dosed their children with acetaminophen, leading to unnecessary emergency visits. Losek and colleagues[34] reported that 22% of acetaminophen dose orders were outside accepted recommendations.

Some investigators have reported studies on immunization errors. Feikema and colleagues,[35] using data from the United States 1997 National Immunization Survey, found that 21% of children were over-immunized for at least one vaccine, and 31% were under-immunized for at least one vaccine. The costs associated with extra vaccination were estimated conservatively at $26.5 million. A study by Butte and colleagues[36] determined that strict interpretation of immunization guidelines contributed to 35.5% of patients having at least one invalid dose. Petridou and colleagues[37] found that there were only 11 reported errors per million immunization doses in Greece in 1999–2000, but the rate of reporting was not noted.

The Learning from Errors in Ambulatory Pediatrics (LEAP) study[25] aimed to learn scope, range, potential causes, and possible solutions to medical errors in pediatric ambulatory care. Among 14 pediatric practice sites, there were 147 medical errors reported during the study period. The largest group of errors was related to medical treatment (37%), but errors were also associated with: patient identification (22%); preventive care including immunizations (15%); diagnostic testing (13%); patient communication (8%); and other less frequent causes. Of the medical treatment errors, 85% were medication errors. The investigators determined that among the medication errors, 55% were related to ordering, 30% to failure to order, 11% to administration, 2% to transcribing, and 2% to dispensing.

Kaushal and colleagues[23] reported a prospective cohort study at six office practices in Boston area over 2 months. They discovered 57 preventable adverse drug events (rate 3%, 95% CI 3%–4%) in the care of 1788 patients. None of the events was determined to be life threatening, but eight (14%) were serious. Forty (70%) were related to parental drug administration. The authors determined that improved communication between providers and parents and between pharmacists and parents were the preventive strategies with the most potential benefit to prevent these errors.[26] Using the same data, they determined that children with multiple prescriptions were at increased risk of preventable adverse drug events, with an odds ratio of 1.46 (95% CI 1.01–2.11).

Leyva and colleagues[38] examined the impact of language barriers on medication errors in New York. They sought to determine how well Bronx Spanish-speaking Latino parents of children 5 years and younger understand written medication instructions. After receiving instructions on administration of ferrous sulfate, only 22% of parents demonstrated correct medication administration (amount and frequency). Subjects who reported comfort when speaking English were more likely to demonstrate correct medication amount to be administered (50% versus 21%, OR 3.8; 95% CI, 1.2–12.2) and correct frequency (93% versus 51%, OR 12.4; 95% CI, 1.5–99.1). Both education (OR 1.22, 95% CI, 1.03–1.45) and comfort speaking English (OR 3.81, 95% CI, 1.13–12.86) independently predicted correct medication dosing.

Neuspiel and colleagues[39] describe a voluntary, anonymous, non-punitive, team-based error reporting system, paired with team-based system analysis, rapid redesign, and monitoring of changes in the setting of a pediatric ambulatory department of an academic hospital in New York City. This system was partly modeled on a project implemented in an academic adult primary care setting in Charlottesville, Virginia.[22] In the New York study in the first year, 80 errors were reported, compared with only 5 errors reported during the prior year via a traditional incident reporting system. Both medication and non-medication errors were included.

Garbutt and colleagues[40] report a survey of 439 attending pediatricians and 118 residents about attitudes and experiences in disclosing errors to patients. Only 39% thought current reporting systems were adequate. Residents were more likely than attending physicians to believe that disclosure would be difficult (96% versus 86%, $P = .004$) and to want disclosure training (69% versus 56%, $P = .03$). Attending pediatricians were less likely than residents to be deterred from disclosing an error if the family was unaware of it (12% versus 26%, $P < .001$), if they thought the family would not want to know about it (20% versus 29%, $P = .04$), or if they thought they might get sued (13% versus 21%, $P = .04$).

What can be concluded from current knowledge on medical errors in ambulatory pediatrics? They are frequent events, often related to medication errors. Receiving multiple medications increases the risk of errors. Improving communication with patients and their parents appears to be a ripe opportunity for reducing errors. Language and cultural barriers in communication are particularly important to overcome to reduce the likelihood of medication errors in children. A nonpunitive, team-based reporting system may improve reporting. There appear to be disjointed attitudes about disclosure of errors to patients between pediatric residents and attending physicians, suggesting a training opportunity in this area.

RESIDENCY COMPETENCIES RELEVANT TO QUALITY IMPROVEMENT AND SAFETY

In 2002, in response to the 2001 *Crossing the Quality Chasm* report, the Institute of Medicine (IOM) convened an interdisciplinary summit to reform health professions education "to enhance patient care quality and safety."[41] The IOM committee report from this summit stated its "new vision for health professions education":

All health professionals should be educated to deliver patient-centered care as members of an interdisciplinary team, emphasizing evidence-based practice, quality improvement approaches, and informatics.

The IOM committee proposed a set of five core competencies that all clinicians should possess:

1. Provide patient-centered care
2. Work in interdisciplinary teams
3. Employ evidence-based practice
4. Apply quality improvement
5. Use informatics

The IOM committee called for accreditation bodies to require training programs for health care professionals to educate students in how to deliver patient care using these core competencies. At the time of this report's publication, evidence for educational activities in quality improvement within the health professions was described as "sparse."

GRADUATE MEDICAL EDUCATION REQUIREMENTS IN PEDIATRICS

The ACGME pediatric residency program requirements, which became effective July 1, 2007, include several sections relevant to addressing the IOM core competences in quality and patient safety (http://www.acgme.org/acWebsite/downloads/RRC_progReq/320_pediatrics_07,012,007.pdf). In the section on practice-based learning and improvement, the requirements state:

Residents must demonstrate the ability to investigate and evaluate their care of patients, to appraise and assimilate scientific evidence, and to continuously improve patient care based on constant self-evaluation and life-long learning.

To achieve this competency, residents must:

- Identify strengths, deficiencies, and limits in their knowledge and expertise;
- Set learning and improvement goals, identify and perform appropriate learning activities;
- Analyze their practice systematically with quality improvement methodology and implement changes to improve their practice;
- Incorporate formative evaluation feedback into daily practice;
- Locate, appraise, and assimilate evidence from publications related to their patients' health problems;
- Use information technology to optimize their learning; and
- Participate in the education of others.

Individual or teams of residents may participate in a quality improvement project to meet part of this competency, or they may be active members of a QI committee, under the supervision of experienced faculty.

The ACGME also calls for competency in systems-based practice:

Residents must demonstrate an awareness of and responsiveness to the larger context and system of health care, as well as the ability to call effectively on other resources in the system to provide optimal health care.

This competency calls for:

- Incorporation of considerations of cost awareness and risk-benefit analysis for patient-and/or population-based care as appropriate;

- Advocacy for quality patient care and optimal patient care systems;
- Working in interprofessional teams to enhance patient safety and improve patient care quality; and
- Participation in identifying system errors and implementing potential system solutions.

The program must ensure that resident education addresses systems approach to examining health care delivery, system errors and system solutions to prevent errors. Each resident must be actively engaged in the identification of system errors and in the development of system solutions, under the guidance of experienced faculty.

ACADEMIC PEDIATRIC ASSOCIATION EDUCATIONAL GUIDELINES

In 2004, the Academic Pediatric Association (APA; formerly the Ambulatory Pediatric Association) published the APA Educational Guidelines for Pediatric Residency. The section of this curriculum on quality improvement defines its goal as: "to understand the importance of and how to use quality improvement methods to monitor and improve the health care that one provides to children."[42] Objectives to fulfill this goal include:

- Explaining the role of regulatory or accreditation programs in monitoring quality in hospital and office based settings;
- Discussing tools used to assess quality in pediatric practice;
- Describing role of standards, such as HEDIS in setting benchmarks for pediatric services;
- Identifying and evaluating literature defining best practices;
- Analyzing one's own practice for factors that promote or inhibit the delivery of high-quality, cost-effective pediatric care;
- Reviewing patient satisfaction results to identify areas for improvement in one's practice;
- Practicing continuous quality improvement in one's practice using the PDSA or similar framework;
- Balancing cost and quality in medical decision-making.

The APA Educational Guidelines also include a section on medical errors and patient safety, the goal of which is "to understand the importance of error reduction in medical practice."[42] The objectives listed to meet this goal include:

- Discussing the impact of medical errors, including how such errors might occur in one's own practice;
- Acknowledging the importance of reducing medication errors in pediatric practice and ways to do so;
- Frankly disclosing when an error has occurred, and determine its contributing causes;
- When a preventable medical error occurs in one's practice, investigate it without assigning blame, distinguish personal from system causes, identify latent conditions that may result in errors and propose interventions to reduce or eliminate such risks, identify how and to whom errors should be reported, and describe methods used to evaluate errors.
- Demonstrating a commitment to systematic error reduction, including self-surveillance to reduce error-prone conditions, such as fatigue.
- Identifying Web sites about patient safety that are useful for physicians.

VALUE OF THE AMBULATORY SETTING FOR LEARNING ABOUT QUALITY AND SAFETY

Pediatric continuity practices present natural opportunities for residents to engage in both practice-based learning and system-based practice while applying quality improvement skills. Residents usually train in the same practice location over a 3-year period. As they are providing continuous care, it is common for them to identify gaps in the delivery of health care at the practice site. Residents are often interested in improvement and the continuity setting may provide both time and real life opportunity to engage in small cycles of change to improve care delivery. While working with a multidisciplinary ambulatory care team, including nursing, medical assistants, registrars, administration and social work, they can create common goals and share ideas for system change. Residents then can participate in real time improvement cycles with members of their continuity practice team. Time may be found during ambulatory block or outpatient rotations to be engaged in long-term design and implementation of ambulatory improvement projects during training.

The ACGME 2007 guidelines call for residents to participate in quality improvement projects, as well as locate, appraise, and assimilate evidence from scientific studies related to their patients' health problems as part of the competency of practice-based learning. During their continuity experience, residents can identify gaps in both knowledge and applied clinical practice, which may be improved by quality improvement methods. Immunization rates, lead screening policies, and asthma management are clinical areas where residents can improve their knowledge about standards of care and work on eliminating the gaps in care delivery.

Because residents spend 10%–20% of their training during residency in their continuity site and in ambulatory block rotations, these are important opportunities to apply quality improvement skills. Gaps in care identified in continuity practices often stimulate the resident's desire to act as a patient advocate and improve the system of health care in which they practice. Their quality improvement work may require that they interface with schools, health insurance administrators, and practice managers, further meeting ACGME competencies.

The American Board of Pediatrics (ABP) has recognized the importance of quality improvement for patient care and safety, reflected in current and future board recertification requirements. They note that pediatricians can be knowledgeable, and yet still have gaps in quality of care. Part four of the "Maintenance of Certification" (see https://www.abp.org/ABPWebSite/) provides activities that allow pediatricians to demonstrate that they can assess, reduce variation, and systematically improve the quality of care they deliver. Physicians can demonstrate competency either by participating in an ongoing ABP-approved structured quality improvement project or by completing internet-based quality improvement activities. Because all residents will be required to participate in quality improvement learning and practice to maintain certification, they will benefit from learning how to improve care delivery and incorporate team strategies in the ambulatory setting.

EXPERIENCE WITH RESIDENT TRAINING IN QUALITY IMPROVEMENT

In 2007, Boonyasai and colleagues[43] reported a systematic review on the effectiveness of educating clinicians on quality improvement. They also sought to determine whether the effectiveness of such curricula is influenced by teaching methodology. Among 39 studies meeting eligibility criteria, 31 were team-based projects, and 37 were combinations of didactic with experiential learning.

The studies evaluated by Boonyasai and colleagues[43] included a range of two to eight out of nine adult learning principles (median = seven). These principles include the following characteristics:

1. enabling learners to be active participants;
2. providing content relating to learners' current experiences;
3. assessing learners' needs and tailoring teaching to their past experiences;
4. allowing learners to identify and pursue their own learning goals;
5. allowing learners to practice their learning;
6. supporting learners during self-directed learning;
7. providing feedback to learners;
8. facilitating learner self-reflection;
9. role-modeling behaviors.

Evaluations of effectiveness included 22 controlled trials (eight randomized; 14 not randomized), and 17 pre/post– or time series measurements. Educational outcomes were described in 14 studies, and 28 studies described clinical process or patient outcomes. Of 10 studies that evaluated knowledge, nine studies reported only positive effects, but most of the assessment tools were not validated. There were mixed results among the six assessments of attitudes. Skill or behavior outcomes were measured in six studies, four of which reported only positive results. Among the 28 studies of clinical outcomes, eight reported only beneficial effects. Mixed or no effects were more frequent in the controlled studies. There were only four studies reporting both educational and clinical outcomes. Boonyasai and colleagues[43] conclude that most published QI curricula employ appropriate adult learning principles and show improvement in the knowledge or confidence of learners to perform QI.

Seven of the 39 studies evaluated by Boonyasai and colleagues[43] involved resident physicians.[44–50] All were in ambulatory sites, combining didactic instruction with participation in QI activities. Five of these were integrated into 4-week rotations, and two had regular weekly or biweekly meetings over a year. Boonyasai and colleagues[43] found that QI curricula among trainees with clinical outcomes reported mostly beneficial improvement in documentation and disease management, but that their study designs were weak, because they were mainly uncontrolled.

EXPERIENCE WITH RESIDENT TRAINING IN PATIENT SAFETY

Battles and Shea report that resident physicians are involved in many medical errors, and that their deficient education in patient safety contributes to the potential harm of patients.[51] These authors called for the use of root-cause analysis with a near-miss reporting system in teaching hospitals to guide needed changes in graduate medical education programs. In a subsequent publication, Sachdeva and colleagues[52] suggested the use of standardized patients in an objective structured clinical examination (OSCE) as a teaching tool in patient safety, using cases derived from actual events. present the results of a national consensus conference on patient safety curricula for surgical residency programs.[53]

Specific experiences with resident patient-safety curricula with relevance to pediatrics have been reported by two family medicine residency programs. Coyle and colleagues[54] evaluated the effectiveness of an educational program to improve medical event reporting attitude and behavior in ambulatory care. They found that attendance at six monthly patient-safety educational conferences was significantly correlated with medical event-reporting attitude and behavior change. Barriers to reporting included lack of time, extra paper work, and concerns about career and personal reputation. Another patient safety curriculum[55] includes introductory workshops for faculty and residents, several didactic courses, individual portfolios, and a series of small group exercises including chart reviews, case presentations and a long-term quality improvement project. These activities are coordinated by a multidisciplinary team. Evaluation of the curriculum includes ongoing assessment of resident performance in the included activities and in an annual OSCE. The program was successfully introduced, although OSCE results were not included in this publication.

EXPERIENCE WITH QUALITY IMPROVEMENT TRAINING IN PEDIATRIC AMBULATORY SETTINGS

Since 2004, the pediatric residency training program at New York Presbyterian Hospital (NYPH) has instituted annual longitudinal quality improvement projects based in the continuity clinic setting. This program trains 60 pediatric residents based at four community-based practice locations. Under the guidance of a faculty mentor, residents select a gap in care and then design and implement improvements using the methodology of the model for improvement.[56] Residents participate in their clinic site-based improvement project during their ambulatory block rotation and hand-off the work to the next resident participating in the longitudinal project.

Projects are driven by ideas for change generated by the pediatric residents, who identify gaps in their knowledge and/or practice and then as a group determine which gap they plan to improve over the course of the academic year. The curriculum includes an overall presentation about quality improvement and the model for improvement as well as four team meetings over the course of the year to discuss AIM statements, "Plan, Do, Study and Act" (PDSA) cycles, measurement and sustaining change as they apply to their current improvement work. In the spring of each academic year, the four projects are presented and evaluated for adherence to the model for improvement, reaching stated goals and potential for sustaining the system changes, which have been incorporated into the practice. This work is unique in that it moves from the hypothetical model of writing a proposal for system changes to actually embedding this work into the clinic setting, performing PDSA cycles, and achieving results with actual system changes.

During their projects, residents are change agents but learn the value of a team model to initiate and sustain change. Faculty mentors oversee participation in the improvement work, while residents choose the gap in care studied and direct the change process. Each resident team reviews and presents the evidence supporting their improvement. Following the dimensions of quality outlined by the IOM, gaps in care have fallen into the categories of effective, safe, patient-centered, efficient, timely and equitable. For example, residents have chosen to improve care in the following areas:

- *Screening*- anemia, lead, tuberculosis, hypertension and asthma
- *Mental Health* – domestic violence and postpartum depression
- *Safety* – home medications and over the counter medications, improving communication between subspecialists and primary care providers
- *System* – redesigning flow of vision and hearing screening
- *Anticipatory Guidance* – dental health, obesity and screen time, and development screening.

Residents have real time opportunities during the rotation to plan and implement a PDSA cycle and suggest the next cycle for the following resident.

An evaluation program has been instituted to assess the quality of the training program. Residents complete knowledge, skills and attitude surveys at the end of their rotations; and faculty mentors also reflect on resident skill and attitude development. Skills recorded include defining the gap in care, developing AIM statements, project measures, conducting tests of change, developing system tools, engaging other members of the improvement team, obtaining feedback from the population of interest, and preparing either a didactic or the final presentation. At the conclusion of this process, all residents are required to complete an email sign-out, which allows the residents to summarize the work completed during their block rotation, and suggest a PDSA cycle for the next resident. In addition, it allows all team members to be informed of the status of their improvement work.

When surveyed, the majority of the residents felt their work on the QI project helped them understand how to evaluate patient care practices, improve quality of care, and develop the ability to effectively use system resources to provide quality care. Of graduating third year residents, 88.5% thought that they were at least somewhat prepared to initiate and implement a quality improvement program using the model for improvement at their next clinical setting. In addition, at the summative presentations of the four longitudinal projects, QI mentors evaluate each project for adherence to the model for improvement, success of improvement work, involvement of team members, and the ability to sustain and spread results. The projects have generally scored high with challenges identified in the area of spreading and sustaining change.[57] Test scores on a knowledge survey demonstrate that, by their third year, residents have obtained a greater QI knowledge than untrained general pediatric faculty members, reinforcing the success for resident training in the combination of curriculum about QI and the practical application of QI skills in the ambulatory setting.[58]

The effectiveness of resident training in quality improvement in a pediatric ambulatory environment has also been reported by Mohr and colleagues[47] This pre-through-post–observational study examined the impact of faculty facilitated improvement team meetings on improving immunization completion by two years of age. The residents' team successfully implemented five changes in clinic processes, associated with an increase in immunization completion from 60% to 86% ($P = .04$).

CHALLENGES TO TEACHING QI AND PATIENT SAFETY IN AMBULATORY PEDIATRICS

Irrespective of the model chosen as a training methodology and improvement tool, the challenges of incorporating a QI curriculum into residency training stem, first, from time constraints. The nearly saturated schedules of residents in programs that strain to meet training requirements while also satisfying clinical care needs may distract from educational programming. New curricular elements may be equally challenged to receive adequate focus and attention.

Furthermore, the training of residents in QI is hampered by the limited number of faculty who understand how to teach these methods and approaches. Although all faculty are able to teach the differential diagnosis of signs and symptoms in their area of clinical expertise, few have received formal instruction in improvement methodologies or have participated in structured improvement efforts that would make them comfortable with teaching these methods to house staff.[58]

In 2008, the Institute for Healthcare Improvement initiated an "Open School" to foster education of health professions students in improvement methods and principles of quality and safety (http://www.ihi.org/IHI/Programs/IHIOpenSchool). This initiative may prove to be an important cross-cutting effort to enhance the education available to current medical, nursing and other health professions students.

In addition, many programs identify needs for data support, curricula, online resources and evaluation. In a survey of 77 New York City[59] primary care residency programs, 69% identified a need for statistical support for data analysis; 62% noted a need for a curriculum guide; and only 10% were resident led projects.[59] The majority of programs reported some resident participation or were faculty-led with resident involvement. Other typical challenges that are reported include: how to engage team members around development and planning cycles of change and the sustainability of work when the champions (ie, residents) are no longer engaged in their QI work.

A key issue for hospital leaders in quality and safety is identifying strategies to align operational improvement needs with faculty members' priorities both in clinical care and academic research or scholarly activity. Quality improvement research has traditionally been viewed differently than other investigational efforts, but in recent years it has become increasingly rigorous; this may lead to greater recognition by promotions committees in universities and academic medical centers. To the extent that clinical improvement work is fostered by physician participation, it is essential that improvement leaders facilitate the opportunity for collaborating faculty to pose investigational questions that are publishable and can contribute to academic advancement, while also improving systems, processes, and outcomes of care.

FUTURE DIRECTIONS

The pediatric ambulatory setting continues to be ripe for improvement in care, as well as a key location for training future pediatricians in quality and safety. The ambulatory setting is also undergoing significant transformation as information technology continues its accelerating penetration into the health care delivery system. The interface between electronic health record implementation and advancing quality and patient safety in ambulatory settings will have a great impact on pediatric care.

Some future goals that are likely to facilitate improvement in both measurement and clinical outcomes include:

- Development of better measures of quality of care by individual providers
- Improved methodology of studies examining the effectiveness of QI interventions
- Further development and more widespread use of common measure sets for pediatric conditions
- Better recognition and measurement of the impact of equity on child health outcomes
- More knowledge of the types of medical errors occurring in ambulatory pediatric settings and effective strategies to prevent them
- Provider training on disclosure of medical errors
- Full integration of training in safety and quality in pediatric residency, particularly in the ambulatory setting, with prioritization of time for this effort
- Evaluation studies of models for teaching quality and safety to pediatric residents
- Faculty development in QI methodology and effective methods to teach it
- Recognition of QI scholarship in the faculty promotions process

The achievement of these goals will bring pediatrics closer to the quality of care that children deserve.

REFERENCES

1. Parkerton P, Smith DG, Belin TR, et al. Physician performance assessment. Nonequivalence of primary care measures. Med Care 2003;41:1034–47.
2. Hofer TP, Hayward RA, Greenfield S. The unreliability of individual physician "report cards" for assessing the costs and quality of care of a chronic disease. JAMA 1999;281:2098–105.
3. American Academy of Pediatrics Steering Committee on Quality Improvement and Management and Committee on Practice and Ambulatory Medicine. Principles for the development and use of quality measures. Pediatrics 2008;121: 411–8.
4. Leawood KS. Pay for performance. American Academy of Family Physicians; 2006. Available at: www.aafp.org/x30307.xml. Accessed December 24, 2008.
5. Thompson JW, Ryan KW, Pinidiya SD, et al. Quality of care for children in commercial and medicaid managed care. JAMA 2003;290:1486–93.
6. Mangione-Smith R, Decristifaro AH, Setodji CM, et al. The quality of ambulatory care delivered to children in the United States. N Engl J Med 2007;357: 1515–23.
7. McGlynn EA, Asch SM, Adams J, et al. The quality of health care delivered to adults in the United States. N Engl J Med 2003;348:2635–45.
8. Dougherty D, Meikle SF, Owens P, et al. Children's Health Care in the First National Healthcare Quality Report and National Healthcare Disparities Report. Med Care 2005;43(Suppl 3):I58–63.
9. Love AS, Spiegel S. The inner-city asthma intervention tool kit: best practices and lessons learned. Ann Allergy Asthma Immunol 2006;97(Supp 1):36–9.
10. Homer CJ, Forbes P, Horvitz L, et al. Impact of a quality improvement program on care and outcomes for children with asthma. Arch Pediatr Adolesc Med 2005; 159:464–9.
11. Miles PV, Miller M, Payne DM, et al. Alliance for pediatric quality: creating a community of practice to improve health care for America's children. Pediatrics 2009;123:S64–6.
12. Committee on Quality of Health Care in America, Institute of Medicine. Crossing the quality chasm: a new health system for the 21st century. Washington, DC: National Academies Press; 2001.
13. Betancourt JR, Green AR, King RR. Improving quality and achieving equity: a guide for hospital leaders; Massachusetts General Hospital. Available at: http://www2.massgeneral.org/disparitiessolutions/z_files/DSC%20Leadership%20Guide%2012.18.08.pdf. Accessed December 24, 2008.
14. Dovey SM, Meyers DS, Phillips RL, et al. A preliminary taxonomy of medical errors in family practice. Qual Saf Health Care 2002;11:233–8.
15. Dovey S, Phillips R, Green L. Medical errors affecting vulnerable primary care patients in six countries: a report of the LINNAEUS Collaboration. Academy for Health Services Research and Health Policy Annual Research Meeting. Washington, DC: AHSRHP; 2002.
16. Elston D, Sieck C, Sullivan R, et al. Developing ambulatory care physician performance measures. J Am Acad Dermatol 2008;59:505–13.
17. Foster A, Murff H, Peterson J, et al. The incidence and severity of adverse events affecting patients after discharge from the hospital. Ann Intern Med 2003;138: 161–7.
18. Gandhi R, Burstin HR, Cook EF, et al. Drug complications in outpatients. J Gen Intern Med 2000;15:149–54.

19. Gandhi T, Weingart S, Borus B, et al. Adverse drug events in primary care. N Engl J Med 2003;348:1556–64.
20. Gurwitz JH, Field TS, Harrold LR, et al. Incidence and preventability of adverse drug events among older persons in the ambulatory setting. JAMA 2003;289: 1107–16.
21. Hammons T, Piland NF, Small SD, et al. Ambulatory patient safety. What we know and need to know. J Ambul Care Manage 2003;26:63–82.
22. Plews-Ogan ML, Nadkarni MM, Forren S, et al. Patient safety in the ambulatory setting: a clinician-based approach. J Gen Intern Med 2004;19:719–25.
23. Kaushal R, Goldmann DA, Keohane CA, et al. Adverse drug events in pediatric outpatients. Ambul Pediatr 2007;7:383–9.
24. McPhillips HA, Stille CJ, Smith D, et al. Potential medication dosing errors in outpatient pediatrics. J Pediatr 2005;147:761–7.
25. Mohr JJ, Lannon CM, Thoma KA, et al. Learning from errors in ambulatory pediatrics. In: Henriksen K, Battles JB, Marks ES, et al, editors. Advances in patient safety: from research to implementation. Washington, DC: Agency for Healthcare Research and Quality; 2005. Available at: www.ahrq.gov/downloads/pub/advances/vol1/Mohr.pdf. Accessed March 5, 2008.
26. Zandieh SO, Goldmann DA, Keohane CA, et al. Risk factors in preventable adverse drug events in pediatric outpatients. J Pediatr 2008;152:225–31.
27. Shaughnessy AF, Nickel RO. Prescription-writing patterns and errors in a family medicine residency program. J Fam Pract 1989;29:290–5.
28. Dill JL, Generali JA. Medication sample labeling practices. Am J Health Syst Pharm 2000;57:2087–90.
29. Ernst ME, Brown GL, Klepser TB, et al. Medication discrepancies in an outpatient electronic medical record. Am J Health Syst Pharm 2001;58:2072–5.
30. Kozer E, Scolnik D, Macpherson A, et al. Variables associated with medication errors in pediatric emergency medicine. Pediatrics 2002;110:737–42.
31. Li SF, Lacher B, Crain EF. Acetaminophen and ibuprofen dosing by parents. Pediatr Emerg Care 2000;16:394–7.
32. McErlean MA, Bartfield JM, Kennedy DA, et al. Home antipyretic use in children brought to the emergency department. Pediatr Emerg Care 2001;17: 249–51.
33. Goldman RD, Scolnik D. Underdosing of acetaminophen by parents and emergency department utilization. Pediatr Emerg Care 2004;20:89–93.
34. Losek JD. Acetaminophen dose accuracy and pediatric emergency care. Pediatr Emerg Care 2004;20:285–8.
35. Feikema SM, Klevens M, Washington ML, et al. Extraimmunization among US children. JAMA 2000;283:1311–7.
36. Butte AJ, Shaw JS, Bernstein H. Strict interpretation of vaccination guidelines with computerized algorithms and improper timing of administered doses. Pediatr Infect Dis J 2001;20:561–5.
37. Petridou E, Kouri N, Vadela H, et al. Frequency and nature of recorded childhood immunization-related errors in Greece. Clin Toxicol 2004;42:273–6.
38. Leyva M, Sharif I, Ozuah P. Health literacy among Spanish-speaking Latino parents with limited English proficiency. Ambul Pediatr 2005;5:56–9.
39. Neuspiel DR, Guzman M, Harewood C. Improving error reporting in ambulatory pediatrics with team approach. Advances in Patient Safety: new Directions and Alternative Approaches, vol. 1. Rockville (MD): Agency for Healthcare Research and Quality; 2008.

40. Garbutt J, Brownstein DR, Klein EJ, et al. Reporting and disclosing medical errors: pediatricians' attitudes and behaviors. Arch Pediatr Adolesc Med 2007; 161:179–85.
41. Greiner AC, Knebel E, editors. Health professions education: a bridge to quality. Washington, DC: Institute of Medicine; 2003.
42. Kittredge D, editor. APA educational guidelines for pediatric residency. McLean (VA): Academic Pediatric Association; 2004.
43. Boonyasai RT, Windish DM, Chakraborti C, et al. Effectiveness of teaching quality improvement to clinicians. JAMA 2007;298:1023–37.
44. Coleman MT, Nasraty S, Ostapchuk M, et al. Introducing practice-based learning and improvement ACGME core competencies into a family medicine residency curriculum. Jt Comm J Qual Saf 2003;29(5):238–47.
45. Djuricich AM, Ciccarelli M, Swigonski NL. A continuous quality improvement curriculum for residents: addressing core competency, improving systems. Acad Med 2004;79(Suppl):S65–7.
46. Holmboe ES, Prince L, Green M. Teaching and improving quality of care in a primary care internal medicine residency clinic. Acad Med 2005;80: 571–7.
47. Mohr JJ, Randolph GD, Laughon MM, et al. Integrating improvement competencies into residency education. Ambul Pediatr 2003;3:131–6.
48. Nuovo J, Balsbaugh T, Barton S, et al. Development of a diabetes care management curriculum in a family practice residency program. Dis Manage 2004;7(4): 314–24.
49. Ogrinc G, Headrick LA, Morrison LJ, et al. Teaching and assessing resident competence in practice-based learning and improvement. J Gen Intern Med 2004;19(5 Pt 2):496–500.
50. Varkey P, Reller MK, Smith A, et al. An experiential interdisciplinary quality improvement education initiative. Am J Med Qual 2006;21(5):317–22.
51. Battles JB, Shea CE. A system of analyzing medical errors to improve GME curricula and programs. Acad Med 2001;76:125–33.
52. Battles JB, Wilkinson SL, Lee SJ. Using standardized patients in an objective structured clinical examination as a patient safety tool. Qual Saf Health Care 2004;13(Suppl 1):i46–50.
53. Sachdeva AK, Philibert I, Leach DC, et al. Patient safety curriculum for surgical residency programs: results of a national consensus conference. Surgery 2007; 141:427–41.
54. Coyle YM, Mercer SQ, Murphy-Cullen CL, et al. Effectiveness of a graduate medical education program for improving medical event reporting attitude and behavior. Qual Saf Health Care 2005;14:383–8.
55. Singh R, Naughton B, Taylor JS, et al. A comprehensive collaborative patient safety residency curriculum to address the ACGME core competencies. Med Educ 2005;39:1195–204.
56. Lane M, Hyman D. Using "The Model for Improvement" to achieve the ACGME competencies of practice based learning and system based practice [abstract]. Pediatric Academic Society Meeting. Toronto (ON), May 2007.
57. Lane M, Hyman D. Strategies for assessing the effectiveness of a resident quality improvement training program [abstract]. Pediatric Academic Society Meeting. Honolulu (HI), May 2008.

58. Lane M, Hyman D. Strategies for assessing the effectiveness of a resident quality improvement training program [abstract]. National Initiative for Children's Healthcare Quality. Dallas (TX), March 2009.
59. NYC Department of Health and Mental Hygiene. New York City Primary Care Residency Program Survey Report Clinical Systems Improvement, April 2008.

The Medical Home–Improving Quality of Primary Care for Children

Steven E. Wegner, JD, MD[a,b,*], Richard C. Antonelli, MD, MS[c],
Renee M. Turchi, MD, MPH[d,e]

KEYWORDS

- Medical home • Quality of care
- Improving quality of primary care for children and youth
- Implementation

The concept of a medical home is not new, but today appears to be a key driver for enhancing the value of health services as care systems are transitioned to meet the ongoing challenges of improving quality and containing costs.[1,2] Initially, the term was put forth to mean the single location for all health information about a patient with special health care needs.[3] It became clear that despite this limited scope, the medical home approach was an important mechanism to support communication and coordinate care with multiple providers. Subsequently, the term was cited in the American Academy of Pediatrics (AAP) 1974 policy statement regarding "Fragmentation of Health Care Services for Children."[4]

Dr. Calvin Sia was successful with his campaign to incorporate the medical home concept into the Child Health Plan in Hawaii in 1978–79.[5] National dissemination began with an AAP conference on the medical home in 1989, culminating in collaboration with the Maternal and Child Health Bureau (MCHB) to establish the National Center of Medical Home Initiatives for Children with Special Needs.[3,6] In 2002 and 2004, the AAP and Medical Home Initiatives for Children with Special Needs Project Advisory Committee published a policy statement outlining operational definitions for the seven characteristics of the medical home, a policy reaffirmed in August 2008.[7,8] In March 2007, the "Joint Principles of the Patient-Centered Medical

[a] AccessCare, 3500 Gateway Centre Boulevard, Suite 130, Morrisville, NC 27560-8501, USA
[b] The University of North Carolina at Chapel Hill, School of Medicine, Department of Pediatrics, USA
[c] Children's Hospital Boston and Harvard Medical School, Division of General Pediatrics, 300 Longwood Avenue, Boston, MA 02115, USA
[d] St. Christopher's Hospital for Children, Erie Avenue at Front Street, Philadelphia, PA 19134, USA
[e] Department of Pediatrics, Drexel University School of Public Health, Philadelphia, PA, USA
* Corresponding author.
E-mail address: sew@ncaccesscare.org (S.E. Wegner).

Pediatr Clin N Am 56 (2009) 953–964
doi:10.1016/j.pcl.2009.05.021 pediatric.theclinics.com

Home" were collaboratively published by the AAP, the American Academy of Family Physicians, the American College of Physicians, and the American Osteopathic Association.[9,10] The medical home policy has also been affirmed by Family Voices and the National Association of Pediatric Nurse Practitioners.[11,12]

The remainder of this article provides an overview of the challenges faced in United States health care delivery systems that affect child health, explains how the medical home might address them, describes methods for measuring quality in medical homes, and identifies barriers to implementation of the model.

CHALLENGES FOR THE UNITED STATES HEALTH CARE DELIVERY SYSTEMS AND PRIMARY CARE

Today, millions of Americans, including children and youth, suffer from preventable illness and chronic diseases that challenge the United States health care systems.[13,14] In 2006, almost 7 million United States children (9%) had asthma, 4.7 million had a learning disability, 9.6 million (13%) took a prescription medication for at least 3 months for a health problem, and 5% missed 11 or more days of school in the previous 12 months because of an illness or injury.[15] Diabetes afflicts more than 150,000 American children and youth under the age of 20; and 13,000 more are diagnosed with type 1 diabetes each year.[16] In addition, technical advancements in health care services have led to dramatic improvements in the survival of premature infants and those with serious health problems, adding to the number of children with complex health needs.[14,17,18] It is estimated that 15% of youth in the United States have a chronic condition that affects daily life[19] and that 22% of households with children have at least one child with a special health care need, based on the 2005 to 2006 National Survey of Children with Special Health Care Needs.[20] Moreover, with advances in medical technology, more youth are surviving into adulthood.[19]

The implications of chronic health problems on the health care system and expenditures are profound. Data from the 2000 Medical Expenditure Panel Survey (MEPS) suggest that children and youth with special health care needs (CYSHCN) incur health care costs three times higher than those without special needs with estimates of costs incurred by CYSHCN ranging from more than 40% to 70% of total costs.[18,20,21]

The United States health care delivery systems are generally structured to address episodic and acute health care problems and are poorly organized for improving the health of populations and managing patients with chronic health problems.[22–24] Children and youth with complex health care problems are often shuffled among numerous health care providers in geographically dispersed settings with limited coordination and communication among providers. Information infrastructures and health data exchanges are underdeveloped.[23] Although the proportion of United States primary care physicians (PCPs) using electronic medical records increased from 17% to 28% between 2001 and 2006, the United States lags far behind leading countries where up to 98% of PCPs use electronic medical records to improve care.

Underinvestment also occurs in the areas of primary care and preventive care.[2,13] Only about 7% of United States health care dollars are spent on primary care; and the median income of specialists was approximately double that of PCPs in 2004.[2,25] Reimbursement for a 30-minute office visit with a patient is approximately one third of that for 30 minutes spent performing diagnostic, surgical, or imaging procedures.[25] Furthermore, expenses related to providing care coordination in primary care offices are generally not reimbursed.[26] With PCPs facing increasing demands, receiving relatively low compensation, and saddled with high educational loan indebtedness, fewer physicians are choosing careers in primary care.[25,27] This poses a significant challenge to an already vulnerable system that lacks capacity to provide sufficient access to high-quality, community-based primary care. Furthermore, when viewed from the perspective of meeting the needs of children and their families, cogent arguments have been put forth to transform the way services are provided in pediatric well-child encounters.[28]

ATTRIBUTES OF CARE PROVIDED IN A MEDICAL HOME

The medical home model may address many of the limitations of the United States health care delivery systems and improve quality of care, reduce cost escalation, foster patient- and family-centered care, and improve coordination of care. The medical home is a strategy for health services delivery that involves providing primary care that is accessible, continuous, comprehensive, family centered, coordinated, compassionate, and culturally effective.[8,29–31] Medical home has been defined by Antonelli and colleagues[29] as "an approach to providing comprehensive primary care in a high-quality and cost effective manner." In a medical home model, the family and PCP are mutually responsible for developing a plan of care and making decisions for a child's or youth's health care and related services.[7,8] The pediatric health care professional is responsible for helping the family navigate the health care delivery systems and supportive services throughout childhood and adolescence and assisting with the transition of care into adulthood. The child/youth receives treatment- and prevention-focused care in a convenient and accessible setting to assist him or her with attaining the highest level of health possible. When necessary, care is coordinated among all involved and needed health care providers and community services, including educational and vocational assistance, community resources, and home-based services.

IMPLEMENTATION OF THE HIGH-QUALITY MEDICAL HOME

Implementation of the medical home model has progressed over time, often incrementally as a continuous process-improvement approach. Some programs have implemented only a select number of model characteristics, while others have been more exhaustive. Data from the 2006 to 2007 National Study of Physician Organizations (NSPO) were used to estimate the extent of adoption of four of seven of the Joint Principles.[24] Approximately one third of responding medical groups use primary care teams at the majority of their practice sites. Two thirds of the practices engaged in some type of quality-improvement initiatives.

Accessible Care

The AAP operationally defines accessible care as care provided in the child's or youth's community, where the child or youth can easily gain access to the practice, where the physician is available to speak directly with families when needed, where all payer sources are accepted, and which meets the Americans with Disabilities Act requirements.[8] The 2008 National Scorecard on US Health System Performance assigned the United States a score of 58 out of 100 possible points on measures of access, specifically related to health insurance coverage and affordability.[23] Data from the 1997 National Survey of America's Families found that the emergency department was a usual source of care for 6.1% of Medicaid respondents, 5.4% of respondents with private insurance, and 24.1% of uninsured respondents with incomes below 200% of the federal poverty level.[32] Having access to a usual source of care within state Medicaid programs has been found to be associated with higher Medicaid provider reimbursement rates, lower prevalence of capitated payment arrangements, and decreased concerns regarding paperwork expectations.[33] Federally qualified health centers and rural health centers are critical elements in the primary care safety net system. This model of health care delivery for children, youth, and adults can improve access for families in areas where access to care is limited and provide quality care to both insured and uninsured adults at a lower cost to the health care system.[34]

Family-centered Care

In *Crossing the Quality Chasm*, the Institute of Medicine (IOM) defined patient-centered care as "providing care that is respectful of and responsive to individual patient preferences, needs, and values, and ensuring that patient values guide all clinical decisions."[22] AAP's concept of "family centered care" resembles more closely MCHB's idea that "family centered care assures the health and well-being of children and their families through a respectful family-professional partnership." Specifically, AAP's organizational principles for family-centered care include:[8]

- Having a medical home PCP who is known to the family;
- Establishing mutual responsibility between the care provider(s) and family with the family being recognized as having the most significant role as caregiver;
- Providing complete information to the family to assist them with sharing responsibility for decision-making with the care provider;
- Supporting the family to enable them to actively coordinate care;
- Recognizing the family as the expert in the child's care and of the youth as an expert in his or her care.

The results of the 1999–2001 National Survey of Children With Special Health Care Needs indicated that an estimated two thirds of families of CSHCN believed that the care received was family centered.[35] While most families report receiving family-centered care, poverty, minority status, lack of insurance, and functional limitations are associated with decreased perception of family–professional partnerships.[36] Engaging all families as partners in caring for children is imperative for ensuring that high-quality, efficient care is delivered.[37]

Continuous Care

Continuous care has been operationally defined by the AAP as:

- Having the same primary pediatric health care professionals available from infancy through young adulthood;
- Providing transition assistance to families, children, and youth by performing developmentally appropriate health assessments and counseling;
- Ensuring that the medical home physician communicates and participates to the fullest extent allowed in care; and
- Providing discharge planning when the child is hospitalized or care is provided at another facility or by another provider.[8]

Comprehensive Care

The AAP operational dimensions for comprehensive care require that:

- Care be delivered or directed by a well-trained physician who is able to manage and facilitate all aspects of care;
- Ambulatory and inpatient care services be available at all times;

Primary prevention services be provided, including health promotion and disease and injury prevention assessments, screenings, and counseling;
Preventive, primary, and tertiary care, as well as educational, developmental, psychosocial, and other service needs be identified and addressed;
Physicians advocate for the family in obtaining comprehensive care;
Information about private and public payers and special financial programs be provided to the family; and
Longer appointment times for CYSHCN be available when needed.[10]

The 1999–2001 National Survey of CSHCN found that almost 80% of respondents reported having had no problems obtaining needed specialty referrals.[35]

Coordinated Care

The concept of coordinated care is defined operationally by the AAP with eight organizational principles.[8] The process of care coordination generally includes identifying needs, making assessments, setting priorities, communicating, networking, educating, advocating for resources, and monitoring.[18] A plan of care is collaboratively developed by the provider, family, and youth; shared with other care providers; and coordinated with community agencies and educational and vocational systems helping to address health needs of the child or youth.[8] Care is coordinated among multiple providers through the medical home. A complete health record is maintained at the primary medical practice; and necessary information is shared with the child or youth, family, and consulting provider(s), including the specific reason(s) for a referral. Families are linked to support groups and other community resources as needed.[8] Coordinating with the child's or youth's educational system is paramount. Often the CYSHCN's medical condition affects his or her functioning at school and individualized education plans need modification or input from the health care team.[37] The benefits of care coordination include clinical and process improvements, reductions in health care costs, and improvement in family satisfaction.[26]

Care coordination is often an essential service for families of CYSHCN,[38] but results of the 2001 National Survey of CSHCN indicated that only 40% of parents of CSHCN believed that effective care coordination was received.[35] In the follow-up National Survey in 2005–2006, only 46% of parents of CSHCN felt they had received effective care coordination when needed, with nearly 32% stating they had not received one or more aspects of care coordination.[39] One of the principal barriers to achieving comprehensive service provision via the pediatric medical home is the multifactorial nature of care coordination needs for children, youth, and families.[40] These investigators present a methodology for medical home teams to measure the activities and outcomes of care coordination, thus enabling practices to document and improve their performance in this critical service model. While many of the costs of managing chronic medical conditions in a medical home setting will be borne by traditional payers, the comprehensive needs of children, youth, and families, not unlike those of geriatric patients, will broaden the potential range of services for which funding must be sought. These include educational, behavioral, vocational, and family support services. Recent work supported by the Commonwealth Fund delineates a multidisciplinary framework and approach to designing care coordination for pediatric systems of care.[41]

Compassionate Care

The AAP organizational principles of compassionate care state that verbal and nonverbal interactions reflect expressions of concern for the well-being of the child or youth and family and suggest that all care providers make efforts to understand and empathize with the feelings and perspectives of the family and child or youth.[8]

Culturally Effective Care

AAP has outlined three operational principles of culturally effective care:

- The family and child/youths' cultural background, including beliefs, rituals, and customs, is recognized, valued, respected, and incorporated into the plan of care.
- Translators or interpreters, a language line, technology, and other mechanisms are used to optimize the understanding of the medical encounter and plan of care.
- Written materials are provided in the family's primary language when appropriate and feasible. [8]

MEASURING QUALITY OF THE MEDICAL HOME

Tools for measuring the level of medical home implementation of physician practices are available from Web site of the Center for Medical Home Improvement (CMHI) and from the National Committee for Quality Assurance (NCQA). The CMHI offers three major assessment tools for primary care practices: The Medical Home Index,[42] The Medical Home Index—Short Version,[43] and The Medical Home Family Index and Survey.[44] The NCQA developed the Physician Practice Connections—Patient-Centered Medical Home (PPC-PCMH) program to assess how practices are functioning as patient-centered medical homes and to recognize physicians who deliver excellent care using the program standards.[27]

Medical Home Index

The Medical Home Index is a validated self-assessment tool that has been designed to measure operational dimensions of the seven broad characteristics defining the medical home: accessibility, continuity, family-centered quality, comprehensiveness, degree of coordination, level of compassion, and cultural effectiveness.[42,45]

The Medical Home Index begins with questions about practice characteristics, such as practice type, number of providers, availability of a care coordinator at the practice, payer mix, and familiarity with the medical home concept and family-centered care. It then queries 25 indicators organized within the following six domains:[42]

- Organizational capacity. This measures communication, access, family access to the medical record, office environment, process for obtaining feedback from families of CYSHCN, cultural competence, and staff education about community resources and CYSHCN.
- Chronic condition management. This measures the processes for identifying CYSHCN, as well as care continuity, continuity across settings, cooperative management between the PCP and specialists, support for the transition into adulthood, and family support.
- Care coordination for CYSHCN and their families. This measures care coordination and role definition; family involvement in care coordination; child and family education activities; assessment of needs of CYSHCN and care planning; resource information and referrals to community, state, and national resources; and advocacy of CYSHCN and their families.
- Community outreach. This is measured using two indicators: community assessment of needs for CYSHCN and community outreach to agencies and schools.

Data management. This measures electronic data support and data retrieval capacity.

Quality improvement/change. This measures the quality standards structures and quality-related activities of the practice.

Practices rate each of 25 medical home quality indicators by selecting the appropriate level achieved by the practice, from level 1 to level 4, with level 4 being the highest.[42,45] The levels are selected based on the descriptions given for each level for each quality indicator. For each measure, the practice assesses whether the level has been partially or completely achieved based on whether the criteria described are fully or partially met.[42] Practices that plan to use the Medical Home Index are asked to inform the Center for Medical Home Improvement in writing of their intentions.

Medical Home Index—Short Version

The Medical Home Index—Short Version consists of 10 of the 25 indicators from the full Medical Home Index and uses a simplified response scale.[43] It is designed to be a quick report card when it is not feasible to complete the full version.

Medical Home Family Index and Survey

Practices that complete the medical home self-assessment are asked to obtain feedback from families of CYSHCN using the Medical Home Family Index and Survey.[42,44] This tool is designed for use with a cohort of families whose CYSHCN have received care at the practice for at least a year. The Family Index and Survey is composed of two major parts: the Family Index and the Center for Medical Home Improvement Family/Caregiver Survey.[44] The Family Index asks 25 questions assessing the care that the child receives from his or her PCP (eg, whether children get needed health care at any time of day, if the PCP listens to concerns and questions, and if the PCP has a care coordinator). The Family/Caregiver Survey asks for information regarding the child's health problems, health status, needed services, health care use, and family's involvement in specific care-coordination activities.

National Committee for Quality Assurance's Physician Practice Connections—Patient-centered Medical Home standards

The PPC-PCMH standards are congruent with the Joint Principles.[27] The program is intended to promote and evaluate nine practice standards: (1) access and communication, (2) patient-tracking and registry functions, (3) care management, (4) patient self-management support, (5) electronic prescribing, (6) test tracking, (7) referral tracking, (8) performance reporting and improvement, and (9) advanced electronic communications. Practices that apply for Physician Practice Connections recognition receive scores for the nine standards based on performance on 30 substandards, and can earn up to 100 points. Ten of the 30 substandards are considered "must-pass elements." To receive recognition as a patient-centered medical home, practices must score at least 25 of 100 points and pass at least 5 of 10 must-pass elements. These must-pass elements include:

- Written standards for patient access and patient communication
- Use of data to show standards for patient access and communication are met
- Use of paper or electronic charting tools to organize clinical information
- Use of data to identify important diagnoses and conditions in practice
- Adoption and implementation of evidence-based guidelines for three chronic conditions
- Active patient self-management support

- Systematic tracking of test results and identification of abnormal results
- Referral tracking using a paper or electronic system
- Clinical and/or service performance measurement by physician or across the practice
- Performance reporting by physician or across the practice[27]

Achieving recognition in the PPC-PCMH program offers some practices the opportunity to meet requirements for other programs or to qualify for additional payments. For example, PPC-PCMH recognition satisfies requirements for the Bridges to Excellence program.[29]

Medical Home Implementation Toolkit

Medical Home Implementation Toolkit, a new tool for assessing organizational progress toward implementing the medical home model, has been developed by AAP. Training was provided via teleconferences from March to June of 2009 (see http://www.medicalhomeinfo.org).

RECENT EXPANSION OF MEDICAL HOME INITIATIVES TO NONPEDIATRIC SETTINGS

Although pediatricians have led the development of medical home definition and implementation, organizations charged with caring or paying for the care of older patients have recognized the value of the medical home approach and moved to adopt it. As noted by Berenson:[2]

> *In Medicaid, the primary care case management model (is) oriented more to helping recipients gain access to care; it has had some success and is being expanded toward more fully conceived Medical Home approaches. For example, Carolina Access…is now being broadened to Community Care of North Carolina for patients with chronic conditions as a complement to the existing focus on patient-centeredness.*

The Commonwealth Fund 2006 Health Care Quality Survey found that when adults have a medical home, their access to needed care, receipt of routine preventive screenings, and management of chronic conditions improve substantially.[46] In contrast, disease and chronic care management programs that operate independently of physician practices tend not to reduce costs or improve quality significantly.[2]

Medicare Medical Home Demonstration Project

The Center for Medicare and Medicaid Services developed the Medicare Medical Home Demonstration Project to test the value of the model among family, internal medicine, geriatrics, general, specialty, and subspecialty practices.[47] The goal is to reward phased implementation of the medical home approach for care of adults with chronic conditions. Implementation will be scored using objective criteria for 28 specific core capabilities organized into six domains. Tier 1 practices must have 17 basic medical home capabilities. After determining the tier in which a practice may fall, per-member per-month case-management fees will be paid for all eligible patients in the practice with fees reflecting relative value units for medical home services and adjustment for patient complexity.[47,48]

A recent randomized trial of care coordination among Medicare beneficiaries in 15 care-coordination programs suggests that programs without strong transitional elements or person-to-person contact yielded little to no impact on health care expenditures and health care quality measures.[49]

Patient-Centered Primary Care Collaborative

The Patient-Centered Primary Care Collaborative (PCPCC) is a nationwide effort by large provider organizations, large employers, health plans, pharmaceutical companies, AARP (formerly the American Association of Retired Persons), the Commonwealth Fund and others to promote adoption of the PCMH.[50] The four leading primary care physician organizations involved agreed to adopt the PCPCC Joint Principles of the PCMH.[9]

BARRIERS TO ACHIEVING THE MEDICAL HOME MODEL

Numerous barriers obstruct the widespread dissemination and implementation of the medical home model of care delivery. These include dysfunctional financing, insufficient infrastructure, lack of interoperable computerized records, the need for provider education and training, demands on time, competing expectations of PCPs, lack of communication among multiple systems caring for CYSHCN, and the overall structure of the United States health care delivery systems, including a lack of integrated systems of care.[3,25,51] The costs associated with implementing the medical home model are significant and will need to be offset in some way.

ACKNOWLEDGMENTS

The authors thank Julie Jacobson Vann, PhD, and Charles G. Humble, PhD, for their many contributions to the early drafts of this manuscript.

REFERENCES

1. American Academy of Pediatrics, Council on Pediatric Practice. Pediatric records and a "medical home." In: Standards of child care. Evanston (IL): American Academy of Pediatrics; 1967. p. 77–9.
2. Berenson RA, Hammons T, Gans DN, et al. A house is not a home: keeping patients at the center of practice redesign. Health Aff 2008;27(5):1219–30.
3. Sia C, Tonniges TF, Osterhus E, et al. History of the medical home concept. Pediatrics 2004;113(5):1473–8.
4. American Academy of Pediatrics, Committee on standards of child health care. Standards of Child Health Care. 3rd edition. Evanston (IL): American Academy of Pediatrics; 1977.
5. Cash C. Role model: the visionary behind the medical home concept looks back on career milestones. AAP News 2007;28(6):24–5.
6. Dolins JC, Tait VF. American Academy of Pediatrics. Medical homes and community pediatrics at the AAP. 2008. Available at: http://www.medicalhomeinfo.org/Dolins%20Tait%20Memo%20-%20October%2008.pdf. Accessed December 29, 2008.
7. American Academy of Pediatrics. Medical Home Initiatives for Children with Special Health Needs Project Advisory Committee. The medical home, policy statement, organizational principles to guide and define the child health care system and/or improve the health of all children. Pediatrics 2002;110(1):184–6 (Reaffirmed: Pediatrics. 2008 (August); 122(2):450 doi:10.1542/peds.2008-1427.
8. American Academy of Pediatrics. Medical Home Initiatives for Children with Special Health Needs Project Advisory Committee. The medical home, policy statement, organizational principles to guide and define the child health care system and/or improve the health of all children. The medical home. Pediatrics 2004;113(5):1545–7.

9. American Academy of Family Physicians. American Academy of Pediatrics, American College of Physicians, American Osteopathic Association. Joint principles of the patient-centered medical home. 2007. Available at: http://www.medicalhomeinfo.org/Joint%20Statement.pdf. Accessed December 28, 2008.
10. American Academy of Pediatrics. What is a medical home? Available at: http://www.medicalhomeinfo.org; 2008. Accessed December 28, 2008.
11. Family Voices. Medicaid policy recommendations. June 2005. Available at: http://www.familyvoices.org/Information/Medicaid_Statement.pdf. Accessed February 23, 2009.
12. National Association of Pediatric Nurse Practitioners. NAPNAP position statement on pediatric healthcare/medical home: key issues on delivery, reimbursement, and leadership. Available at: http://www.napnap.org/userfiles/File/Pediatric Healthcare.pdf. Accessed February 23, 2009.
13. Trust for America's Health. Blueprint for a healthier America, modernizing the federal public health system to focus on prevention and preparedness. 2008. Available at: http://healthyamericans.org/report/55/blueprint-for-healthier-america. Accessed December 26, 2008.
14. Palfrey JS, Sofis LA, Davidson EJ, et al. The pediatric alliance for coordinated care: evaluation of a medical home model. Pediatrics 2004;113(5):1507–16.
15. Centers for Disease Control and Prevention. US Department of Health and Human Services, National Center for Health Statistics. Summary health statistics for US children: national health interview survey. 2006. 2007, Series 10, Number 234. Available at: http://www.cdc.gov/nchs/fastats/children.htm. Accessed December 26, 2008.
16. Centers for Disease Control and Prevention. National Center for Chronic Disease Prevention and Health Promotion. Diabetes projects. 2008. Available at: http://www.cdc.gov/DIABETES/projects/cda2.htm. Accessed December 26, 2008.
17. Nolan KW, Carter Young E, Baltus Hebert E, et al. Service coordination for children with complex healthcare needs in an early intervention program. Infants Young Child 2005;18(2):161–70.
18. American Academy of Pediatrics (5), Council on Children with Disabilities. Care coordination in the medical home: integrating health and related systems of care for children with special health care needs. Pediatrics 2005;116(5):1238–43.
19. Harvey J, Pinzon J. Care of adolescents with chronic conditions. Paediatr Child Health 2006;11:43–8.
20. Maternal and Child Health Bureau, Health Resources and Services Administration, US Department of Health and Human Services. The national survey of children with special health care needs chartbook 2005–2006. Rockville (MD): US Department of Health and Human Services. 2008. Available at: http://mchb.hrsa.gov/cshcn05. Accessed December 9, 2008.
21. Brock Martin A, Crawford S, Probst JC, et al. Medical homes for children with special health care needs. J Health Care Poor Underserved 2007;18(4):916–30.
22. Institute of Medicine. Crossing the quality chasm: a new health system for the 21st century. 2001. Available at: http://books.nap.edu/html/quality_chasm/reportbrief.pdf. Accessed December 16, 2008.
23. The Commonwealth Fund Commission on A High Performance Health System. (2008). Why not the best? Results from the national scorecard on US health system performance. 2008. Available at: http://www.commonwealthfund.org/publications/publications_show.htm?doc_id=401577. Accessed September 24, 2008.

24. Rittenhouse DR, Casalino LP, Gillies RR, et al. Measuring the medical home infrastructure in large medical groups. Health Aff 2008;27(5):1246–58.
25. Bodenheimer T. Primary care—Will it survive? N Engl J Med 2006;355(9):861–4.
26. Antonelli RC, Antonelli DM. Providing a medical home: the cost of care coordination services in a community-based, general pediatric practice. Pediatrics 2004;113(5):1522–8.
27. NCQA. Standards and guidelines for physician practice connections—patient-centered medical home (PPC-PCMH). 2008. Available at: http://www.ncqa.org/tabid/629/Default.aspx. Accessed December 17, 2008.
28. Schor EL. Rethinking well-child care. Pediatrics 2004;114:210–6.
29. Antonelli RC, Stille CJ, Freeman LC. Enhancing collaboration between primary and subspecialty care providers for children and youth with special health care needs. Georgetown University Center for Child and Human Development. 2005. Available at: http://gucchd.georgetown.edu/topics/special_health_needs/object_view.html?objectID=6582. Accessed December 20, 2008.
30. Homer CJ, Klatka K, Romm D, et al. A review of the evidence for the medical home for children with special health care needs. Pediatrics 2008;122(4):e922–37.
31. American Academy of Pediatrics. Medical home. Available at: http://www.aap.org/healthtopics/medicalhome.cfm. Accessed November 26, 2008.
32. Dubay L, Kenney GM. Health care access and use among low-income children: Who fares best? Health Aff 2001;20(1):112–21.
33. Berman S, Dolins J, Tang S, et al. Factors that influence the willingness of private primary care pediatricians to accept more Medicaid patients. Pediatrics 2002;110(2):239–48.
34. National Association of Community Health Centers (NACHC). America's Health Centers: making every dollar count. Available at: http://www.nachc.com/client/documents/issues-advocacy/policy-library/research-data/fact-sheets/Cost-Effectiveness-Fact-Sheet-12-06.pdf. Accessed February 18, 2009.
35. Strickland B, McPherson M, Weissman G, et al. Access to the medical home: results of the National Survey of Children with Special Health Care Needs. Pediatrics 2004;113(5):1485–92.
36. Denboba D, McPherson MG, Kenney MK, et al. Achieving family and provider partnerships for children with special health care needs. Pediatrics 2006;118(4):1607–15.
37. Turchi RM, Gatto M, Antonelli R. Children and youth with special healthcare needs: There is no place like (a medical) home. Curr Opin Pediatr 2007;19(4):503–8.
38. Liptak GA, Revell GM. Community physician's role in case management of children with chronic illnesses. Pediatrics 1989;84(3):465–71.
39. National Survey of Children with Special Health Care Needs. Available at: http://cshcndata.org/dataquery/SurveyAreas.aspx?yid=2. Accessed February 23, 2009.
40. Antonelli RC, Stille CJ, Antonelli DM. Care coordination for children and youth with special health care needs: a descriptive, multisite study of activities, personnel costs and outcomes. Pediatrics 2008;122:e122–216.
41. Antonelli R, McAllister J, Popp J. Developing care coordination as a critical component of a high performance pediatric health care system: forging a multidisciplinary framework for pediatric care coordination. The Commonwealth Fund, 2009, in press.
42. Center for Medical Home Improvement. The Medical Home Index, measuring the organization and delivery of primary care for children with special health

care needs. 2006. Available at: http://www.medicalhomeimprovement.org/assets/pdf/MHI-FullV_2006CMHI.pdf. Accessed December 17, 2008.
43. Center for Medical Home Improvement. The Medical Home Index—Short Version: measuring the organization and delivery of primary care for children with special health care needs. 2006. Available at: http://www.medicalhomeimprovement.org/assets/pdf/MHI-ShortV_2006CMHI.pdf. Accessed December 17, 2008.
44. Center for Medical Home Improvement. The medical home family index and survey. 2006. Available at: http://www.medicalhomeimprovement.org/assets/pdf/FamilyMHFI_Survey2006.pdf. Accessed January 3, 2009.
45. Cooley SC, McAllister JW, Sherrieb K, et al. The Medical Home Index: development and validation of a new practice-level measure of implementation of the medical home model. Ambul Pediatr 2003;3(4):173–80.
46. Beal AC, Doty MM, Hernandez SE, et al. Closing the divide: how medical homes promote equity in health care. Commonwealth Fund publication no. 1035. Available at: www.commonwealthfund.org. Accessed January 29, 2009.
47. Mathematica, Inc. Medicare medical home demonstration (MMHD): overview. Baltimore: Medicare and Medicaid Services; 2008.
48. Pope GC, Kautter J, Ellis RP, et al. Risk adjustment of Medicare capitation payments using the CMS-HCC model. Health Care Financ Rev 2004;25(4): 119–41.
49. Peikes D, Chen A, Schore J, et al. Effects of care coordination on hospitalization, quality of care, and health care expenditures among Medicare beneficiaries. JAMA 2009;301(6):603–18.
50. Patient-centered Primary Care Collaborative. Available at: http://www.pcpcc.net. Accessed January 30, 2009.
51. McAllister JW, Presler E, Cooley WC. Practice-based care coordination: a medical home essential. Pediatrics 2007;120(3):e723–33.

The Role of Health Information Technology in Quality Improvement in Pediatrics

Alan E. Zuckerman, MD[a,b,*]

KEYWORDS

- Health information technology • Quality improvement
- Pediatrics • Children • Interoperability

Health information technology (HIT) will play an important role in most efforts to improve the quality of pediatric medicine, as evident from the range of investigations and projects discussed in this volume. The importance of using information technology as an integral component of quality initiatives was identified early in the development of electronic medical records (EMR) in the classic paper by Clement McDonald, "Protocol-Based Computer Reminders, the Quality of Care and the Non-Perfectability of Man,"[1] That paper, published in 1976, demonstrated the need for computerized reminders in a crossover study in an internal medicine clinic. The role of HIT in quality improvement is not limited to tools integrated into EMR, but that remains an important strategy. Today, much attention is focused on interoperability of clinical systems that integrate and share data from multiple sources. There are also additional freestanding quality-improvement tools that can be used without an EMR. This article explores the many roles of HIT in quality improvement from several perspectives.

IDENTIFYING ROLES FOR HEALTH INFORMATION TECHNOLOGY WITHIN THE INSTITUTE OF MEDICINE DEFINITION OF QUALITY

In its 2001 report, *Crossing the Quality Chasm*, the Institute of Medicine set forward a six-part definition of quality and closely aligned each dimension of quality to the

[a] Department of Family Medicine, Georgetown University Hospital, 3800 Reservoir Rd NW # PHC2, Washington, DC 20007, USA
[b] Department of Pediatrics, Georgetown University Hospital, 3800 Reservoir Rd NW # PHC2, Washington, DC 20007, USA
* Department of Pediatrics, Georgetown University Hospital, 3800 Reservoir Rd NW # PHC2, Washington DC 20007.
E-mail address: aez@georgetown.edu

Pediatr Clin N Am 56 (2009) 965–973
doi:10.1016/j.pcl.2009.05.018 pediatric.theclinics.com

use of HIT.[2] Since that time, several pediatric investigators, most recently Spooner,[3] have expanded on this framework and illustrated its application. While it is easy to see how information technology directly affects safety, effectiveness, timeliness, and efficiency of care, the dimensions of equity and patient-centeredness are more elusive and harder to illustrate in meeting the quality-assurance needs of children. Equity is best represented as the use of HIT to reduce health disparities in children. Patient-centeredness represents the task of delivering patient care in the context of the patient's family and values. This has long been a quality goal for pediatric practice and an essential component of a medical home.[4] In 2009, a new report in the Institute of Medicine *Quality Chasm* series, *Computational Technology for Effective Health Care: Immediate Steps and Strategic Directions,* raises the challenge of "crossing the health care IT chasm" and creates a vision for twenty-first century health care and wellness through patient-centered cognitive support.[5]

FUNCTIONAL STRATEGIES FOR QUALITY IMPROVEMENT

Functional strategies separate systems that play an active, passive, or reporting role in quality improvement. A primary role of HIT is to help visualize data in an EMR. Documentation of care is often the focus of information system design. But attention should also be given to improving access to information in the record by making information more readily available and displaying that information in a way that can be understood quickly to support informed decision-making in a time-constrained patient-care environment. An important strategy for visualization is to aggregate and integrate data from multiple sources through interoperability among computer systems. Evaluation of growth and obesity, for example, is facilitated by extraction of all growth measurements and graphical display.[6] This function is more effective if measurements from other practices are combined with data in the current record. Complete immunization histories can be assembled by immunization registries[7] and aggregated medication histories are available through prescription benefit claims histories and data exchange among the inpatient, emergency, and ambulatory settings. Computer systems that deliver content and guidelines to the point of care assist quality improvement by integrating visualization of patient data with expert- and evidence-based guidelines. The Health Level 7 (HL7) information buttons enable integration of these external links into electronic record applications.

Systems that provide active clinical decision support represent a key goal for HIT and a national strategy and roadmap has been proposed by American Medical Informatics Association.[8] Such decision support may involve simple reminders for tasks that the clinician must perform or specific computer-generated orders and plans of care that can be implemented with a single click. Alternative HIT architectures for clinical decision support include self-contained decision-support modules used on the clinician's workstation or through access to a Web site. Interoperable clinical guidelines distribute decision logic using a rule-writing syntax, such as the Arden Syntax or GuideLine Implementability Appraisal,[9] that allows the EHR to run the rules on individual patient records at the time of care and generate advice that can be implemented during the visit. Because of the complexity and variability of decision-support requirements, focus has shifted to interoperable clinical data formats and Web services that separate the patient-care activities of the clinician (who may use a variety of computer systems) from the decision-support activities that can be performed at a central site independent of the site of patient care. Use of centralized Web-based decision support requires the use of deidentified data so that only the responsible clinician knows the patient identification and the decision recommendations. The development of the HL7 Decision Support Service[10] has created a framework for this type of Web service, which has the potential to make decision support widely available. It eliminates the need for each vendor or each health care institution to develop its own version of the same decision-support tool because data from diverse systems and organizations can share a single provider of decision support. Immunization forecasting (reviewing the vaccine history to assess what additional vaccines are required or recommended) has been one of the greatest decision-support needs for children and also has been a very complex task to implement in multiple environments. Through the work of Integrating the Healthcare Enterprise, standard profiles for sending immunization data[11] are now available and standard Web services are under development that can be shared by multiple EHR vendors and provided by multiple decision-support providers.

The newest role for HIT is to extract data for external quality reporting by providing an automated alternative to manual chart review. This task is most challenging because quality measures are more complex than the types of chart abstraction tools used for clinical research chart review. Many quality measures are population based and call for reports of percentages of children receiving appropriate services. Many others are time based and seek to identify status and outcomes at a point following initial diagnosis or treatment. Exclusion and inclusion criteria must be considered and some may require a minimal sample size. The Agency for Healthcare Research and Quality and the National Quality Forum are working to develop templates for automating chart review and quality reporting. The needs of children must be included.[12]

TYPES OF HEALTH INFORMATION TECHNOLOGY TOOLS FOR QUALITY IMPROVEMENT

Tools that are integrated into an EMR have become the standard approach to the use of HIT at the point of care, but other approaches should be considered. Tools that provide interoperability among information systems address the task of aggregating and assembling data for quality care decisions. Such tools are important in the care of children because of the need to monitor longitudinal data and be aware of events in other provider settings, particularly when a child is not accompanied by the parent who may have brought the child to an emergency room or to another encounter. Tools that are freestanding and used separately from the process of documenting care, are important because of the low EHR adoption rate in pediatrics.[13] Freestanding quality assurance is usually performed with Web-based tools and applications for mobile or handheld devices, such as cell phones and personal digital assistants. The mobile Internet browser on a cell phone is merging the two technologies of handheld applications and Web access in a single device. Tools for data mining and information discovery can use practice records to seek evidence for quality initiatives, evaluate specific needs of a practice for quality improvement, and generate patient-specific reminders for deficiencies, such as missing immunizations or screening tests. The use of service-oriented architecture (SOA) or Web services is an important strategy for sending patient data to a Web service that reviews the data and returns assessments and advice. SOA can also be used as a strategy to extract specific data elements from a practice information system through queries that select patients and return only the information needed for quality measurement or improvement, thus protecting patient privacy by excluding data not needed for the current analysis.

FEDERAL STRATEGIES FOR USING HEALTH INFORMATION TECHNOLOGY FOR QUALITY IMPROVEMENT

The Decade of Health Information, which began with the executive order creating the Office of the National Coordinator for Health Information Technology on April 27, 2004, has a 10-year goal for computerizing medical records for most Americans.[14] It was inspired by "Revolutionizing Health Care Through Information Technology,"[15] a report of the President's Information Technology Advisory Committee, and a later report, "Ending the Document Game," from the Congressional Commission on Systemic Interoperability.[16]

The federal strategy for using HIT for quality improvement, articulated through the strategic plans of the Office of the National Coordinator for Health Information Technology, involves a five-step process: (1) setting priorities for breakthroughs or transformations in health care than can be achieved through use of HIT, (2) development and harmonization of standards, (3) certification of EHR based on use of standard criteria, (4) creation of the Nationwide Health Information Network, and (5) monitoring of implementation and adoption. Throughout this process, attention is also given to protection of privacy of personal health information and to governance of networks and information exchange with goals of improving transparency of information while improving safety, increasing effectiveness, and reducing cost through quality improvement.

The setting of priorities began with the American Health Information Community and its workgroups and is now moving to successor organizations and advisory committees. The Health Information Standards Panel[17] has been responsible for standards harmonization and the Commission for Certification of Health Information Technology[18] has been the certification body. Several trial implementations of the Nationwide Health Information Network have demonstrated the breakthrough priorities in a variety of communities.[19] Many federal agencies have played a role in using HIT for quality improvement in children. The Agency for Healthcare Research and Quality[20] has funded a range of related projects, called Transforming Healthcare Quality Through Information Technology, and the Health Resources and Services Administration[21] has developed an HIT Toolkit to assist community health center networks in deploying HIT to improve quality. The National Institutes of Health has launched several translational research network projects to gather evidence for quality improvement, including the Newborn Screening Translational Research Network.[22] The Centers for Disease Control and Prevention has established the Public Health Information Network and provides important child health data on its Web site.[23]

A review of activities from the Office of the National Coordinator for Health Information Technology shows that use cases initiated under the federal HIT initiatives cover a wide range of quality-improvement targets:[24]

Consumer Empowerment: Registration & Medication History

This is a core summary record that transfers critical data from a personal health record or another EHR that might otherwise come from a waiting room clipboard and allows updates at each visit. Its use for children is an important strategy for supporting safe electronic prescribing in the context of past and current problems, medications, and allergies along with administrative assistance with demographics, insurance, and usual pharmacy.

Electronic Health Record: Laboratory Result Reporting

This assures that results are correctly transcribed into an EHR for review by a provider and for comparison with previous values. The challenges of result management in pediatrics have been identified as a quality-improvement target in pediatrics suitable for HIT interventions.[25]

Bio-Surveillance: Visit, Use, and Lab Result Data Remote Monitoring

This was intended as a tool for uncovering patterns of disease in the community, which could then inform providers of the risk of problems they might not otherwise expect. The target measures for bio-surveillance are designated by a separate data committee and transmitted using a standard set of electronic messages to capture data about visits or laboratory tests. The intended setting is primarily the emergency room, but the methods can also be applied to ambulatory visits in sentinel practices or to hospital admission. Separate tools are used to analyze and identify patterns in the data, which are reported on a continuous and timely basis.

Emergency Responder Electronic Health Record

This represents an attempt to improve quality through delivery of essential medical data in the field at times of accidents or disasters so as to maintain continuity of care and to avoid medication errors in emergencies. Data are moved from a previous medical summary to first-responder records, to emergency department records, and to definitive care, and are available to future primary care providers.

Consumer Empowerment: Consumer Access to Clinical Information

This extended the original use case to include a broader view of personal health records and their use to inform patients about their care. Children with special needs and chronic conditions can benefit as well as parents of all children. Adolescents create special privacy concerns as well as the need to assess their readiness to review their own laboratory results.

Medication Management

This addresses the medication reconciliation process at times of changes in providers, such as on admission and discharge from the hospital.

Quality

This is a use case for automated extraction of quality measures from an electronic health record based on a query template. Like bio-surveillance, the use case provides tools for sending data. Other committees must generate the targets of what data to send.

Patient Provider Secure Messaging

This extends encounters for patients with chronic conditions by messaging between office visits.

Personalized Healthcare

This brings genomic information to the provider through the collection of family health histories that can be transferred between systems and used as input for risk-analysis programs. The use case also provides a means of storing genetic testing data in an EHR. Genomic data carry lifelong significance and use of genetic testing and family history data should be part of quality child health care.

Consultations and Transfers of Care

This uses a structured medical summary to replace letters and can improve the sharing of data between primary care and specialists, thus facilitating better comanagement. Electronic documents that conform to the HL7 Clinical Document Architecture have a header section that allows automated filing of the letter into the correct patient chart with annotation of subject, type of document, and clinical encounter that generated the letter. Such electronic documents represent an improvement over dictated letters scanned into an

EHR. Clinical Document Architecture documents also include optional discrete coded data fields extracted from the human readable text. These make it possible for such data as diagnoses and codes, medication and doses, laboratory results, and vital signs to be extracted from the letter and copied into the patient's EHR for reuse and graphical display.[26]

Public Health Case Reporting

This sends electronic messages to health departments for reportable diseases.

Immunizations & Response Management

The most important use case for children, this enables sharing of immunization records between practices and immunization information systems or immunization registries.

Newborn Screening

This is a use case that addresses the mandatory interoperability that must occur among hospitals, public health workers, consumers, and ambulatory practices both for the initial screening as well as confirmatory testing and referral for management and follow-up of conditions detected. These data exchanges occur on paper and by phone if HIT tools are not mobilized to assure the completion of the process.

Medical Home: Problem Lists & Practice-Based Registries

This identifies key EMR enhancements required to deliver HIT support for a pediatric medical home model through enhanced problem lists and practice-based registries that allow tracking of services and guideline compliance for patients with chronic diseases and other special needs.

Maternal and Child Health

This addresses data integration issues among various providers and public health agencies needed to deliver available services to pregnant women and their infants.

Additional use cases, gaps, and extensions

Additional use cases, gaps, and extensions under development include those related to general laboratory orders, order sets medication gaps, clinical note details, common device connectivity, long-term care—assessments, consumer adverse event reporting, scheduling, prior authorization in support of treatment, payment, and operations.

STATE STRATEGIES FOR USING HEALTH INFORMATION TECHNOLOGY FOR PEDIATRIC QUALITY IMPROVEMENT

State strategies for using HIT for quality improvement are of special importance to children because of the role states have in controlling Medicaid and State Children's Health Insurance Programs and in integrating quality monitoring requirements into those programs. In October 2008, the State Alliance for e-Health issued its first report to the nation, *Accelerating Progress: Using Health Information Technology and Electronic Health Information Exchange to Improve Care*.[27] The report addresses recommendations on the state role in using HIT and health information exchange, including making a patient-centered, interoperable, and portable EHR available for every child by 2014. Medicaid Transformation Grant Programs have the potential to support new quality initiative infrastructures for children and many focus on improving data integration among diverse systems for Early and Periodic Screening Diagnosis and Treatment programs, immunization registries, and lead screening. School health programs represent another opportunity for quality improvement outside of conventional practice settings. Payer strategies for using HIT for pediatric quality improvement are often referred to as pay for performance. Projects within state Medicaid programs also have private-sector counterparts that may share criteria. Consumer strategies for using HIT for pediatric quality improvement include personal health records and efforts to improve transparency of quality and cost though health value exchanges.

Health information exchange strategies for using HIT for pediatric quality improvement may include placing HIT in practices so they can communicate with each other. The New York City Department of Health has installed electronic health records in over 1000 practices. MassShare, the state-level health information exchange for Massachusetts, is engaged in similar community-wide HIT implementations.

Section 1139A(d)(1)(D) and 1139A(f) of the Children's Health Insurance Program Reauthorization Act of 2009 calls for a project to demonstrate the impact of a model EHR format for children as part of quality measures for child health. This format will "allow interoperable exchanges that conform with Federal and State privacy and security requirements," will be "structured in a manner that permits parents and caregivers to view and understand the extent to which the care their children receive is clinically appropriate and of high quality," and will be "capable of being incorporated into, and otherwise compatible with, other standards developed for electronic health records." Newborn screening and newborn hospital discharge summaries could be a foundational component.

PRIVATE SECTOR STRATEGIES FOR USING HEALTH INFORMATION TECHNOLOGY FOR PEDIATRIC QUALITY IMPROVEMENT

The private sector has also developed strategies for using HIT for pediatric quality improvement through initiatives of professional societies and the work of organizations that advocate for the health of children. The Alliance for Pediatric Quality brings together several professional societies working on quality care for children.[28] The American Academy of Pediatrics Partnership for Policy Implementation seeks to create computable guidelines that will allow HIT to be mobilized to implement guidelines for care.[29] The special pediatric requirements for use of HIT have been well articulated in a policy statement from American Academy of Pediatrics[30] and in the HL7 EHR functional model for children. Children's hospitals have played an important role in advancing the use of HIT for quality improvement and also in providing personal health records for the children they serve to help maintain continuity of care among children with special needs and chronic diseases.[31] The use of HIT to reduce health disparities in children remains a frontier where HIT may be able to exert a leveling influence to improve quality and health outcomes.

DISASTER PREPAREDNESS AND USING HEALTH INFORMATION TECHNOLOGY FOR PEDIATRIC QUALITY IMPROVEMENT

Experiences of children following Hurricane Katrina have created a new awareness of the vulnerability of children.[32] The disruption of newborn screening programs and management of children with genetic disorders is a problem that HIT might address by helping to maintain continuity of services. The joint policy on emergency information forms for children with special needs developed jointly by The American Academy of Pediatrics and the American College of Emergency Medicine should be applied to all children. Forms are available on the Web and families are encouraged to keep these forms available when emergency care is needed. HIT can address this need and improve transfer of data from electronic records.

ON THE HORIZON

On February 17, 2009, President Obama signed the economic stimulus package, the American Recovery and Reinvestment Act, which provides $19 billion for health care information technology. The funds will be Medicare and Medicaid incentives for the adoption of the EHR and support for health information exchanges, EHR adoption, and other HIT efforts that depend on the evolving definition of "Meaningful Use".[33]

SUMMARY

HIT holds great promise for supporting quality-improvement efforts in pediatrics. Activities will continue to include a variety of strategies to make more data available when care decisions are made, to make guidelines on appropriate care available at the point of care, to automate the decision process and reminder process through clinical decision support, and to monitor the need for targeted intervention through quality reporting. Quality-improvement and monitoring activities based on the use of paper charts are resource intensive and can reach only a limited population. The use of HIT tools for quality improvement can integrate quality improvement into routine care for all children and make continuous quality improvement feasible.

REFERENCES

1. McDonald CJ. Protocol-based computer reminders, the quality of care and the non-perfectability of man. N Engl J Med 1976;295(24):1351–5.
2. Institute of Medicine, Committee on Quality of Health Care in America. Crossing the quality chasm. A new health system for the 21st century. Washington, DC: National Academy Press; 2001.
3. Spooner SA, Classen DC. Data standards and improvement of quality and safety in child health care. Pediatrics 2009;123(1):S74–9.
4. American Academy of Pediatrics, Medical Home Initiatives for Children with Special Needs Project Advisory Committee. Policy statement: the medical home. Pediatrics 2002;110(1):184–6, Reaffirmed May 2008.
5. Stead WW, Lin HS, editors. Computational technology for effective health care: immediate steps and strategic directions. Washington, DC: The National Academies Press; 2009.
6. Rattay KT, Ramakrishnan M, Atkinson A, et al. Use of an electronic medical record system to support primary care recommendations to prevent, identify, and manage childhood obesity. Pediatrics 2009;123(1):S100–7.
7. Fiks AG, Grundmeier RW, Biggs LM, et al. Impact of clinical alerts within an electronic health record on routine childhood immunization in an urban pediatric population. Pediatrics 2007;120(4):707–14.
8. Osheroff JA, Teich JM, Middleton B, et al. A roadmap for national action on clinical decision support. J Am Med Inform Assoc 2007;14(2):141–5.
9. Shiffman RN, Dixon J, Brandt C, et al. The GuideLine Implementability Appraisal (GLIA): development of an instrument to identify obstacles to guideline implementation. BMC Med Inform Decis Mak 2005;5:23.
10. Kawamoto K, Lobach D. Proposal for fulfilling strategic objectives of the US Roadmap for National Action on Decision Support through a service-oriented architecture leveraging HL7 services. J Am Med Inform Assoc 2007;14(2):146–55.
11. Integrating the Health Care Enterprise. Immunization profile page. Available at: http://www.ihe.net. Accessed April 7, 2009.
12. National Quality Forum. Project pages. Available at: http://www.qualityforum.org. Accessed April 7, 2009.

13. Kemper AR, Uren RL, Clark SJ. Adoption of electronic health records in primary care pediatric practices. Pediatrics 2006;118(1):e20–4.
14. Thompson TG, Brailer DJ. The decade of health information technology: framework for strategic action: delivering consumer-centric and information-rich health care. Washington, DC: Department of Health and Human Services; 2004.
15. President's Information Technology Advisory Committee. Revolutionizing health care through information technology. Washington, DC: National Coordination Office for Information Technology Research and Development; 2004.
16. Commission on Systemic Interoperability. Ending the document game: connecting and transforming your healthcare through information technology. Washington, DC: Government Printing Office; 2005.
17. Health Information Technology Standards Panel. Available at: http://www.hitsp.org. Accessed April 7, 2009.
18. Commission for Certification of Health Information Technology. Available at: http://www.cchit.org. Accessed April 7, 2009.
19. Office of the National Coordinator for Health Information Technology. Nationwide health information network pages. Available at: http://www.hhs.healthit/nhin. Accessed April 7, 2009.
20. Agency for Healthcare Research and Quality. Health information technology pages. Available at: http://www.ahrq.gov. Accessed April 7, 2009.
21. Health Resources and Services Administration. Maternal & child health pages. Available at: http://www.hrsa.gov. Accessed April 7, 2009.
22. National Institute of Child Health and Human Development. Newborn screening translational research network pages. Available at: http://nichd.nih.gov. Accessed April 7, 2009.
23. Center for Disease Control. Public health information network pages. Available at: http://www.cdc.gov. Accessed April 7, 2009.
24. Office of the National Coordinator for Health Information Technology. Use case pages. Available at: http://healthit.hhs.gov under Standards and Certification. Accessed June 19, 2009.
25. Ferris TG, Johnson SA, Co JPT, et al. Electronic results management in pediatric ambulatory care: qualitative assessment. Pediatrics 2009;123:S85–91.
26. Dolin RH, Alschuler L, Boye S, et al. HL7 clinical document architecture, release 2. J Am Med Inform Assoc 2006;13(1):30–9.
27. National Governors Association Center for Best Practices. State alliance for e-health pages. Available at: http://www.nga.org/center/health. Accessed April 7, 2009.
28. Miles PV, Miller M, Payne DM, et al. Alliance for Pediatric Quality. Alliance for Pediatric Quality: creating a community of practice to improve health care for America's children. Pediatrics 2009;123(1):S64–6.
29. American Academy of Pediatrics. Partnership for policy implementation pages. Available at: http://www.aap.org/qualityimprovement. Accessed April 7, 2009.
30. Spooner SA, Council on Clinical Information Technology. Special requirements of electronic health record systems in pediatrics. Pediatrics 2007;119:631–7.
31. Menachemi N, Brooks RG, Schwalenstocker E, et al. Use of health information technology by children's hospitals in the United States. Pediatrics 2009;123:S80–4.
32. Rath B, Donato J, Duggan A, et al. Adverse health outcomes after Hurricane Katrina among children and adolescents with chronic conditions. J Health Care Poor Underserved 2007;18(2):405–17.
33. Blumenthal D. Stimulating the adoption of health information technology. N Engl J Med 2009;360(15):1477–9.

Nursing: Key to Quality Improvement

Susan R. Lacey, PhD, RN[a,b,c,*], Karen S. Cox, RN, PhD[a,c]

KEYWORDS

• Nursing • Quality • Nurse-sensitive indicators • NQF • NDNQI

In the past two decades, a great deal of evidence generated through empirical findings has suggested that nurses and effective nursing care contribute to quality patient outcomes;[1–5] however, most of these findings have been based on large-scale studies that have not included institutions that exclusively care for children. In addition, the Institute of Medicine has published several key documents that demonstrate strong links between nursing and patient quality.[6,7] Patients who are admitted to inpatient settings are there primarily for 24-hour surveillance of health care status (ie, vital signs, improvements, deterioration), to receive therapeutic regimens prescribed by physicians, as well as to receive nursing interventions driven by the patient's condition. All other types of care can be delivered in an outpatient setting. Disentangling nursing care and interventions linked to specific patient outcomes is complicated by two factors: (1) clinical or health information systems or electronic charting systems do not systematically collect nursing interventions in discreet data fields for adequate analysis, similar to how physician diagnoses and orders are captured for billing (eg, International Classification of Disease codes and diagnosis-related groups); and (2) nursing care has traditionally been included in the daily charge rate for reimbursement, which creates no real incentive for organizations to collect individual nursing actions.[8] In the coming months, these barriers must be addressed or organizations stand to lose millions in reimbursement because the Centers for Medicare and Medicaid Services have indicated reduced or no reimbursement for "never events," that is, adverse events that occur in the inpatient setting, many of which are nurse sensitive[9] as follows:

Object inadvertently left in after surgery
Air embolism
Blood incompatibility

[a] Bi-State Nursing Workforce Innovation Center, UMKC School of Nursing, 2464 Charlotte Street, Room 3413, Kansas City, MO 64108, USA
[b] Nursing Workforce and Systems Analysis, UMKC School of Nursing, 2464 Charlotte Street, Room 3413, Kansas City, MO 64108, USA
[c] Children's Mercy Hospitals and Clinics, 2401 Gillham Road, Kansas City, MO 64108, USA
* Corresponding author. Children's Mercy Hospitals and Clinics, 2401 Gillham Road, Kansas City, MO 64108.
E-mail address: srlacey@cmh.edu (S.R. Lacey).

Pediatr Clin N Am 56 (2009) 975–985
doi:10.1016/j.pcl.2009.05.004 pediatric.theclinics.com
0031-3955/09/$ – see front matter

Catheter-associated urinary tract infection
Pressure ulcer (decubitus ulcer)
Vascular catheter-associated infection
Surgical site infection—mediastinitis (infection in the chest) after coronary artery bypass graft surgery
Certain types of falls and trauma
Surgical site infections following certain elective procedures, including certain orthopedic surgeries, and bariatric surgery for obesity
Certain manifestations of poor control of blood sugar levels
Deep vein thrombosis or pulmonary embolism following total knee replacement and hip replacement procedures

Although only a few of these current never events translate to the pediatric population, it is clear that this trend of not paying for adverse events will continue to enter the health care payment structure and undoubtedly include other payer types and adverse events.

Two key studies have used pediatric patient outcomes and nurse staffing. Both found that units with better staffing (eg, a lower nurse-to-patient ratio) had better quality outcomes.[10,11] Absent of additional studies using pediatric settings exclusively, there is no reason to assume that the same link between nurse staffing and patient outcomes does not exist. This article explains in detail the importance of nursing care in the quality agenda and explores the existing gaps in this field of science. In addition, key stakeholders and groups that advocate and focus on specific quality agendas within the field of pediatrics are briefly described. Pediatric health care uses a multidisciplinary model of delivery with physicians and nurses as key drivers of that care; however, each discipline uses specific domains of knowledge and interventions, making it difficult to separate them when evaluating patient outcomes. Much work needs to be conducted using health services research approaches that link and partition the overall and combined contribution of discipline-specific providers.

REGISTERED NURSES AND PATIENT OUTCOMES

The findings of numerous large-scale studies are very clear—greater numbers of registered nurses (RNs) positively impact the quality of patient care. The Agency for Healthcare Research and Quality published a meta-analysis of 94 studies that found an increased number of RNs was associated with decreased mortality, a shorter length of stay, and a lower risk of adverse events.[5] Most of these studies used staffing variables identified as RN full-time equivalents or a percentage concentration of RNs to other type of licensed and nonlicensed nursing personnel associated with specific types of gross patient outcomes such as mortality. A portion of these studies used patient outcomes aggregated at the hospital level, with a small group of studies using the nursing "unit" as the level of analysis. More refined studies have sought to understand the relationship between nurse staffing and specific patient outcomes deemed "nurse sensitive." Nurse-sensitive outcomes are those in which the actions (or lack of actions) of nurses impact patient outcomes. Experts who study this area of outcomes research have suggested a list of key indicators that are most likely nurse sensitive. They are urinary tract infections, pneumonia, shock, hemorrhage in the upper gastrointestinal tract, the length of stay in medical patients, and the failure to rescue in surgical patients.[4]

NURSING PREPARATION AND PATIENT OUTCOMES

A growing body of literature suggests that units staffed with nurses who have predominantly completed programs of study at least at the baccalaureate (BSN) level (4-year programs) have better patient outcomes when compared with those staffed primarily with graduates of 3-year diploma (hospital-based programs) or 2-year associate degree programs. These studies have included gross and specific patient outcome measures.[12,13] What is not understood is how the nurses' role is improved given more education. The logic is that a more comprehensive education produces an RN with better surveillance, critical thinking, and technical skills, but these specific relationships have not yet been defined by this program of research. More refined work needs to be conducted to help clarify this phenomenon, as well as more funding allocated to do so.

NURSING SKILL MIX AND PATIENT OUTCOMES

In addition to good evidence suggesting that education and the concentration of RN full-time equivalents are important to quality, the skill mix of nursing personnel (including RNs, licensed vocational/practical nurses [LVN, LPNs], and nursing assistants [NAs]) impacts quality outcomes. Research has found that hospital units where more RNs are employed in comparison with LPNs and NAs have better outcomes than when this mix of staff is reversed.[14,15]

A detailed comprehensive reference for the link between nurse staffing and patient outcomes is provided in a key resource document from the Agency for Healthcare Research and Quality partially funded by the Robert Wood Johnson Foundation. The text, entitled "Patient Safety and Quality: An Evidence-Based Handbook for Nurses," can be obtained from the agency or downloaded from their Web site.[16,17] In addition, the chapter on pediatric safety is a valuable resource for children's care in general as well as key nursing issues.[18]

TWO KEY STUDIES

Two studies have used pediatric patients exclusively when examining the link between nurse staffing and patient outcomes.[10,11] The first study was conducted in 2003 with administrative data from seven academic, not-for-profit children's hospitals, including 16 medical/surgical, 5 oncology, and 12 intensive care units.[10] The study looked at the association between staffing and five outcomes: medication errors, central line infections, blood stream infections, intravenous infiltrations, and patient or family complaints. The findings indicated a strong inverse relationship between a greater concentration of RN hours to other types of nursing providers on units and the rates of central line and blood stream infections.

Other key findings offered insight into the use of "agency" or "float" nurses. Lower blood stream infections occurred when there were lower concentrations of these types of RNs on the unit. Agency nurses are those who are not employed by the hospital but rather contracted through a third-party staffing vendor. They may or may not know the hospital, its policies, or protocols.

Nurses who "float" are those who are hired to work on one particular unit but due to patient census are pulled to unfamiliar units to work shifts to complete the staffing rosters. They are disadvantaged in that they know less about the unit in terms of policies, patient diagnoses, and even where supplies are kept. In an emergency, knowing where equipment is kept may be a matter of life or death. We know little about the impact of agency and float nurses. As the nursing shortage grows and hospitals are forced to fill the gaps with these types of alternative providers, it will be imperative that we have better data to understand this potential impact on patient outcomes.

It is unreasonable to assert that any nurse can work any unit on any given day. The practice analogy for physicians is that a gastroenterologist can easily move to a cardiovascular unit to take a patient load, which would be unthinkable. Yet this practice is performed on a regular basis in settings with nursing personnel. This type of administrative practice will be tested in the next few years as the need for more staff nurses increases due to the aging baby boomers and their increased consumption of health care goods and services. It is unclear through empirical studies how this impacts overall patient outcomes (adverse events) specifically, and much of this uncertainty is thought to be due to issues related to reporting these events, but, again, the paucity of evidence makes this an assumption and not a fact.

The second pediatric study examined mortality and other complications in children using a large administrative data set of 3.65 million hospital discharges from 288 general and children's hospitals within the state of California.[11] The methods used to describe RN staffing were more sensitive in this study in that they used the Medstat's Resource Demand Scale index (RDScale) calculated for each patient rather than the standard calculation of RN staffing which relies on the Centers for Medicare and Medicaid Services case mix method. The case mix method has been the predominant way in which these large-scale studies have been designed.

The findings from this study suggested that greater resource-adjusted RN care was related to significant reductions in postoperative blood infections, postoperative pneumonia, and pulmonary complications. There was also evidence of lower urinary tract infections but only within institutions with higher adjusted RN care. There was no significant relationship between adjusted RN care and mortality in this study.

MAGNET HOSPITAL DESIGNATION AND PATIENT OUTCOMES

The Magnet Recognition Program is sponsored by the American Nurses Credentialing Center.[19,20] Magnet status has been referred to as the gold standard of practice environments for nursing personnel. It is the only recognition program that focuses exclusively on nursing practice issues and culture. Hospitals that obtain Magnet designation do so after a rigorous application process followed by an intense site visit by professional Magnet appraisers, and not all hospitals that apply obtain this distinction. The criteria for evaluation include demonstrated excellence in nursing practice which includes, but is not limited to, nursing autonomy, nursing research, and the opportunity for professional development through credentialing in specialty areas.

Research over the past 2 decades indicates that hospitals with Magnet designation have better nursing outcomes (turnover and satisfaction) as well as better patient outcomes.[2,21,22] Again, the assertion is that when nurses have more input in their professional practice environments and can implement research or quality improvement projects, patients are likely to benefit from this level of engagement.

INTERDISCIPLINARY TEAMS

Although nursing personnel represent the largest group of caregivers within the health care setting, the keys to success in improvement and quality regardless of the population are the collective efforts of nurses, physicians, and the wide range of provider types that support the pediatric client through the continuum of care. No single group of providers can do this work alone. It is an accurate assertion that physicians write the orders for medical care that must be administered to move the patient from illness to wellness or safe passage in palliative care; however, without nurses performing the interventions linked to these orders while continually monitoring the patients' reactions to them, there can be little hope that the patient and family will have safe passage through the systems of care. In addition, nurses have their own unique body of knowledge and nursing interventions that are based on the condition of the patient. This intersection of medical and nursing interventions is imperative to create the environment needed to improve patient outcomes. Interdisciplinary teams and strong communication among patients, families, and providers are critical. The nurse, who spends more time with the patient than physicians, is the caregiver who can collect appropriate patient data (eg, test results, reactions to therapies) and monitor physician (eg, orders and protocols) and nursing inputs (medical and nursing interventions and the response to these interventions) to create a clear picture of the current status of the patient as well as facilitate discussions for subsequent orders that must be included in the plan of care.

Critical Communication Between Providers

In 2005 a report by the Joint Commission found that the root cause of 70% of more than 2400 sentinel events was communication failure between providers or between family and providers. In those 70% of events, 75% of the patients died due to this type failure.[22] Children are even more vulnerable because staff rely heavily on surrogates (eg, parents or advocates) to communicate for them about their history or reactions to certain drugs and therapies.[23]

Many studies suggest the importance of good communication between providers, even in settings where there is a more hierarchical nature (physician over the RN). To achieve the best outcomes for patients, critical communication in the culture of the unit or hospital must include the ability of provider exchange to get the person's attention, express concern, state the problem, propose an action, and reach a decision.[24] These actions must be conducted in a mutually respectful atmosphere without fear of retribution. The nature of trust, although not a part of this discussion, is paramount to the overall interchange required to ensure the patient does not get caught in the middle of dysfunctional communication between providers.

In an effort to address this critical communication between providers, a system called situation background assessment recommendation (SBAR) has been introduced into hospital systems. Although we are still determining the success of this system, it is far better than having no specific plan of action in transferring information, particularly when patient status is rapidly deteriorating and time is of the essence.[25]

PEDIATRIC-SPECIFIC EFFORTS

All specialty areas by population within health care have attempted to carve out unique contributions to move the quality agenda forward. The same is true for pediatric clients. Absent of a few, most of these groups are interdisciplinary in nature, if not by design then by implementation. For example, the American Academy of Pediatrics[26] has created standards of care for certain patient conditions, but without the implementation of these standards by nurses (or other types of providers such as physical, occupational, or respiratory therapists) in the day-to-day care of patients, there would be little opportunity to actualize these standards at the bedside or clinic environment. Likewise, most organizations that create standards of care have input from a wide variety of providers as well as consumers to ensure the standards are applicable in today's complex health care systems and with the current state of primary and third-party payers.

NURSING INITIATIVES

National Quality Forum

The National Quality Forum (NQF) is a not-for-profit group with strong private-public partnerships that seeks to improve quality for all citizens across the continuum of care.[27] Nursing quality is part of their agenda, with the full understanding that nurses are principal caregivers in today's health care environment. In addition, the NQF recognizes that nurses act as follows:

> *...as the principal caregivers in any healthcare system, directly and profoundly affect the lives of patients and are critical to the quality of care patients receive. However, patient acuity and shorter lengths of stay, the nursing shortage, changing technology, expansion of public and community health services, and higher patient expectations have produced a greater demand for care, mounted financial pressure, and limited nursing resources. Today's nurses practice in a constrained environment that tests the core of their contribution to quality.*

National Quality Forum–endorsed National Voluntary Consensus Standards for Nursing-sensitive Care

The NQF has framed a variety of important issues when recognizing, reporting, and enriching the data that can be generated by nursing practice:[28,29]

> *As "nursing-sensitive," these consensus standards include measures of processes and outcomes—and structural proxies for these processes and outcomes (eg, skill mix, nurse staffing hours)—that are affected, provided, and/or influenced by nursing personnel—but for which nursing is not exclusively responsible.*
>
> *These consensus standards are intended for use by the public and other healthcare stakeholders to evaluate the extent to and ways in which nurses in acute care hospitals contribute to patient safety, healthcare quality, and a professional work environment.*

Three domains of nurse-sensitive measures reflect the proximity and types of nursing actions and inputs to the specific outcome group: (1) patient-centered measures, which focus on specific patient outcomes; (2) nursing interventions, which focus on the fundamental teaching and interventions for preventable adverse events linked to comorbid conditions; and (3) system-centered outcomes, which evaluate the provision of nursing care in terms of quantity and skill mix by the organization. The list in **Box 1** outlines these specific measures within each of these domains.[28]

As previously indicated, numerous studies have explicated the link between the educational level of RNs and patient outcomes.[12,13] This emerging science offers great opportunity to strengthen nurses. One additional key initiative for the nursing profession is to find ways to infuse quality language and education into nursing education, which has been by and large absent from accreditation standards in the past. The NQF advocates for the following:[28]

> *...recognizes the contribution of nurses to patient safety and healthcare outcomes. While measurable outcomes have been associated with higher levels of education it is difficult to determine the extent that variations in earnings, perception of health, smoking rates, voting patterns, and other outcomes are solely attributable to education and how much to other factors.*

National Database for Nursing Quality Indicators

The National Database of Nursing Quality Indicators (NDNQI) is a proprietary database of the American Nurses Association.[30] The database collects and evaluates unit-specific, nurse-sensitive data from diverse hospitals across the United States.

Hospitals that are part of the Magnet Recognition Program must participate in a national database to compare their patient outcomes with those of similar units.

Box 1
Three domains of nurse-sensitive measures

Patient-centered outcome measures

Death among surgical inpatients with treatable serious complications (failure to rescue): percentage of major surgical inpatients who experience a hospital-acquired complication and die

Pressure ulcer prevalence: percentage of inpatients who have a hospital-acquired pressure ulcer

Falls prevalence: number of inpatient falls per inpatient days

Falls with injury: number of inpatient falls with injuries per inpatient days

Restraint prevalence: percentage of inpatients who have a vest or limb restraint

Urinary catheter-associated urinary tract infection for ICU patients: rate of urinary tract infections associated with use of urinary catheters for ICU patients

Central line catheter-associated blood stream infection rate for ICU and high-risk nursery patients: rate of blood stream infections associated with use of central line catheters for ICU and high-risk nursery patients

Ventilator-associated pneumonia for ICU and high-risk nursery patients: rate of pneumonia associated with use of ventilators for ICU and high-risk nursery patients

Nursing-centered intervention measures

Smoking cessation counseling for acute myocardial infarction: percentage of patients with a history of smoking within the past year who received smoking cessation advice or counseling during hospitalization

Smoking cessation counseling for heart failure: percentage of patients with a history of smoking within the past year who received smoking cessation advice or counseling during hospitalization

Smoking cessation counseling for pneumonia: percentage of patients with a history of smoking within the past year who received smoking cessation advice or counseling during hospitalization

System-centered measures

Skill mix: percentage of RN, LVN/LPN, unlicensed assistive personnel, and contracted nurse care hours to total nursing care hours

Nursing care hours per patient day: number of RNs per patient day and number of nursing staff hours (RN, LVN/LPN, and unlicensed assistive personnel) per patient day

Practice Environment Scale–Nursing Work Index: composite score and scores for the five subscales of (1) nurse participation in hospital affairs; (2) nursing foundations for quality of care; (3) nurse manager ability, leadership, and support of nurses; (4) staffing and resource adequacy; and (5) collegiality of nurse-physician relations

Voluntary turnover: number of voluntary uncontrolled separations during the month by category (RNs, advanced practice nurses, LVN/LPNs, NAs)

The NDNQI is primarily the database to which the majority of these institutions contribute information on the following nurse indicators:[30]

- Nurse turnover
- Patient falls/injury falls
- Hospital- and unit-acquired pressure ulcers
- Physical/sexual assault
- Pain assessment/intervention/reassessment cycle

- Peripheral intravenous infiltration
- Physical restraints
- Nosocomial infections
  - Catheter-associated urinary tract infections
  - Central line–associated blood stream infections
  - Ventilator-associated pneumonia
- Staff mix
  - RNs
  - LPNs/LVNs
  - Unlicensed assistive personnel
- Nursing care hours provided per patient day
- RN education/certification
- RN survey
  - Practice Environment Scales option
  - Job Satisfaction Scales option
  - Job Satisfaction Scales–Short Form option

Translating Care at the Bedside

The Translating Care at the Bedside (TCAB) program is a funded initiative started by the Robert Wood Johnson Foundation and the Institute of Medicine.[31] This program focuses on nurse-driven identification of problem areas of care (patient outcomes) or process issues (eg, workflow). Front-line staff nurses are more likely to be attuned to the issues that involve their care environment and often know best how to solve their own problems. Hospitals and units are selected for funding by this initiative, but their selection is met by substantial resources, training, and continued coaching and mentoring of the TCAB nurses in order for them to succeed with their projects. To date, there are ten hospitals participating in this important initiative, and the reporting of outcomes is in progress. For a snapshot of this work, the reader may review the TCAB Web site or a series of articles in the *American Journal of Nursing*.[32]

PLANNING FOR THE PEDIATRIC HEALTH CARE WORKFORCE

It is difficult to imagine that if there was a pressing need to determine how many pediatric nurses there were in the United States one would not be able to do so; however, in 2008 Lacey and colleagues[33] found that there is no formal tracking of nurses who work in pediatric settings within any entity that collects nursing data. They presented a call to action for finding ways to determine a sound methodology for tracking the supply-demand chain of pediatric nurses to meet the demands of the future, which looks perilous as more children are diagnosed with chronic diseases and funding for children's health lacks stability. In addition, national nursing organizations must collaborate with physician groups to have the right provider with the right patient at the right time in their care, including pediatric patients.

SUMMARY

In light of the current and potentially long-term financial crisis in the United States, there will be significant competing demands for how the nation's budget is spent. Although the authors understand the need to shore up our financial and business markets, it is critical that we simultaneously address our crippled health care system. Economic experts agree that this must be part of the overall solution for fiscal health. If we do not have children who have adequate and appropriate access to health care not only for disease states but for prevention, we will fail to produce a viable and thriving workforce that can contribute to the tax base and national productivity of goods and services to make us competitors in the world economy. It will take a collective effort not only by advocates for children but also by advocates for all citizens to move a different, more innovative agenda forward. Only then will we see a significant return on investment for human capital that will again put the United States on the road to prosperity and health for years to come.

Most importantly, those who care for all Americans must be taught basic concepts and application of quality improvement techniques.[34,35] We have continued for too long to add on to the list of concepts we must teach our students in nursing, medicine, as well as other professional programs of study. These curricular elements are as fragmented as our health care system. There is no perfect science in quality improvement, but basic understanding of core concepts is critical to address our current and future practice settings. Quality improvement is not for one department. It is incumbent on all of us to know these basic tenets and their application in health care. Perhaps it is time to form a common group of concepts, techniques, and language to be included across professional curricula so that all can function proficiently together regardless of the diagnosis or symptom each may encounter and across the continuum of care.

ACKNOWLEDGMENTS

The authors thank Adrienne Olney, MS, at the Bi-State Nursing Workforce Innovation Center for support with this manuscript.

REFERENCES

1. Aiken LH, Clarke SP, Sloane DM, et al. Nurses' reports of hospital quality of care and working conditions in five countries. Health Aff 2001;20:43–53.
2. Aiken LH, Smith HL, Lake ET. Lower Medicare mortality among a set of hospitals known for good nursing care. Med Care 1994;32:771–87.
3. Blegan MA, Goode CJ, Reed L. Nurse staffing and patient outcomes. Nurs Res 1998;47:43–50.
4. Needleman J, Buerhaus P, Mattke S, et al. Nurse-staffing levels and the quality of care in hospitals. N Engl J Med 2002;346:1715–22.
5. Kane RL, Shamliyan TA, Mueller C, et al. The association of registered nurse staffing levels and patient outcomes: systematic review and meta-analysis. Med Care 2007;45(12):1195–204.
6. Committee on Quality of Health Care in America, Institutes of Medicine. Crossing the quality chasm. Washington (DC): National Academies Press; 2001.
7. Committee on Quality of Health Care in America, Institutes of Medicine. Keeping patients safe: transforming the work environment of nurses. Washington (DC): National Academics Press; 2004.
8. Lacey SR, Cox KS, O'Donnell R. Flying the murky skies: the roles nurses can play in solving "never events." Mod Healthc 2008;38(26):26.
9. Centers for Medicare and Medicaid Services. Available at: www.cms.hhs.gov. Accessed January 15, 2009.
10. Stratton KM. The relationship between pediatric nurse staffing and quality of care in the hospital setting [dissertation]. Denver (CO): University of Colorado Health Sciences Center; 2005. Dissertation Abstract International, 66(11). DAI-B. (UMI No. AAT 3196584).
11. Mark BA, Harless DW, Berman WF. Nurse staffing and adverse events in hospitalized children. Policy Polit Nurs Pract 2007;8(2):83–92.

12. Aiken LH, Clarke SP, Cheung RB, et al. Education levels of hospital nurses and patient mortality. JAMA 2003;290:1617–23.
13. Blegan MA, Vaughn T, Goode CJ. Nurse experience and education: effect on quality of care. J Nurs Adm 2001;31:33–9.
14. Jarman BS, Cault S, Alves B, et al. Explaining differences in English hospital death rates using routinely collected data. Br Med J 1999;318:1515–20.
15. Aiken LH, Clarke SP, Sloane DM, et al. Hospital nurse staffing and patient mortality: nurse burnout and job dissatisfaction. JAMA 2002;288:1987–93.
16. Clarke SP, Donaldson NE. Nurse staffing and patient care quality and safety. In: Hughes RG, editor. Patient safety and quality: an evidence-based handbook for nurses. Rockville (MD): Agency for Healthcare Research and Quality; 2008.
17. The Robert Wood Johnson Foundation. Health and health care improvement. Available at: www.rwjf.org. Accessed January 15, 2009.
18. Lacey S, Smith JB, Cox K. Pediatric safety and quality. In: Hughes RG, editor. Patient safety and quality: an evidence-based handbook for nurses. Rockville (MD): Agency for Healthcare Research and Quality; 2008.
19. American Nurses Credentialing Center. Available at: http://www.nursecredentialing.org/Magnet.aspx. Accessed January 15, 2009.
20. McClure ML, Hinshaw AS. The future of magnet hospital. In: McClure ML, Hinshaw AS, editors. Magnet hospitals revisited. Washington (DC): American Nurses Association Publishing; 2002. p. 117–27.
21. Mark BA, Salyer J, Wan TT. Professional nursing practice: impact on organizational and patient outcomes. J Nurs Adm 2002;33:224–34.
22. Joint Commission on Accreditation of Healthcare Organizations. Sentinel event statistics. Available at: http://www.jointcommission.org/SentinelEvents/Statistics. Accessed January 15, 2009.
23. Agency for Healthcare Research and Quality. 20 tips to help preventmedical errors in children. Rockland (MD): AHRQ; 2002. Publication No. 02–P034.
24. Leonard M, Graham S, Bonacum D. The human factor: the critical importance of effective teamwork and communication in providing safe care. Qual Saf Health Care 2004;13:i85–90.
25. Institute for Healthcare Improvement. SBAR technique for communication: a situational briefing. Available at: http://www.ihi.org/IHI/Topics/PatientSafety/SafetyGeneral/Tools/SBARTechniqueforCommunicationASituationalBriefingModel.htm. Accessed January 15, 2009.
26. American Academy of Pediatrics. Available at: www.aap.org. Accessed January, 2009.
27. National Quality Forum (NQF). Available at: www.qualityforum.org. Accessed January, 2009.
28. Nursing Care Quality at NQF. Available at: www.qualityforum.org/nursing/#measures. Accessed January 15, 2009.
29. National Quality Forum. Nurses' educational preparation and patient outcomes in acute care: a case for quality. Available at: www.qualityforum.org/pdf/nursing-quality/FinalNursesEdPreparation.pdf. Accessed January 15, 2009.
30. National Database of Nursing Quality Indicators (NDNQI). Available at: www.nursingquality.org. Accessed January, 2009.
31. Transforming Care at the Bedside. Available at: www.ihi.org/IHI/Programs/TransformingCareAtTheBedside. Accessed January 15, 2009.
32. American Journal of Nursing. Available at: http://www.nursingcenter.com/search/search.asp?query=TCAB&R1=V2&section=0&searchAll=1henursingcenter.com. Accessed January 15, 2009.

33. Lacey SR, Kilgore M, Yun H, et al. Secondary analysis of merged American Hospital Association (AHA) data and US Census data: beginning to understanding the supply-demand chain in pediatric inpatient. J Pediatr Nurs 2008;23(2):161–8.
34. Cronenwett L, Serwood G, Barnsteiner J, et al. Quality and safety education for nurses. Nurs Outlook 2007;55(3):122–31.
35. Voss JD, May NB, Schorling JB, et al. Changing conversations: teaching safety and quality in residency training. Acad Med 2008;83(11):1080–7.

Maintenance of Certification: The Role of the American Board of Pediatrics in Improving Children's Health Care

Paul V. Miles, MD

KEYWORDS

• Quality • Quality improvement • Maintenance of certification • Professional development

Board certification in American health care began in 1911 and grew out of the *Flexner Report*, which addressed major concerns about the quality of medical education. The American Board of Pediatrics (ABP) was one of the first boards formed. The ABP was created in 1933 by the American Academy of Pediatrics, the American Pediatric Society, and the pediatric section of the American Medical Association to address the issue of who should be called a "pediatrician."[1] At the time, some physicians with little or no training in children's care were calling themselves pediatricians. The ABP was created to answer the question: "What education and training should be required of physicians to provide the best care for children and warrant the title of pediatrician?" The concern about physician quality continued to spread to other clinical areas and eventually led to the establishment of the American Board of Medical Specialties (ABMS), which now has 24 members across all specialties. No other country has a similar voluntary process for defining and assessing physician expertise in specialty care. Pediatric certification initially addressed only general pediatric care. Subspecialty certification began with pediatric cardiology in 1961 and there are now 14 certified pediatric subspecialties, the newest being child abuse pediatrics, which was created in 2007. Over the years, the ABP has certified over 90,000 pediatric generalists and subspecialists. Today, the almost 250 pediatric leaders from around the country who make up the ABP set standards and develop tools to help pediatricians assess their level of knowledge and skills to deliver quality care.

The model for assessing physician quality for the first 7 decades was based on demonstrating medical knowledge: "The more you know, the better the care you

The American Board of Pediatrics, 111 Silver Cedar Court, Chapel Hill, NC 27514, USA
E-mail address: pvm@abpeds.org

Pediatr Clin N Am 56 (2009) 987–994
doi:10.1016/j.pcl.2009.05.010
pediatric.theclinics.com

deliver." In the beginning, certification involved passing an oral examination. This was eventually augmented with a written examination. Oral examinations at initial certification were given until 1988, but were eliminated when it was determined that performance on the written examination accurately predicted who would pass the oral examination. Initially, pediatric certification was a one-time examination of knowledge at the end of training and certification was a lifetime designation. There are still almost 20,000 "permanent" certificate holders who have lifelong certification, but this is no longer considered the gold standard. In 1952, the first randomized clinical trial was conducted and, as both basic and clinical research grew, the knowledge base for pediatrics increased exponentially. It became apparent that the standard of a one-time assessment of medical knowledge at the end of training was not sufficient to assure the public of the ongoing quality of certified pediatricians. As a consequence, in 1988, recertification was introduced and diplomates were required to pass a comprehensive examination of medical knowledge every 7 years to be recertified. Certification has been a continuously evolving process.

American health care is now engaged in a second quality revolution even more profound than the Flexner revolution. The current revolution is focused on the quality and safety of clinical care and is international in scope. As early as the mid-1970s, studies began to appear documenting significant gaps in quality and safety of care at every level of care. In the mid-1970s, John Wennberg[2] published his first study showing significant unexplained variation in health care. This work eventually led to the *Dartmouth Atlas of Healthcare*. Wennberg[3] has shown that even among well-trained, well-intentioned board-certified physicians, variations in quality, cost, and use of care are significant. Using the Medicare national database, Fisher and colleagues[4] showed that increased spending and increased use of specialists do not necessarily translate into better outcomes. In fact, the opposite appears to be true.

By the late 1980s and early 1990s, the tools and methods of quality improvement that had been developed for manufacturing and production in industry were introduced into health care[5] and it became possible to define quality of care. The commonly used definition of "the gap between the care that could be delivered using evidence-based medicine and best practices and the care that is actually delivered" became widely accepted. Two seminal Institute of Medicine (IOM) reports were published in 1999 and 2000. *To Err is Human*[6] documented significant gaps in patient safety and *Crossing the Quality Chasm*[7] documented the broader problems with quality in health care and called for the systematic redesign of health care and the use of quality improvement. In the *Chasm* report, the IOM noted that quality care should have six characteristics. It should be (1) safe, (2) timely, (3) effective, (4) efficient, (5) equitable, and (6) patient centered. The IOM reports have focused primarily on system failures as the source of most of the quality problems in American health care. However, there has been increasing interest in the role that physicians play in the delivery of quality care. It became apparent to some health leaders that the model of a medical knowledge as the only physician competency for delivering quality care was not adequate. As a result, Leach, Batalden, and colleagues[8] proposed an expanded set of core physician competencies that they felt were necessary to deliver quality care. The six core competencies of (1) patient care, (2) medical knowledge, (3) communication, (4) professionalism, (5) practice-based learning and improvement, and (6) system-based practice were endorsed by the Accreditation Council for Graduate Medical Education (ACGME) in 1999 and became the standard for resident and fellowship training in medicine.

In 2000, this profound shift in addressing physician quality spread when the ABMS endorsed the same core competencies for board certification and moved from a periodic assessment of medical knowledge as the standard for assessing physician quality to a more continuous ongoing assessment of the six competencies. This ongoing assessment is called Maintenance of Certification (MOC),[9] which consists of four parts:

Part 1. Maintaining a valid license to practice
Part 2. Demonstrating a lifelong commitment to learning through ongoing knowledge self assessment
Part 3. Passing a periodic secure examination of medical knowledge
Part 4. Demonstrating the ability to assess and improve the quality of practice performance

To be called a board-certified pediatrician under the MOC framework requires a level of training, competence, and knowledge that can only be achieved by completing a rigorous, defined, closely monitored, ACGME-approved training program and then demonstrating a level of knowledge comparable to established standards by passing the initial certifying examination. Once this landmark baseline threshold is reached, the emphasis shifts to demonstrating lifelong professional development and the ability to deliver quality care and to continually improving that care through MOC.

Part 1 of MOC requires a diplomate to maintain a valid unrestricted license to practice. Previously, restrictions on licenses were difficult to track across 70 different state and territorial medical licensing boards. The electronic notification system recently developed by the Federation of State Medical Boards provides real-time national sharing of any restriction placed on a medical license by any licensing boards. This has led to an increase in the number of revocations of board certification related to restricted or revoked licenses. MOC Part 2 requires diplomates to demonstrate a career-long commitment to learning by completing a series of open-book knowledge self-assessment activities every 5 years. The American Academy of Pediatrics' Pedialink system is an example of an ABP-approved Part 2 program. For Part 3, diplomates will be required to demonstrate current knowledge to practice by passing a secure examination of medical knowledge in each area of certification every 10 years.

Quality improvement is at the heart of Part 4 of the ABP's new MOC program. In a real sense, all of MOC, but especially Part 4, applies the principles of quality improvement to career-long professional development in a series of assessments and self assessments and in improvement activities around the six core physician competencies adopted by the ACGME and the ABMS. Beginning in 2010 and then for 6 years, more than 60,000 pediatricians will be required to demonstrate competence in quality improvement as they progress through the new version of MOC.

The focus on quality improvement is appropriate as gaps in quality are present in pediatrics. Mangione-Smith and colleagues[10] have demonstrated that children receive only 46% of recommended care in the United States. With the ability to define quality and to systematically improve care using the science of quality improvement, physicians have the professional obligation to actually measure whether the care they deliver is safe, timely, evidence-based, efficient, equitable, and meets patients' needs. If there is a gap in quality, physicians have the professional obligation to improve care.

There are two options for Part 4 of MOC by which pediatricians can meet the ABP requirement that they assess and improve practice performance. The first option is to use Web-based improvement modules, such as the Electronic Quality Improvement in Pediatric Practice (EQIPP) modules developed by the American Academy of Pediatrics, the Patient Safety Improvement Program developed by the ABMS, or Performance Improvement Modules (PIMs) developed by the ABP. These modules guide pediatricians through the basic process of measuring and improving quality of care for a small sample of patients from their clinical practice using evidence-based guidelines. Participating pediatricians can compare their performance to peers and to national standards. The format is straightforward. The diplomate measures the quality of care his or her care team delivers for a small sample of patients (usually 10 consecutive patients). The measures are developed from evidence-based or consensus-based guidelines and the process allows a physician or group of physicians to assess and compare their results against those of peers both locally and nationally and against benchmark best practices. If process measures are used, there has to be strong evidence that the processes are tightly linked to outcomes. Once baseline data are completed, the physician or team reflect on their gaps in quality and decide how they could improve care. They are provided with a short list of changes that have worked for other practices. They can choose from among these for implementation or they can develop their own unique strategy. They are encouraged to form a team within their practice to implement change and to include patients wherever possible. After the change has been implemented, they are required to remeasure their care to determine if improvement has occurred. If improvement has occurred, they are encouraged to incorporate the changes into their ongoing delivery of care. They are required to complete at least one cycle of remeasurement and are strongly encouraged to continue testing additional changes. Some of the Web-based modules require more than one improvement cycle to receive credit for MOC Part 4. Many physicians are stimulated by this experiential learning to become more knowledgeable about quality improvement science and practice redesign and go on to spread this knowledge to the rest of their practice. To address the competencies of communication and professionalism, activities are being developed that enable diplomates to assess their ability to communicate with patients and peers and to assess the impact of their own professional behavior on care.

The other option for MOC Part 4 involves diplomates receiving credit for participating in an ABP-approved established quality-improvement project. Over 20% of physicians are currently involved in a local, regional, or national improvement effort that involves the patients in their practice.[11] The ABP has established standards for what it considers are valid quality improvement projects that it will approve for Part 4 credit. The standards have been adapted from published formal recommendations, such as SQUIRE (Standards for Quality Improvement Reporting Excellence), and address such methodological issues as having a well-defined aim; clearly identifying the domains of quality being addressed; having appropriate measures; identifying appropriate benchmarks of performance; proposing tests of change that are evidence based or have strong evidence to support their being tested; defining the sampling method being used; addressing issues of sample size and data quality; addressing privacy and patient protection; and identifying appropriate methods for analysis, display, and reporting of results. (Standards are available at https://www.abp.org/abpwebsite/moc/performanceinpractice/approvedq1projects/approved/qi_project_standards). The ABP has also developed standards for meaningful participation by a diplomate in an approved quality improvement project to receive MOC Part 4 credit. So far, the ABP has approved over 20 projects and continues to receive additional applications at an increasing rate. The ABP has focused on approving projects from larger, established organizations that have a greater chance of sustainability over time and has discouraged applications from individuals or small practices. However, small practices are not excluded from this option, as many of the projects that have been approved are hospital, regional, state, and national quality improvement initiatives that involve solo and small practices. Most of these projects are designed to help individual physicians and practices collect measurement data. Most provide coaching or education on improvement science and practice redesign. The approved projects showing the most rapid and dramatic improvements involve collaborative open sharing of performance data across practices so that practices can learn rapidly from each other about what works. The physicians and practices in these collaboratives all test the same change ideas simultaneously. This allows larger sample sizes and creates the ability to determine what actually works at a much faster pace than can be achieved by individual practices. This approach resembles the pediatric cancer oncology networks of the past 30 years, one of the most successful long-term examples of systematically improving outcomes for children.[12] The Cystic Fibrosis Foundation quality improvement collaborative is particularly notable for its willingness to share center-specific quality-performance data on its public Web site as a way for cystic fibrosis centers to identify and learn from centers that are demonstrating benchmark improvements in care.[13] Participation in the cystic fibrosis collaborative has been approved by the ABP for Part 4 credit. Another ABP-approved project is the national collaborative sponsored by the National Association of Children's Hospitals and Related Institutions to eliminate catheter-associated infections in pediatric intensive care units. Within 18 months, 29 units have demonstrated a greater than 50% reduction in line infections with greater than 600 infections prevented, over 60 deaths prevented, and an estimated $20 million reduction in costs. The collaborative was successful in recruiting a second wave of 32 units and is beginning to recruit for the third wave. The goal is to spread this effort to all 300-plus pediatric intensive care units nationally in the next several years. This would result in an estimated 500 prevented deaths and between $70 and $100 million in cost reductions. A unique feature of this collaborative is the use of factorial design that allows various units to test more than one set of changes at a time in a quasi-experimental design that begins to blend quality improvement with outcomes research.[14] The ABP has helped promote similar multicenter improvement efforts for Part 4 and has approved for MOC credit projects in neonatal care, access to care, prevention of blood stream infections in pediatric intensive care units, asthma, and immunizations. Additional applications are pending. These projects represent a model for improving outcomes while reducing costs and waste by reducing unwanted variation in care, especially in pediatric subspecialty care. The numbers of children affected each year across the United States by most complex problems are relatively small, making it difficult if not impossible for any one practice or center to have a large enough number of patients to be able to determine on its own what constitutes quality care, especially care related to clinical effectiveness. There is a significant opportunity to integrate data collection in these projects with emerging electronic health records so that the data can be used not only for daily delivery of care and quality improvement but also for longitudinal studies and clinical trials. The ultimate goal is one-time data entry during the delivery of quality care that can be used to improve care, guide professional development, and generate new knowledge so that "we learn from every child we treat."

The ABP is working with the National Association of Children's Hospitals and Related Institutions, the American Academy of Pediatrics, the Child Health Corporation of America, and with specialty societies and other organizations through the Alliance for Pediatric Quality (www.kidsquality.org) to spread successful existing quality improvement projects and to promote or help create new national projects to improve children's health care through shared data, collaborative practice, and application of quality improvement science. All of these efforts are intended to integrate the ABP's MOC process into daily practice.

The requirement that all diplomates measure and improve quality of care calls for a different approach to assessment and standard setting than the assessment of medical knowledge. Several health services researchers[15,16] have pointed out the inherent difficulties in trying to distinguish whether one individual physician's clinical performance differs from another in a valid, statistically significant manner. Issues of small sample size, how much of a patient's care can be attributed to any one individual physician, and how to adjust for confounding factors, such as severity of illness, makes measuring individual physician clinical quality a difficult task. In addition, the problem of clinical quality in American health care is not that a few physicians or hospitals provide low-quality care, but rather that there is a significant gap between the mean performance of the majority of providers and optimum care. The ABP and other boards are creating maintenance of certification programs that help physicians close the quality gap. The ABP standard for MOC Part 4 requires diplomates to demonstrate with data the quality of the care they deliver, to compare their quality to peers and to benchmarks, and, where gaps exist, to systematically improve care over time. This approach represents a shift from searching for a small number of low-performing "bad apples" to a focus on improving the performance of the majority of physicians, the "good apples." The challenge is to help all physicians and their care teams deliver better care no matter where they are rather than trying to change only a few low-performing physicians (**Fig. 1**). In doing this, the ABP and the other ABMS boards have become drivers for changing physician practice behavior to improve quality of care.

For physicians, the practice of medicine is rapidly changing and there are both internal and external forces driving the need to assess and improve quality of care.

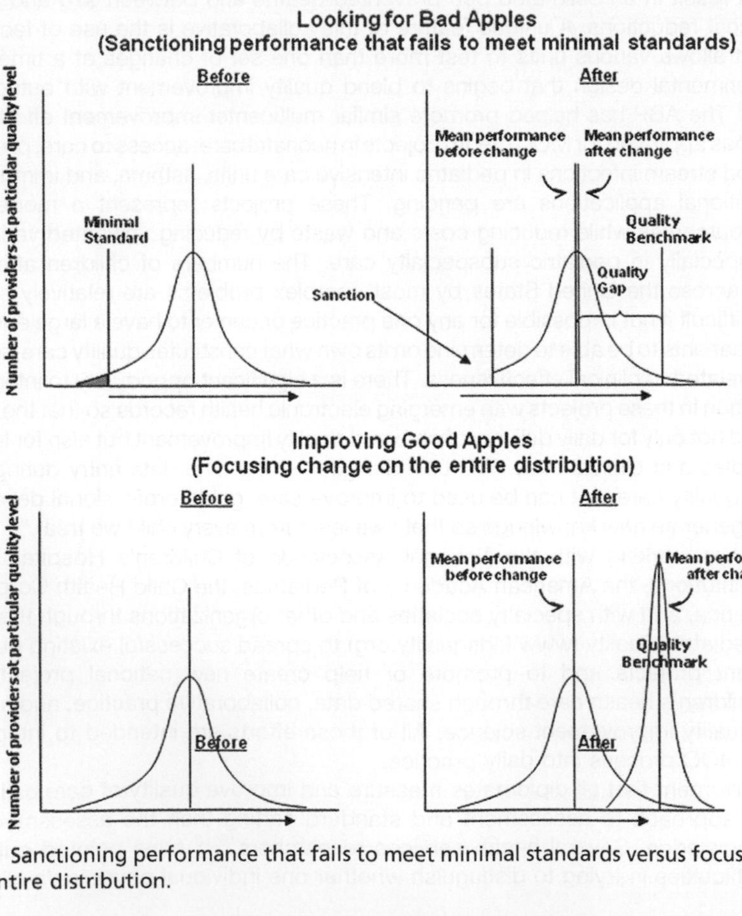

Fig. 1. Sanctioning performance that fails to meet minimal standards versus focusing change on entire distribution.

For almost 75 years, the ABP has been committed to assuring the public that certified pediatricians possess the knowledge, skills, and experience needed to provide high-quality care in pediatrics. In 1933, the year the ABP was formed, Sir William Osler, referring to the Flexner revolution, wrote:

> *I am sorry for you, young men of this generation. You will do great things. You will have great victories, and standing on our shoulders, you will see far, but you can never have our sensations. To have lived through a revolution, to have seen a new birth of science, a new dispensation of health, reorganized medical schools, re-modeled hospitals, a new outlook for humanity, is not given to every generation.*[17]

We are now engaged in another quality revolution. The ABP has added the assessment and improvement of practice performance to the critical assessment of medical knowledge in the new MOC program and in doing so has become a major force in helping pediatricians close the quality gap in children's health care.

REFERENCES

1. Halpern S. American pediatrics. Los Angeles (CA): University of California Press; 1988. p. 102.
2. Wennberg JE. Understanding geographic variations in health care delivery. N Engl J Med 1999;340(1):52–3.
3. Wennberg JE. Variation in use of Medicare services among regions and selected academic medical centers: is more better?. New York: New York Academy of Medicine; 2005.
4. Fisher ES, Wennberg DE, Stukel TA, et al. Variations in the longitudinal efficiency of academic medical centers. Health Aff (Millwood) 2004;23.
5. Banks NJ, Palmer RH, Berwick DM, et al. Variability in clinical systems: applying modern quality control methods to health care. Jt Comm J Qual Improv 1995; 21(8):407–19.
6. IOM (Institute of Medicine). To error is human: building a safer health system. Washington, DC: National Academies Press; 2000.
7. IOM (Institute of Medicine). Crossing the quality chasm: a new health system for the 21st century. Washington, DC: National Academies Press; 2001.
8. Accreditation Council for Graduate Medical Education. 2001. Available at: http// wwe.acgme.org. Accessed January 14, 2009.
9. Horowitz SD, Miller SH, Miles PV. Board certification and physician quality. Med Educ 2004;38(1):10–1.
10. Mangione-Smith R, DeCristofaro AH, Setodji CM, et al. The quality of ambulatory care delivered to children in the United States. N Engl J Med 2007;357(15): 1515–23.
11. Audet AM, Doty MM, Shamasdin J, et al. Measure, learn, and improve: physicians' involvement in quality improvement. Health Aff (Millwood) 2005;24(3): 843–53.
12. Simone JV. The evolution of cancer care for children and adults. J Clin Oncol 1998;16:2905–6.
13. Cystic fibrosis foundation improvement collaborative. Available at: http//www.cff.org.
14. NACHRI catheter associated blood stream infection collaborative. Available at: http//www.nachri.org.
15. Landon BE, Normand SL, Blumenthal D, et al. Physician clinical performance assessment: prospects and barriers. JAMA 2003;290(9):1183–9.

16. Greenfield S, Kaplan SH, Kahn R, et al. Profiling care provided by different groups of physicians: effects of patient case-mix (bias) and physician-level clustering on quality assessment results. Ann Intern Med 2002;136(2):111–21.
17. Cushing H. The life of Sir William Osler. London: Oxford University Press; 1940. p. 1036.

A Pediatrician's Opinion

Richard Lander, MD

KEYWORDS

• Art of medicine • Quality issues • Managed care

Top quality health care available to every American is a lofty yet attainable goal and one we must strive to reach in our lifetime. Quality care leads to improved patient health which, in turn, decreases the expenditure of health care dollars. With this in mind, insurers have or are setting up quality improvement goals they have called pay for performance. Pediatricians who reach the established goals will be better paid for their services. Each pediatrician must decide whether increased payment warrants the increased work involved and whether these goals are ones with which the pediatrician is in agreement. Also important to consider is what to do if an insurer changes the rules of the game part way through. Do you still stay under contract with the insurer? At what point does a pediatrician decide that it is no longer worth his or her participation?

If the practice of medicine were pure science, pay for performance would be both feasible and advantageous. Tables of "quality care" would be established with input from varied sources such as payers, employers, and pediatricians represented by the American Academy of Pediatrics.

Pediatricians who demonstrate compliance with the established norms would be rewarded with higher ratings and therefore higher pay. The problem with this model is that while medicine is indisputably science it is also art. Pay for performance does not recognize the elegance of diagnostic skill. Patients and their conditions do not always fit into an established table. A capable diagnostician must evaluate a patient's condition bearing in mind that this particular condition might deviate from the normal definition of standard guidelines. This evaluation is where the art of medicine comes into play.

Of particular concern to pediatricians are the problems associated with vaccinating the patient population. These problems might cause deductions in both rating and payment. Current Healthcare Effectiveness Data and Information Set (HEDIS) recommendations suggest that an infant be fully immunized by 24 months of age. Will the pay for performance programs take into consideration the multiple manufacturer vaccine shortages which prohibit compliance or the increasing vaccine refusal rate that American practitioners have been experiencing? How will pay for performance

Essex Morris Pediatrics Group, 203 Hillside Avenue, Livingston, NJ 07039, USA
E-mail address: rl@empg.pcc.com

Pediatr Clin N Am 56 (2009) 995–996
doi:10.1016/j.pcl.2009.05.003
pediatric.theclinics.com

reward the time spent educating patients regarding the risk versus benefits of vaccines and will it recognize if a family is willing to accept vaccines but only on a delayed schedule? Should that pediatrician receive credit not only for improving the quality of care for that child who otherwise would not have been protected against multiple infectious diseases but also for improving the safety of the community in which he or she lives?

True quality of care can only be achieved when physicians possess a thorough grounding in the science of medicine coupled with the artistic ability to apply that science to diagnosis and treatment. Pay for performance may be well able to compensate the science of medicine but it is ill equipped to recognize or compensate the art. Guidelines will work if they are just that, guidelines, but pay for pediatricians must never be tied to them. It is imperative to recognize that the treatment of patients does not fit into boxes. If we are truly committed to excellence of care, we must expect more from the providers of that care than to force them into providing pediatrics from column A or B. We want to achieve a healthy outcome for our patients whether we follow a cookbook recipe or individualize management to that patient's needs. Pay for performance rewards standard care; America's children deserve excellent care.

Pay for Performance: Quality- and Value-Based Reimbursement

Norman (Chip) Harbaugh, Jr., MD[a,b,c,d,e,f,*]

KEYWORDS

- Quality-driven health care • Quality initiatives
- Health care quality • Health care reform
- Performance incentives • Physician initiatives
- Physician payment

The quality of current health care is of vital concern nationally, and the structural arrangements of health care have been evolving rapidly to respond to increasing financial pressures and demands to ensure quality. The United States spends more on health care than any other nation—nearly $2.3 trillion annually.[1] This amount is 16.7% of the gross domestic product (GDP) and is expected to grow to 20% of GDP by 2015.[1] The United States can provide its citizens with a first-class health care system for less. As much as $700 billion per year in health care services are delivered in the United States that do not improve health outcomes.[2] With health care costs spiraling out of control despite suboptimal quality of care, it is imperative that all stakeholders involved in health care (physicians, patients, payers, and purchasers) collaborate to explore new models of health care delivery and reimbursement to address some of these challenges. This article reviews the past, present, and possible future models of physician payment for health care delivery.

Current physician payment systems are not designed to promote quality outcomes. The Institute of Medicine has recognized the need to reform physician payment. In its report entitled "Crossing the Quality Chasm,"[3] it recommended that fair payment should be given for good clinical management. Physicians should share in the benefits of quality improvements. Purchasers should have the opportunity to recognize quality

[a] Children's Medical Group, 1875 Century Boulevard, Suite 150, Atlanta, GA 30345, USA
[b] Kid's First Independent Practice Association, GA, USA
[c] Steering Committee on Quality Improvement and Management, American Academy of Pediatrics, USA
[d] Section on Administration and Practice Management, Executive Board, American Academy of Pediatrics, USA
[e] Child Healthcare Financing Committee, American Academy of Pediatrics, USA
[f] United Healthcare Physician Advisory Committee
* Children's Medical Group, 1875 Century Boulevard, Suite 150, Atlanta, GA 30345.
E-mail address: chipharb@comcast.net

Pediatr Clin N Am 56 (2009) 997–1007
doi:10.1016/j.pcl.2009.05.006 pediatric.theclinics.com

differences between health care providers. Financial incentives should align with implementation of care processes based on best practice and better coordination of care leading to better patient outcomes.

EVOLUTION OF PHYSICIAN PAYMENT MODELS

Fee for service, the traditional physician payment system, essentially pays for production and rewards volume and intensity rather than value.[4] In the early 1990s, the spread of capitation, with its incentive to reduce patient access to health care services and thereby reduce costs, raised concerns about its effect on quality of care.[5] These concerns led to the development of multiple quality measures that are common today because capitation does not align compensation with outcomes. New methods of paying physicians are needed so that doctors are rewarded for providing high quality care at the best value.

Pay for performance (P4P) is arguably the most striking change in the US health care system since the inception of managed care. P4P is the use of incentives to encourage health care delivery processes (eg, the use of evidence-based practices) that promote better outcomes as efficiently as possible.[6] P4P is not an all-encompassing solution but one method among many that are targeted at different levels of the health care system.

Although the adoption of P4P has been rapid, there remains considerable uncertainty about how best to design and implement it.[7] The report entitled "Rewarding Provider Performance"[8] released by the Institute of Medicine concluded that early experience with P4P has been promising, yet its effectiveness has received mixed reviews. Some physicians argue that P4P data are not perfect and should not be released to the public or used for evaluation. Nevertheless, public and private purchasers, frustrated by lackluster physician leadership, are not willing to let "the perfect stand in the way of the good."[9] The need for reform is so great that the Institute of Medicine panel has cautiously endorsed moving forward with P4P initiatives.

CONTROVERSIES ABOUT PAY FOR PERFORMANCE

Health outcomes are not the result of medical care alone but of many other determinants. Factors such as the social environment (education, income, and occupation), physical environment (air and water quality), individual behavior, and genetics affect outcomes; therefore, the physician community cannot be held wholly accountable for broad health outcomes.[10] Attempts at aligning physician payment with outcomes need to be multifaceted and require collaboration among the four main stakeholders—physicians, patients, purchasers, and payers.

THE STAKEHOLDERS IN PAY FOR PERFORMANCE

Physicians

Physicians have been reluctant to embrace P4P as a method of public accountability for quality and efficiency for many reasons. On any given report card issued, a physician can appear better than, on par with, or worse than his or her peers; however, most patients believe that their doctors and hospitals are better than average. With report cards, the risk of losing patients' confidence is higher than average.[11] Insurance companies also mine and post data on quality, which doctors allege are produced from poor quality claims data as well as inadequate risk adjustment; health plans subsequently use these data to reward or penalize physicians. Because of these concerns, Congress desires to see more physician involvement in quality reporting before committing to major payment reform,[12] and developing adequate levels of buy-in from physicians and their organizations will be critical to the long-term viability of the P4P program.[13]

Many physicians argue that the only reliable source of information for patients is their doctor; however, providers need to recognize that patients have a right to review and compare the clinical aspects of their medical care. Physicians should acknowledge that information, flawed as it is, is not inherently bad and is dangerous only if improperly used. Doctors need to partner with payers to improve the quality of the tools used in evaluating them. Health care providers would be well served by giving up the role of critic for that of coauthor.[11]

Patients

Employers and payers have focused their efforts on profiling physicians and subsequently publicly reporting their performance data with the hope that professionalism and organizational pride will drive quality improvement. Payers also hope that patients will "vote with their feet and select the highest quality physician."[14] Public disclosure of a physician's rating sends the public a positive message that doctors are willing to be accountable for their performance;[15] however, despite advances in quality measurement and reporting, studies of patients' choices of health care providers continue to show that patients fail to use available information on quality to make informed choices, even when quality measures appear to be highly salient.[16–19] This observation notwithstanding, patients deserve clear and complete explanations about the quality of their care; increasing experience with public reporting of quality metrics will enable patients to make more appropriate decisions.[11] Recently, employers have also begun tying financial incentives for patients to preferential use of providers with higher quality ratings. An example of this is varying a patient's health plan contributions or copayments according to the provider's quality ratings.[14]

From the perspective of physicians, public reporting sometimes seems counterintuitive.[11] Most adults in the United States read at the eighth grade level,[20] and many patients have difficulty understanding comparative information and using it to make informed health care decisions. Many health care plans have dropped patient satisfaction measurements because of consistently high scores with lack of variation across providers, and the expense of collecting patient survey data has been burdensome.[14] Improving comprehension of quality information presented may help patients make better choices.[21]

An important but sometimes under recognized factor in improving health care outcomes is patient responsibility for their own health. While P4P attempts to change physician behavior, encouraging patient self-management via individual and societal education about health and medical care would go a long way toward engaging the consumer of health care services as an active partner.

Purchasers

Employers have been reluctant to participate in health care solutions, and many offer health care coverage simply because their competitors do.[22] They remain skeptical that their corporate interests will be served by solutions arising from the physician, the payer, or the government.[23] Employers are alarmed at the pace of rising health care insurance premiums and are motivated to develop solutions for cost control.[23] It is intuitive that healthier employees spend less money on health care and are more productive. Their goal is to receive the highest level of health care at the lowest cost. Above all, purchasers want predictability and control of their bottom lines as it relates to health care expenditures.[23]

After the suboptimal experience of managed care, which gave a one-time savings, employers expressed interest in getting out of sponsoring health benefits but were reluctant to stop for fear of public backlash. Surveys show that the majority of people with employer-sponsored health care are satisfied with their coverage.[24] Their fate thus sealed, purchasers believe that patient (employee/consumer) choice is an essential lynchpin in improving quality and controlling cost.

Payers

Health plans occupy a unique place within the health care system in having access to a variety of clinical and financial data that can be used in quality improvement activities. Health plans manage care in three ways: (1) through selective contracting and credentialing processes, (2) by developing programs that support care and are made available to associated physicians, and (3) by implementing rules and structures that affect the provision and use of services.[25] Health plans also manage information, most importantly by claims processing. The information obtained becomes a source for physician profiling and feedback. Use review requires information flow from physician to health plan and back to physician; such information can provide physicians with new perspectives on treatment processes.[25]

Health plans manage the cost and quality of care in a difficult environment, facing multiple and sometimes even conflicting objectives. Most plans wish to provide appropriate care[26] and to satisfy patients (employees) who value access and quality more than cost. They also try to satisfy the purchasers (employers), who may care greatly about cost and demand documentation of value and quality.[25] Health plans implement care management and P4P programs to help them achieve these sometimes conflicting objectives; if incorrectly designed or overzealously applied, they can be detrimental.

High quality health plans can create high quality health care.[27] The Institute of Medicine defines this as "the degree to which health services for individuals and populations increase the likelihood of positive health outcomes and are consistent with current professional knowledge."[27] Physicians can provide unique and important information on health plan quality as they observe the effect of health plan practices.[25] Investments in quality improvement by one plan can accrue benefits to other health plans because of overlapping networks. One plan alone may have minimal effect on quality because inadequate data sample size and insufficient incentives may not excite all involved stakeholders. A consortium of plans in a community that cooperates on the design and implementation of P4P is more likely to affect a large enough share of physician income to produce real change.

MEASUREMENT FOR PAY FOR PERFORMANCE

Most P4P measurement is performed by health plans that determine what outcome measures are monitored, such as intermediate and long-term results of health care and changes in health status, functional status, and well-being.[28] Although improving patient outcomes is the most important goal of health care, physicians have voiced concerns about being held accountable for health changes for which their intervention has little direct effect.[28] Determining outcomes accurately is the greatest challenge. Many measures require patient reports and surveys, whereas others rely on laboratory results and clinical measures as well as claims data[28] and may incur significant data collection costs. The health care industry must realize that these outcome measures are nascent programs; without proper scrutiny, the measures may result in increased instead of lowered health care costs.[29]

Currently, the most ubiquitous and least expensive data collection process in the US health care system is the billing process.[29] Hundreds of billions of claims are processed each year and can yield valuable information;[29] however, claims data are created for paying bills and not for research into health care services. Studies of the accuracy of medical claims are discouraging.[30] If claims data are often inaccurate, but randomly so, analyses based on them are biased toward the null hypothesis, which would tend to make excellent physicians and sub par physicians drift into the middle of the pack.[11]

Claims for billing are based on diagnosis codes (International Classification of Diseases, North Revision ICD-9) or procedures (Current Procedural Terminology [CPT]). Research has shown that coding of chronic diseases and coexisting conditions as secondary diagnoses is highly variable, leading to counterintuitive findings.[31] ICD-9 contains diagnosis codes yet fails to differentiate variation within a code. CPT designation allows little to no specificity among multiple codes. Category II CPT codes have been issued that allow coding of clinical values and facilitate performance measures through coding, but these have yet to be widely adopted.[29]

The alternative to using claims-based data is using the clinical data in medical records; however, abstraction of paper records consumes time and resources, and electronic health records have been adopted by only 15% to 20% of office-based physicians.

Analysis of commonly used physician quality measures has revealed that only a handful have significant clinical and financial utility; these measures are not routinely found in claims data. This observation questions the validity of large claims-based data aggregations when compared with clinical medical record data.[29] Despite the many reasons why measurement for P4P is imperfect, physicians should not let "the perfect stand in the way of the good."[10]

Use of Guidelines for Pay for Performance

Clinical practice guidelines (CPGs) are based on clinical evidence and expert consensus to help decision making about treating specific diseases.[32] They help define the standard of care and focus efforts on improving quality. Because most CPGs address single diseases in accordance with medicine's focus on disease pathophysiology, difficulty arises in patients with multiple diseases.[32] Compliance with CPGs has been used for P4P; however, limitations of single-disease CPGs may be highlighted by the growth of P4P initiatives which reward physicians for specific elements of care. This approach may create incentives for ignoring the multidimensional approach required for patients with multiple chronic diseases and also dissuade physicians from caring for sicker or more complex patients. Quality of care standards based solely on these CPGs may also lead to unfair and inaccurate judgments of physicians caring for this sicker population.[32] An additional problem with using CPGs for P4P is that patients do not randomly distribute themselves to their physicians. There needs to be an adjustment for differences in patient mix to minimize the effects of risk selection that may be unfair to patients and physicians. In some reports, the use of risk adjustment for patient health status increased by nearly 50% the number of physicians who felt positively about the usefulness of incentives.[33]

TYPES OF INCENTIVES FOR PAY FOR PERFORMANCE

Various incentive models have been used for P4P. These models include financial incentives such as bonuses or increased fee schedules and nonfinancial incentives such as performance profiling, public reporting, and reduction in administrative requirements.

Financial Incentives

In programs that use financial rewards, some provide true bonuses (ie, additional new money), whereas others redistribute a percentage of payments that were withheld by the payer.[33] In the early phases of P4P, programs based on positive, rather than negative, financial incentives may be more useful to develop adequate levels of physician buy-in to the process to ensure the program's success.[15]

Bonus programs may be competitive or noncompetitive. This structure determines how rewards are allocated across physicians. In competitive programs, doctors compete for bonuses and there are winners and losers, whereas in noncompetitive programs bonuses are based on meeting targets or improving on previous performance. Competitive bonus programs are thought to provide a stronger incentive to improve performance because even those with high baseline performance face the threat of not being rewarded if other physicians have higher relative improvement in performance. Noncompetitive programs, in which all physicians have the opportunity to reach a fixed target to obtain a share of the reward pool, may provide less of an incentive to improve quality. Targets based on improvement over baseline, rather than meeting a specified goal, provide greater incentive for those with very low baseline quality.[14]

Nonfinancial Incentives

Nonfinancial incentive models include performance profiling, public reporting of performance, and reducing administrative requirements. Some health plans offer incentives by ranking physicians into tiers based on cost or quality criteria. Each tier has its own level of physician compensation, copayments and deductibles for the patient, or both. For example, higher performing physicians have lower copayments for patients to encourage patients to use them.[28]

Performance data for profiling and public reporting may relate to access to care, clinical quality, patient satisfaction, patient safety, and patient outcomes. Performance profiling should be across similar groups of physicians, taking into account any significant differences in volume and characteristics of patient populations. Results of internal performance comparisons are presented to physicians for educational purposes, whereas in public reporting data on physician performance is disclosed to the public. Both methods aim to motivate physicians to improve their performance.[33] Public recognition for quality of care may be a stronger incentive than bonus payments, which in the past have been too small to garner much attention from physicians. Such transparency also promotes accountability to the public.[28]

Although public reporting has gained some momentum, current P4P programs are experimental, and public reporting has its limitations regarding data accuracy. The measurement of performance remains narrow in scope and methodologically imperfect, and there are important differences between measures developed for internal improvement and those intended for public release. Public display of results may not be appropriate for programs with unstable measures, inadequate sample size, or an insufficient provider-exception reporting processes. It might also be advisable to establish an adequate duration of provider comment period so that physicians can comment on measures and make initial adjustments before making the results public.[20]

UNINTENDED CONSEQUENCES OF PAY FOR PERFORMANCE

Assigning a monetary value to every aspect of a physician's time and effort may actually reduce productivity, impair the quality of performance, and even increase costs. Some studies have shown that even the suggestion of money promotes behavior marked by selfishness and lack of collegiality.[34] In one such study, primed subjects were consistently less willing to extend themselves to those in need of assistance when money was at stake.[35]

One way to possibly restore the balance between communal and market exchange in health care may lie in the "patient centered medical home." The term suggests an emphasis on social as opposed to economic models in a "compassionate partnership in which the primary care physician coordinates care for the patient's ongoing problems and increases attention to prevention." Health care payers reward the physician with a set fee for each patient cared for in the medical home to provide the most optimal outcomes. This payment accommodates for the time spent on wellness and preventive care that is currently nonreimbursed time. Experts suggest that substantial cost savings are likely to result from such coordination of care.[35]

Health care payers should use great caution as they develop P4P models. Both quality and efficiency measures should be included. Payers need to engage practicing physicians as well as specialty societies in measure development and implementation of their P4P programs. Collaboration among all stakeholders is important in the development of systems of public reporting and accountability. These investments of resources and time can truly improve health care if the various stakeholders do not view each other as adversaries.

EXAMPLES OF CURRENT PAY FOR PERFORMANCE PROGRAMS

Health care quality yardsticks are being developed everyday. There are public, federal, private, or payer-funded programs. In an ideal world there would be one agreed source of quality measures and one place to send data with one set of reports. The following sections describe some examples of ongoing P4P programs.

Centers for Medicare and Medicaid Services

Although the United States does not have a single national health care system, Medicare and Medicaid are by far the single biggest payers for health care services. The Centers for Medicare and Medicaid have several quality measurement projects. The Physician Quality Reporting Initiative is a P4P experiment that involves physicians submitting quality-of-care indicators along with their claims forms. For 2008, there were 119 possible measures that could be submitted; a practice submitting a minimum of three measures for at least 80% of relevant situations could receive a 1.5% increase in reimbursement. This program is basically a "pay for reporting" initiative and is currently voluntary.

National Committee on Quality Assurance

The National Committee on Quality Assurance (NCQA) has two major quality metrics. The Health Effectiveness Data and Information Set (HEDIS) is used by 90% of US health plans to measure performance. Physician Practice Connections, which addresses the effective use of clinical information systems, and the Patient Centered Medical Home are NCQA's recognition programs. In areas where insurers offer P4P, NCQA recognition can lead to higher reimbursement. NCQA certification is a prerequisite for participating in the Bridges to Excellence (BTE) program. BTE is a program in which employers pay physicians a premium for providing superior care in one or more of three areas: diabetes, cardiac, or spine care. BTE is not active everywhere but is one of the few existing P4P programs in which the rewards—up to 10% of the physician's income—are worth the efforts. BTE borrows most of its standards from the physician recognition programs of NCQA.[36]

Integrated Health Care Association

The largest P4P sponsor today is the California-based Integrated Health Care Association (IHA). IHA's collaboration among all stakeholders has allowed it to gain a relevant market share of 60% of practices,[14] and because IHA's members are concentrated in one state, the effective leverage of each program is higher. This model best addresses both efficiency and quality. Measurement areas include clinical performance, patient satisfaction, and investment in information technology. The clinical measures are similar to HEDIS criteria. Patient satisfaction measures include communication with the physician, timely access to care, specialty care, and overall rating. Measures of technology investment include population management as well as clinical decision support via electronic connection with the pharmacy.[37]

These prototypical examples of P4P provide a context for future projections of health care delivery models where quality and efficiency peacefully coexist.

APPROACH TO FUTURE PAY FOR PERFORMANCE MODELS

The effectiveness of existing P4P programs has been evaluated in several studies, and the conclusions regarding its impact have been mixed. The need for payment reform is so great that the medical community continues to seek better answers.

An ideal P4P program of the future would include features of the various models described previously. Community-wide participation has the best potential to transform health care within a geographic region. A consortium of plans associated with physician organizations that have an ongoing open dialogue with purchasers and patient groups might create the right mix to catalyze this process. The emergence of regional physician organizations to manage health information exchange holds the promise of automating clinical data collection and aggregation.[38] Communities of medical specialties such as pediatrics should consider developing common data pools that aggregate information across payers, purchasers, and physicians to have a uniform method for assessing and reporting performance. A common set of national pediatric metrics and their implementation would enable communities to coordinate their efforts across organizations. Without community- or specialty-wide participation, P4P faces a higher risk of failure due to the large burden placed on physicians and their practices.

Physician organizations are more likely than individual practices to alter the infrastructure of the practice milieu in ways that promote better care delivery. Improved information technology that enables organizations to sample patients crossing many practices will increase statistical and clinical significance of performance data. Another benefit of community-wide or regional organizations as the accountable entity would be that physicians tend to respond better to peer-to-peer reputation incentives rather than external payer pressure. Physician organizations will be more likely to take community-based measures and develop internal implementation guidelines that are ideally suited to the local market. Because enforcement is delegated to the physician organization, it is physician to physician. This approach is more likely to promote a shared sense of accountability for a given patient population. It also allows for a closer alignment between local physician preferences and program design. In such a program, it would be more logical to disburse P4P payments to physician organizations rather than individual physicians.

INTERNATIONAL PAY FOR PERFORMANCE EFFORTS

Other societies are experiencing health care quality issues similar to the United States and have P4P models comparable to the US health care system. For example, the UK's Quality and Outcomes Framework (QOF) is one of the world's most ambitious P4P programs to date.[39] The UK's National Health Service (NHS) began in 1948. Its problems included long waiting times as well as gaps in performance between the best and worst physicians. Political pressure led to the new "patient led NHS" resulting in the formation of the QOF in 2004. This change was to be "self improving, in which performance was driven by patients' choice, money following the patient, and competition among physicians."[40] The UK P4P trends toward more active monitoring of physician performance rather than placing implicit trust in health care professionals.[41] Primary Care Trusts, statutory bodies responsible for local health care delivery, were later added to provide financial incentives to motivate behavior change. These Primary Care Trusts organized physician practices to help design quality measures, collect data, and implement procedures and guidelines to ensure better outcomes. In the United States, providers (both hospitals and physicians) can organize themselves in a similar way to achieve these goals in a proactive manner.

Studies from the United Kingdom, consistent with previous work, show that financial incentives can change physician behavior,[42] and that patients receive higher quality care in geographic areas where performance measures and monitoring have been established.[43] The UK's QOF models competition, patient choice, and payment for results. Its basic premise is that interaction between these three elements will produce the dynamics required for greater efficiency and quality. Shifting of care into the community via PCTs substantiates the principles of consortium and community-wide participation. The United Kingdom seems to be ahead of the United States in the adoption of financial incentives to improve the quality of health care.

SUMMARY

There is urgent need for change in the US health care delivery and payment system. P4P is still in its infancy; it will follow its natural progression into some future delivery model. Collaboration among all stakeholders as well as investment of capital, both financial and intellectual, can significantly increase the odds of success of P4P programs. Promoting the emergence of regional physician organizations or trusts to help develop measures, aggregate data, implement quality improvement initiatives, and police their enforcement will allow us to better achieve quality improvement and efficiency. The final solution should be physician driven, patient centered, employer sponsored, and payer administered, with the primary goal of improving the quality of care.

REFERENCES

1. New England Healthcare Institute. Waste in health care: a $700 billion opportunity. Available at: www.nehi.net. Accessed January 9, 2009.
2. Aaron HJ. Waste, we know you are out there. N Engl J Med 2008;359(18):1865–7.
3. Institute of Medicine. Crossing the quality chasm: a new health system for the twenty first century. Washington (DC): National Academies Press; 2001.

4. Rosenthal M. Beyond pay for performance: emerging models of providers—payment reform. N Engl J Med 2008;359(12):1197–200.
5. Berenson R. Capitation and conflict of interest. Health Aff (Millwood) 1986;5(1): 141–6.
6. Casalino L, Gilles RR, Shortell SM. External incentives, information technology, and organizational processes to improve health care quality for patients with chronic diseases. J Am Med Assoc 2003;289:434–41.
7. Leapfrog Group. Incentive and reward compendium guide and glossary 2005. Available at: http://www.leapfroggroup.org/leapfrog_compendium. Accessed July 31, 2007.
8. Institute of Medicine. Rewarding provider performance: aligning incentives in Medicare. Washington (DC): National Academics Press; 2007.
9. Galvin R, Milstein A. Large employers' new strategies in health care. N Engl J Med 2002;347:939–41.
10. Kindig D. A pay-for-population health performance system. JAMA 2006;296: 2611–6.
11. Lee T, Meyer G, Brennan T. A middle ground on public accountability. N Engl J Med 2004;350:2409–12.
12. Glendinning D. Medicare eases quality reporting, warns of annual battles over pay. American Medical News 2006;49(3):1–2.
13. Glendinning D. Pay for performance benefits are unproven, panel says. American Medical News 2006;5:7.
14. Rosenthal M, Fernandopalle R, Song H, et al. Pay for quality: providers' incentives for quality improvement. Health Aff 2004;23(2):127–41.
15. Forrest C, Villagra V, Pope J. Managing the metric vs managing the patient: the physician's view of pay for performance. Am J Manag Care 2006;12(2):83–5.
16. Schneider EC, Epstein AM. Use of public performance reports: a survey of cardiac surgery patients. JAMA 1998;279(20):1638–42.
17. Beaulieu ND. Quality information and consumer health plan choice. J Health Econ 2002;21(1):143–63.
18. Scanlon DP, Chernew M, Sheffler S, et al. Health plan report cards: exploring differences in plan ratings. Jt Comm J Qual Improv 1998;24(1):5–20.
19. Chernew M, Scanlon DP. Health plan report cards and insurance choice. Inquiry 1998;35(1):9–22.
20. Baker G, Delbanco S. Pay for performance: national perspective. 2006 Longitudinal survey results with 2007 market updates. Presentation for Medvantage and Leapfrog Group, December 2007.
21. Greene J, Peters E, Mertz CK, et al. Comprehension and choice of a consumer-directed health plan: an experimental study. Am J Manag Care 2008;14(6): 369–75.
22. Blumenthal D. Employer-sponsored health insurance in the United States: origins and implications. N Engl J Med 2006;355:82–8.
23. Galvin R. Still in the game—harnessing employer inventiveness in US health care system. N Engl J Med 2008;359(14):1421–3.
24. Fronstin P, Collins SR. The 2nd Annual EBRI/Commonwealth Fund Consumerism in Health Care Survey, 2006: early experience with high-deductible and consumer-driven health plans. New York: Commonwealth Fund; 2006.
25. Whaley D, Christianson J, Finch M, et al. Evaluating health plan quality 1: a conceptual model. Am J Manag Care 2003;9(2):S53–64.
26. Kenagy JW, Berwick DM, Shane MF. Service quality in health care. JAMA 1999; 281:661–5.

27. Campbell SM, Roland MO, Buetow SA. Defining quality of care. Soc Sci Med 2000;51:1611–25.
28. Outcomes-based compensation: pay for performance design principles. Presented at the 4th Annual Disease Management Outcomes Summit, Rancho Mirage, California, November 11-14, 2004.
29. De Brantes F, Wickland P, Williams J. The value of ambulatory care measures: a review of clinical and financial impact from an employer/payer perspective. Am J Manag Care 2008;14(6):360–8.
30. Iezzoni LI, Burnside S, Sickles L, et al. Coding of acute myocardial infarction: clinical and policy implications. Ann Intern Med 1988;109(9):745–51.
31. Iezzoni LI, Foley SM, Daley J. Comorbidities, complications, and coding bias: does the number of diagnosis codes matter in predicting in-hospital mortality? JAMA 1992;267:2197–203.
32. Boyd C, Darer J, Boult C, et al. Clinical practice guidelines and quality of care for older patients with multiple comorbid diseases. JAMA 2005;294(6):716–24.
33. American Medical Association. How physician incentives are used to impact medical practice. Chicago: American Medical Association Press; 2003.
34. Vohs KD, Mead NL, Goode MR. The psychological consequences of money. Science 2006;314:1154–6.
35. Hartzband P, Groopman J. Money and the changing culture of medicine. N Engl J Med 2009;360(2):101–3.
36. Rosenthal M, De Brantes F, Senaiko A, et al. Bridges to Excellence—recognizing high quality care: analysis of physician quality and resource use. Am J Manag Care 2008;14(10):670–7.
37. Integrated Healthcare Association. Available at: http://www.iha.org/. Accessed January 9, 2009.
38. De Brantes F, Emery DW, Overhage JM, et al. The potential of HIE as intermediaries. J Healthc Inf Manag 2007;21(1):69–75.
39. Galvin R. Pay for performance: too much of a good thing? A conversation with Martin Roland. Lessons learned from the UK experience with pay for performance. Health Aff 2006;25(5):w12–9.
40. Klein R. The troubled transformation of Britain's National Health Service. N Engl J Med 2006;355(4):409–15.
41. Campbell S, Reeves D, Kontopanletis E, et al. Quality of primary care in England with the introduction of pay for performance. N Engl J Med 2007;357(2):181–90.
42. Gosden T, Forland F, Kristiansen IS, et al. Impact of payment system on behaviour of primary care physicians: a systematic review. J Health Serv Res Policy 2001;6:44–55.
43. Asch SM, McGlynn EA, Hogan MM, et al. Comparison of quality of care for patients in the Veterans Health Administration and patients in a national sample. Ann Intern Med 2004;141:938–45.

How Health Policy Influences Quality of Care in Pediatrics

Lisa A. Simpson, MB, BCh, MPH*, Gerry Fairbrother, PhD

KEYWORDS

- Policy • Quality • Medicaid • CHIP
- Improvement • Measurement

The primary focus of child health policy for the last twenty years has been to improve access to care for children, either through expansions of public coverage through medicaid or State Child Health Insurance Program (SCHIP) or through the funding of direct service programs, such as community health centers; however, two trends are broadening this historical emphasis. First, the growing recognition that the health of children, and ultimately the health of the adults that they will become, depends much more on factors outside the clinical domain.[1] Social determinants and the pervasive inequities that exist in the United States are driving outcomes as varied as birth outcomes, obesity, asthma morbidity, and children's ability to enter school ready to learn or leave school ready to work.[2] The second trend is the increasing focus on the value of health care as health care costs have continued to grow.[3]

Although having health insurance coverage continues to be a first order priority, the policy dialog has become richer by now asking about: to what does the coverage provides access; what the effectiveness and quality of those services are; and the outcomes they produce. This article reviews the important domains of health policy relevant to quality; highlights important trends which have altered the policy landscape over the last decade; and ends by focusing on the Child Health Insurance Program Reauthorization Act (CHIPRA) of 2009, the most important policy investment in quality of care for children in the history of public financing for children's health care.[4]

WHY WORRY ABOUT QUALITY OF CARE IN PEDIATRICS?

As the preceding articles in this volume have made clear, far too often children and adolescents fail to receive care that is of high quality or consistent with clinical

This article was written with support from the Cincinnati Children's Hospital Research Foundation.
Child Policy Research Center, Department of Pediatrics, Cincinnati Children's Hospital Medical Center, 3333 Burnet Avenue, MLC 7014, Cincinnati, OH 45229, USA
* Corresponding author.
E-mail address: lisa.simpson@cchmc.org (L.A. Simpson).

Pediatr Clin N Am 56 (2009) 1009–1021
doi:10.1016/j.pcl.2009.05.014
pediatric.theclinics.com
0031-3955/09/$ – see front matter

recommendations and many opportunities exist to improve the quality of health care for children and adolescents (see **Table 1**).[5,6] Although poor quality care is widespread in the United States and internationally, and although poor quality care affects all dimensions of care, including preventive, acute, chronic and rehabilitative services, the burden of poor quality falls disproportionately on certain populations of children. These disparities have been well documented across types of insurance (public versus private), family income groups (low income versus higher income), race/ethnicity, and primary language spoken at home.[7–9] Public policy has a responsibility to address these particularly vulnerable groups as was so eloquently stated by Hubert Humphrey "[...] the moral test of Government is how that Government treats those who are in the dawn of life, the children; those who are in the twilight of life, the elderly; and those who are in the shadows of life, the sick, the needy and the handicapped."

THE SCOPE OF HEALTH POLICY IN CHILD HEALTH

When health professionals think about health policy, they tend to think primarily of programs that either pay for care (eg, Medicaid or SHIP) or deliver health care services (eg, community health centers). However, many other sectors of policy have an impact on children's lives and their health. In fact, children and their health are disproportionately affected by public policy due in large part to the fact that a large proportion of children live in low income families and they are therefore eligible for publicly funded programs, which are largely means tested. Children are also the beneficiaries of one universal public program, ie, public education, and observers are increasingly realizing the impact of the educational setting on children's health and well-being. Most notably, the childhood obesity epidemic has raised policy-maker awareness at the national and state levels about the importance of focusing on the environments in which children "live, learn and play" and how those environments can prove toxic to healthy choices and lifestyles.[10] Thus, the scope of health policy goes well beyond the financing and delivery of health care services and includes such issues as the foods that can be purchased from food stamps, what food options school provide children, and the presence of walking paths and bike trails in children's neighborhoods.

THE SCOPE OF HEALTH POLICY AND THE QUALITY OF CHILDREN'S HEALTH CARE

Turning from broad policy domains affecting children' health to the quality of health care provided to children and families, the choices made in health policy at the federal and state levels can significantly improve or impede society's ability to move toward improved quality. Combined, Medicaid and SCHIP programs finance care for an estimated 30 million children.[11] This number is equivalent to nearly one of three of America's nearly 73 million children ages 0 to 17 years and up to 40 percent of all children under age 6 years in many states. As dominant payers for children's health services, SCHIP and Medicaid play powerful roles in shaping the health care market as well as health care organizations, such as children's hospitals.[12] At the same time, the majority of children's health care is provided in private offices, clinics, and hospitals that accept both public and private payers.[13] Strategies to improve quality for publicly insured children have been shown to also improve the quality of care for privately insured children.[14,15]

In 2000, Eisenberg and Power articulated the challenges to achieving high quality care as a series of "voltage drops" reducing patients' opportunities to receive the care they need.[16] This framework was used by Chung and Schuster in 2004 to examine how these barriers affect children's health care.[17] This framework is further adapted here to reflect the growing understanding of the steps needed to achieve high quality (**Fig. 1**). This graphic clearly indicates that for children to be able to have even the opportunity for high quality care, they must first have access to health insurance, have that insurance cover a comprehensive range of benefits and providers, have access to a medical home and an appropriate set of services in the community, and have providers equipped with evidence and a capacity to continually measure and improve the quality of care they are providing.

At the same time, this cascade of steps occurs within a larger health system, the features of which are also shaped by health policy decisions. In 2006, the Commission on a High Performance Health System identified four characteristics of a high performing system: (1) high quality, safe care; (2) access to care for all people; (3) efficient, high value care; and (4) system capacity to improve.[18] For children and families, two additional features are critical: the integration of services across type, setting, and time; and the partnerships between funders, systems, families, and providers.[19] Health policies can directly promote these features by requiring or promoting certain activities on the part of private health plans, states, and providers.[20] Ultimately, the result of high performance at the program and system levels is the provision of health care to children and youth that is safe, effective, child- and family-centered, timely, efficient, and equitable, and that results in improved child health and development.

Health Insurance Coverage (Voltage Drops One and Two)

In 2005, the majority (60%) of children were still covered through their parents' employment,[9] 28% were covered by Medicaid or CHIP, and of the over 8 million uninsured, fully two-thirds were eligible for public coverage.[21] The current economic crisis is likely to change this picture resulting in many children losing private coverage, either because their parents lose their employment or their parents' employers stop providing coverage, or transfer the costs to the parents, making it unaffordable for many.[22] Numerous studies have shown that children who have a stable source of insurance are more likely to have a usual source of care, well-child visits, and preventive care and consequently have fewer unmet medical and medication needs and experience fewer delays in care.[23,24] In addition, recent publications have summarized the large volume of evidence on the impact of the SCHIP program.[25–27] The successes include: enrolling the target population and reducing the rate of uninsured children; increasing access to and use of care; giving parents peace of mind about their children's health care; and reducing racial/ethnic disparities in health care coverage.

More recently, policymakers are recognizing that retention of children in their insurance program is almost as great a challenge, particularly for SCHIP and Medicaid, and it is increasingly recognized as crucial for quality care.[28–30] Lack of stable coverage, even if there are only short spells without insurance, adversely affects families' access to and use of services and leads to delays in care and unmet needs.[31] Continuously insured children are less likely to use high-cost emergency medical services or to be hospitalized for such conditions as asthma.[32]

Appropriate Covered Benefits and Providers (Voltage Drop Three)

Once children have insurance coverage and remain stably enrolled, it is essential that the insurance benefit packages provide access to appropriate services and a stable provider network, including both primary and specialty care providers, so that the covered benefits are actually delivered. However, many health plans in the private sector model their benefit package on an adult model of care that is not appropriate for children.[33] This difference was recognized over 40 years ago when the "Early and Periodic Screening, Diagnosis, and Treatment" (EPSDT) program was

Table 1
Quality of Care for Children and Adolescents in the United States: A National Snapshot

	Nationwide Estimate of Population	% Nationwide (95% CI)
Physical and Dental Health		
Indicator 1.1: Children ages 0–17 yrs whose overall health status is excellent or very good	61,141,289	84.1 (83.6–84.5)
Indicator 1.2: Children ages 1–17 yrs whose teeth are in excellent or very good condition overall	46,829,724	68.5 (67.9–69.0)
Indicator 1.4: Children ages 0–17 yrs who are overweight based on Body Mass Index-for-age	4,607,912	14.8 (14.2–15.4)
Indicator 1.6: Children ages 6–17 yrs who missed 11 or more days of school because of illness or injury in the past 12 mos	2,486,464	5.2 (4.9–5.5)
Indicator 1.7: Young children ages 0–5 yrs who have had injuries requiring medical attention during the past 12 mos	2,237,344	9.4 (8.9–9.9)
Indicator 1.9: Children ages 0–17 yrs who currently have health conditions described as moderate or severe by their parents	5,721,482	7.9 (7.6–8.2)
Indicator 1.10: Children ages 0–17 yrs who experienced one or more asthma-related health issues during the past 12 mos	5,841,485	8.1 (7.8–8.4)
Indicator 1.12: Children ages 0–17 yrs who were hospitalized for asthma during past 12 mos (national level data only)	374,282	0.5 (0.4–0.6)
Emotional and Mental Health		
Indicator 2.2: Young children ages 0–5 yrs with moderate or higher risk for developmental, behavioral, or social delay	4,913,967	24.5 (23.6–25.4)
Indicator 2.6: Children ages 6–17 yrs who often exhibit problematic behaviors	3,814,253	7.8 (7.4–8.2)
Indicator 2.7: Children ages 2–17 yrs who have ADD or ADHD and currently take medication for it	2,475,667	3.8 (3.6–4.0)
Indicator 2.8: Children ages 0–17 yrs who have been told by a doctor or health professional that they have autism (national level data only)	332,294	0.5 (0.4–0.5)
Health Insurance Coverage		
Indicator 3.1: Children ages 0–17 yrs who have health care insurance	66,217,390	91.2 (90.9–91.6)
Indicator 3.2: Children ages 0–17 yrs who have had consistent health care coverage during the past 12 months	61,646,174	85.1 (84.6–85.5)
Indicator 3.3: Children ages 0–17 yrs who are currently covered by publicly funded health insurance	19,940,300	27.7 (27.2–28.2)
Health Care Access and Quality		
Indicator 4.1: Children ages 0–17 yrs who had one or more preventive medical visits during the past 12 months	55,995,030	77.8 (77.3–78.2)
Indicator 4.2: Children ages 1–17 yrs who received all needed preventive dental care during the past 12 mos (children who needed preventive dental care)	47,616,245	92.9 (92.5–93.2)

Indicator 4.3: Children ages 0–17 yrs who received both medical and dental preventive care visits during the past 12 mos	41,975,020	58.8 (58.2–59.3)
Indicator 4.4: Children ages 0–17 yrs who went to a hospital emergency room about their health two or more times during the past 12 months	4,133,147	5.7 (5.5 - 6.0)
Indicator 4.5: Children ages 1–17 yrs who received needed mental health care or counseling during the past 12 mos (children who needed mental health care)	2,712,215	58.7 (56.5–61.0)
Indicator 4.6: Children ages 0–17 yrs who received all needed medical care during the past 12 mos	61,412,687	98.5 (98.3–98.7)
Indicator 4.7: Children ages 0–17 yrs who received all needed prescription medicine during the past 12 mos (children who needed prescription medication)	43,675,766	98.8 (98.6–98.9)
Indicator 4.8: Children ages 0–17 yrs who receive health care that meets the American Academy of Pediatrics definition of Medical Home	33,118,954	46.1 (45.6–46.7)
Indicator 4.9: Children ages 0–17 yrs who have personal doctor or nurse (PDN), a health professional who is familiar with the child and the child's health history	60,397,981	83.3 (82.9–83.8)
Indicator 4.10: Children ages 0–17 yrs who have a personal doctor or nurse (PDN) who communicates well and spends enough time with them	47,442,122	65.6 (65.0–66.1)
Indicator 4.11: Children who consistently get needed care quickly from their personal doctor or nurse (PDN) during the past 12 mos (ages 0–17 yrs who have a PDN and needed phone advice and/or urgent care)	29,192,058	91.7 (91.2–92.1)
Indicator 4.12: Children who had problems getting specialty care or services recommended by their personal doctor or nurse (PDN) during the past 12 mos (ages 0–17 yrs who have a PDN and needed specialty care, services, or equipment)	2,561,525	15.5 (14.7–16.3)
Indicator 4.13: Children whose personal doctor or nurse (PDN) follows ups with the family after the child receives specialty care or services (ages 0-17 yrs who have a PDN and needed specialty care, services, or equipment)	9,398,838	57.8 (56.7–58.8)
Indicator 4.14: Young children ages 0–5 yrs whose parents were asked by a doctor or other professional about concerns they may have about the child's learning, development, or behavior during the past 12 mos	8,863,726	37.6 (36.7–38.5)
Indicator 4.15: Young children ages 0–5 yrs whose parents got information to address their concerns about the child's learning, development, or behavior, from a doctor or health professional in the past 12 mos (children whose parents are highly concerned)	1,310,727	43.3 (40.6–45.9)

Note: Shaded estimates do not meet the National Center for Health Statistics standard for reliability or precision. The relative standard error is greater than 30%. *Adapted from* CAHMI/Data Resource Center, 2003 National Survey of Children's Health; (www.childhealthdata.org).

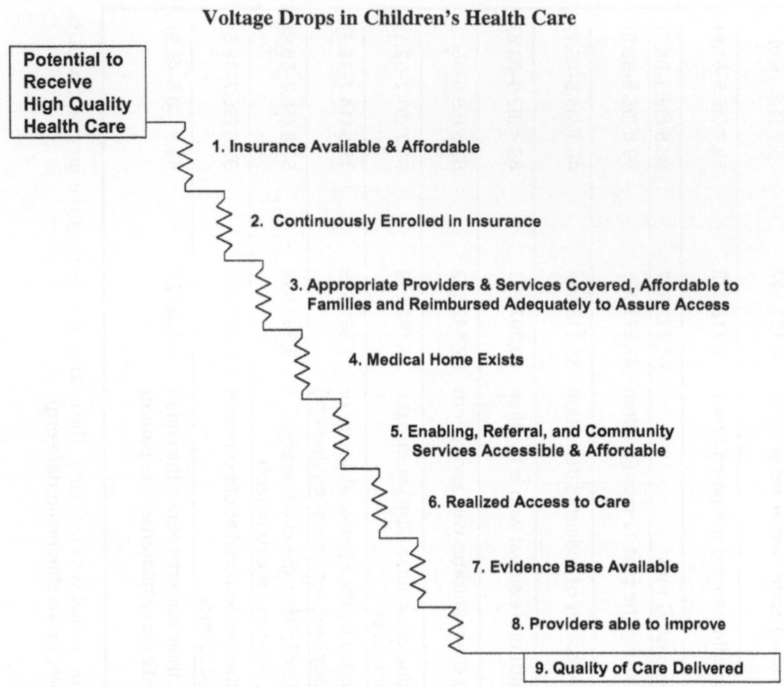

Fig. 1. Voltage drops in children's health care. (*Adapted from* Eisenberg JM, Power EJ. Transforming insurance coverage into quality health care: voltage drops from potential to delivered quality. JAMA 2000;284(16):2100–7; with permission.)

established within Medicaid.[34] Covered services should also promote the development of optimal physical and mental health and social functioning into adulthood.

Several of the benefits guaranteed to Medicaid children through EPSDT are optional under SCHIP, putting those children at risk of not receiving them.[34] Commercial insurance benefit design has become the standard in SCHIP, in effect applying an adult standard to children and hence removing key features essential to addressing the unique health needs of children.[35] Another recent issue is coverage for obesity-related services. Although coverage is becoming more common for adult care, there is substantial variation among public and private sector health plans as to what, if any, obesity-related services will be covered for children.[36]

In addition to stable insurance and a robust benefit package, there need to be sufficient providers to deliver a full range of preventive and primary care services, as well as dental and mental health services and pediatric specialty care. However, access to these services varies substantially by the child's sociodemographic characteristics.[7] In most states, Medicaid reimbursement rates remain substantially lower than the market rate[37] The combination of low reimbursement rates, paperwork requirements, and the increased number of capitated patients deters many private physicians from accepting Medicaid and SCHIP children as patients, or have them accepting only a few.[38]

Realized Access to Comprehensive, Coordinated Services (Voltage Drops Four, Five and Six)

After children have achieved "realized" access to care, children need to receive care that serves the full range of their needs and that is coordinated across providers and community organizations. In 2003, only 46% of children ages 0–17 years received health care that met the American Academy of Pediatrics definition of a medical home (see **Table 1**). A medical home is an approach to providing high-quality, cost-effective health care in which the primary care physician works in partnership with the family, other health care providers, and community to ensure health care is accessible, family-centered, continuous, comprehensive, coordinated, compassionate, and culturally effective.[39] Historically, a medical home has been determined simply by the presence of a usual or primary source of care, such as a pediatrician or family physician. However, thanks to national surveys, it is now possible to operationalize this concept more fully and reflect more of the dimenions of medical home through measurement.[40]

Several key aspects of realized access and medical home can be influenced by public policy. For example, the simple act of obtaining and maintaining health insurance is associated with realized access and improve quality of life.[41] For limited English-language proficient parents, the availability of interpreters is crucial if safe, family-centered care is to be provided.[42,43] However, only a handful of states have set up programs to provide direct Medicaid/SCHIP reimbursement for language services.[44] Similarly, care coordination is critical for children with special health care needs, but the availability of these services varies by insurance type[45,46] Together, these features determine whether children have a medical home that provides continuous primary and preventive health services, as well as health services for illnesses and injuries.

Evidence Base Available (Voltage Drop Seven)

The provision of evidence-based, effective care is a central component of high quality care. However, it is well recognized that the evidence base for pediatric services is lacking in many ways.[47,48] This problem is the end result of longstanding challenges with the appropriate inclusion of children in research, as well as the lack of pharmaceutical company attention to conducting studies in children.[49] In addition, an examination of research funding at the National Institutes of Health between fiscal year 1998 to fiscal year 2003 revealed that, although overall pediatric research increased, its proportion of total NIH spending went down.[50]

Thus, pediatric advocates have worked hard over recent years to increase funding for pediatric research. These efforts have led to several policy changes to support the evidence base in pediatrics, including the creation of the Pediatric Research Initiative in 2000, the Better Pharmaceutical for Children Act and Pediatric Research Equity Act of 2007, and the funding of the National Children's Study, a 20-year, longitudinal cohort study of 100,000 children. More recently, the American Recovery and Reinvestment Act of 2009 (ARRA, also called the "stimulus bill") included $1.1 billion for comparative effectiveness research, which is also a critical dimension of what evidence is missing for improving the quality of care. However, another aspect of the evidence needed to improve quality is evidence about the improvement approaches themselves.[51–54] Funding for this type of research is most lacking.

Capacity to Improve (Voltage Drop Eight)

Over the last decade, significant efforts have been made to help practitioners, organizations, and systems of care improve the quality and safety of care for various populations, including children and adolescents. Notably, the National Initiative for Children's Healthcare Quality is reaching its tenth anniversary and continues to work with practices, states, and health plans to improve care.[55] The American Academy of Pediatrics has had a steering committee on quality improvement and management since 2001. In addition, dozens, if not hundreds, of studies have been published reporting on various efforts to improve quality of care. However, many of these are single-site, one-time efforts that require significant time and effort on the part of participating practices. Although organizations such as hospitals and integrated systems are able to establish an ongoing program dedicated to improving quality, most physician practices can not do so. This situation has led to the recognition that another strategy is needed to assist practitioners. One possible model is an "improvement partnership" within a state or region. The longest standing improvement partnership is the Vermont Child Health Improvement Program (VCHIP), which has been successful in measurably improving care in many areas, including immunizations, perinatal care, and care provision in foster care.[14]

THE FUTURE IMPACT OF POLICY ON QUALITY

The first bill signed into law by President Obama, the Child Health Program Reauthorization Act of 2009, includes a number of provisions that will address most – if not all – of the voltage drops described above. In addition to providing funding for health coverage for over four million more children, it also includes the most significant federal investment in pediatric quality to date. Historically, many state Medicaid programs have had longstanding quality initiatives in place and all states are required by federal law to address performance measurement and quality in a variety of ways. These efforts have been limited by substantial variation across states, which have hampered the ability to understand which populations are experiencing quality challenges or which approaches are proving effective at improving quality. For example, no common quality measure was consistently available from all 50 SCHIP programs in 2006.[56]

These limitations were the impetus for a group of individuals and organizations to collectively educate Congress on what is needed. As a result, policymaker understanding of the gaps in quality for all, as well as for children in particular, has grown in the years preceding the bill's signing. The result is that the CHIPRA legislation contains detailed provisions related to quality of care and funding of $225 million over 5 years, specifically to address pediatric quailty and outcomes. These provisions cover investments in quality measurement, demonstrations on strategies to improve quality for children, health information technology (HIT), and accountability. They are summarized briefly here, and the article about HIT also provides some information about some additional relevant policy changes through the ARRA. Policymakers defined quality beyond technical, clinical quality and included the quality of the Medicaid program and the quality and stability of the insurance coverage as part of the legislation's framework.

Quality Measurement

Quality measurement is a prerequisite to any improvements in quality.[57] The field of quality measurement and improvement has matured significantly since 1997, when SCHIP was first created. Modest investments in research, innovation, and improvement in child health care have produced numerous quality measures and some effective improvement strategies.[54,58] However, many gaps remain in the quality measures available and the scope, effectiveness and reach of improvement efforts.[59,60] The CHIPRA bill has three main provisions related to quality measures: (1) the development of a core set of quality measures for state reporting; (2) a quality measures development program; and (3) demonstrations on using the quality measures. The core measure set must include measures related to the quality of the insurance coverage, the availability of a full range of services, and a full range of quality domains, including effectiveness, family experiences of care, and disparities. The quality measures development program was included in response to the need for new measures and should go a long way toward expanding the available set of validated, evidence based measures. The demonstrations are for using the new measures. The development of the core measure set and the new measures development program must be done in consultation with a broad array of stakeholders, including pediatric providers and experts in quality measurement. These provisions are a major step forward; however, Congress stopped short of requiring states to report using these measures. Consequently, it remains to be seen how many will be actually used.

Demonstrations

The ability to improve the quality of care for children and youth has grown in the last 5 years. However, much remains unclear as to the effectiveness and relative effectiveness of various improvement approaches. The CHIPRA legislation recognizes this and allocates $100 million over 5 years to demonstrations that are focused in the following areas: (1) adoption and use of new pediatric measures (see above); (2) the role of HIT in improving care; (3) provider delivery models that improve care, especially for children with chronic illnesses; and (4) use of a model pediatric electronic health record.

Health Information Technology

HIT is a key tool for improving the quality and efficiency of care. HIT includes: electronic health records, personal health records, use of personal digital assistants, health information exchange, computerized order entry systems, e-prescribing, and disease-specific or population-based registries.[61] Policy efforts on HIT to-date have historically ignored child health needs, despite the fact that children, and child health providers, have unique issues when it comes to HIT. Here again, the child health community has dedicated significant energy and time over the last 5 years to raising the profile of the needs of children to policymaker attention through such efforts as the AAP's Council on Information Technology. The CHIPRA legislation dedicates $5 million to the development of a model pediatric electronic health record.

In addition, the ARRA provides $19 billion for health information technology, an investment that many call a "game changer" in the adoption of electronic health records.[62] The majority of these funds go to funding incentives through Medicare and Medicaid for hospitals and physicians, including pediatricians, to adopt certified electronic health records.[63] Physicians are eligible for the Medicaid incentives if at least 30 percent of their patient load is covered by Medicaid. This requirement means that physicians may receive a maximum Medicaid payment of $75,000 over 6 years. Pediatricians with a Medicaid caseload of 20 percent are eligible for incentive payments, but their total payment is limited to two-thirds of what they would otherwise receive. The stimulus bill also establishes several programs to train health professionals in health informatics and to provide technical assistance to providers to implement HIT.

Accountability

The final aspect of the CHIPRA legislation that is likely to be instrumental in shaping Medicaid and SCHIP policy in the coming years is the focus on transparency and accountability. States continue to be required to report on performance, including quality performance, and the secretary of US Departmet of Health and Human Services (HHS) can design incentives to promote the use of the core measure set. In addition, the HHS secretary must report to Congress on the quality of care provided to children through these two programs. Finally, the legislation establishes for the first time a national Medicaid and CHIP Access and Payment Advisory Committee (MACPAC). This independent committee will have representation from pediatric providers and is charged with examining and reporting to Congress on the degree to which the Medicaid and CHIP programs are assuring access to care and quality of care.

SUMMARY

The next 5 years are likely to see dramatic changes in the way pediatric care is delivered, changes which hopefully will result in significant improvements in the safety and quality of care for children and adolescents. The significant infusion of funds through CHIPRA and ARRA will enable states to launch new programs to both expand access and improve quality. The explicit emphasis in CHIPRA on quality measurement, demonstrations of improvement efforts, HIT, and accountability together will work to shape deployment of these and other health care funds to enhance quality.

In addition, the emphasis on quality measurement and quality improvement in the current legislation is likely to inform the larger health reform initiatives and likely to get underway, aimed at dramatically enhancing health care coverage opportunities, containing costs and increasing value in health care. Thus, the policy framework to improve quality expressed through CHIPRA may be the underpinnings of a larger framework to improve quality in children's health care in health reform. Pediatricians at the local, state and national levels have an opportunity to be involved in this change to ensure the best possible implementation. Pediatricians and other health professionals have been, and will continue to be, active in shaping the policy dialog and through education, research and advocacy working to improve children's health care.

REFERENCES

1. Halfon N, Hochstein M. Life course health development: an integrated framework for developing health, policy, and research. Milbank Quarterly;80(3):433–79.
2. Wise P. The transformation of child health in the United States. Health Aff (Millwood) 2004;23(5):9–25.
3. The Commonwealth Fund Commission on a High Performance Health System. Framework for a high performance health system for the United States. New York: The Commonwealth Fund; 2006.
4. Child health insurance program reauthorization act. February, 2009. Kaiser Commission on Key Facts. Available at: http://www.kff.org/medicaid/upload/7863.pdf. Accessed on April 11, 2009.
5. Leatherman S, McCarthy D. Quality of care for children and adolescents: a chartbook. New York: The Commonwealth Fund; 2004.
6. Mangione-Smith R, DeCristofaro AH, Setodji CM, et al. The quality of ambulatory care delivered to children in the United States. N Engl J Med 2007;357(15):1515–23.
7. Flores G, Tomany-Korman SC. Racial and ethnic disparities in medical and dental health, access to care, and use of services in us children. Pediatrics 2008;121:e286–98; originally published online Jan 14, 2008.
8. Flores G, Tomany-Korman SC. The language spoken at home and disparities in medical and dental health, access to care, and use of services in US children. Pediatrics 2008;121:e1703–14.
9. Owens PL, Zodet MW, Dougherty D, et al. Health care for children and youth in the united states: annual report on patterns of coverage, utilization, quality, and

expenditures in emergency departments for injury. Ambul Pediatrs 2008;8: 219–40.
10. Levi J, Vinter S, Laurent R, et al. F as in fat: how obesity policies are failing in America. Trust for America's Health (TFAH), 2008. Available online at: http://healthyamericans.org/reports/obesity2008/Obesity2008Report.pdf. Accessed July 16, 2009.
11. Duchon L, Smith V. Quality performance measurement in medicaid and SCHIP: results of a 2006 national survey of state officials. Arlington (VA): National Association of Children's Hospitals; 2006.
12. Institute of Medicine. Leadership by example: coordinating government roles in improving health care quality. Washington, DC: National Academies Press; 2002.
13. Hing E, Burt CW. Characteristics of office-based physicians and their practices: United States, 2003–04. Vital Health Stat 13, 2007;13(164):1–34.
14. Shaw JS, Wasserman MC, Barry S, et al. Statewide quality improvement outreach improves preventive services for young children. Pediatrics 2006;118(4): e1039–47.
15. Margolis PA, Lannon CM, Stuart JM, et al. Practice based education to improve delivery systems for prevention in primary care: randomized trial. BMJ 2004;328: 388.
16. Eisenberg JM, Power EJ. Transforming insurance coverage into quality health care: voltage drops from potential to delivered quality. JAMA 284(16):2100–07.
17. Chung PJ, Schuster MJ. Access and quality in child health services: voltage drops. Health Aff (Millwood) 2004;23(5):77–87.
18. Gauthier A, Schoenbaum SC, Weinbaum I. Toward a high performance health system for the United States. New York: The Commonwealth Fund; 2006.
19. Halfon N, DuPlessis H, Inkelas M. Transforming the U.S. child health system. Health Aff (Millwood) 2007;26(2):315–30.
20. Landon BE, Schneider EC, Tobias C, et al. The evolution of quality management in medicaid managed care. Health Aff (Millwood) 2004;23(4):245–54.
21. Fairbrother G, Schuster J, Simpson L. What do we know about the effect of insurance expansions for children? Child Policy Research Center; 1(1):3–19.
22. Schoen C, Davis K, How SKH, et al. U.S. Health system performance: a national scorecard. Web Exclusive. Health Aff (Millwood) 2006;25:w457–75.
23. Wooldridge J, Hill I, Harrington M, et al. Interim evaluation report: congressionally mandated evaluation of the State Children's Health Insurance Program. Mathematica Policy Research I. Washington, DC: U.S. Department of Health and Human Services, Office of the Secretary, Assistant Secretary for Planning and Evaluation; 2003.
24. Damiano PC, Willard JC, Momany ET, et al. The impact of the Iowa SCHIP program on access, health status, and the family environment. Ambul Pediatr 2003;3:263–9.
25. Kenney G. The impact of the State Children's Health Insurance Program on children who enroll: findings from ten states. Health Serv Res 2007;42(4): 1520–43.
26. Kenney G, Yee J. SCHIP at a crossroads: experiences to date and challenges ahead. Health Aff (Millwood) 2007;26(2):356–69.
27. Lambrew JM. The State Children's Health Insurance Program: past, present, and future. New York: The Commonwealth Fund; 2007.
28. Cassedy A, Fairbrother G, Newacheck PW. The impact of insurance instability on children's access, use and satisfaction with health care. Ambul Pediatrs 2008; 8(5):321–8, Epub 2008 Jun 16.

29. Schoen C, DesRoches CM. Uninsured and unstably insured: the importance of continuous insurance coverage. Health Serv Res 2000;35(1 Pt 2):187–206.
30. Duchon L, Schoen C, Doty MM, et al. Security matters: how instability in health insurance puts U.S. workers at risk: findings from the Commonwealth Fund 2001 Health Insurance Survey. New York: The Commonwealth Fund; 2001.
31. Olson LM, Tang S, Newacheck PW. Children in the United States with discontinuous health insurance coverage. N Engl J Med 2005;353:382–91.
32. Szilagyi P, Dick A, Klein J, et al. Improved asthma care after enrollment in the State Children's Health Insurance Program in New York. Pediatrics 2006;117(2): 486–96.
33. Child and Family Policy Center, Improving children's healthy development through SCHIP reauthorization: synopsis and considerations from an expert panel meeting, Dec. 2006.
34. Rosenbaum S, Wise P. Crossing the medicaid–private insurance divide: the case of EPSDT. Health Aff (Millwood) 2007;26(2):382–93.
35. Simpson L, Fairbrother G, Hale S, et al. Reauthorizing SCHIP: opportunities for promoting effective health coverage and high-quality care for children and adolescents. New York: The Commonwealth Fund; 2007.
36. Simpson LA, Cooper J. Paying for obesity: a changing landscape. Pediatrics Forthcoming, June 2009.
37. Johnson P. Medicaid: provider reimbursement—2005, end of year brief. Washington, DC: Health Policy Tracking Services; 2005.
38. Berman S, Dolins J, Tang SF, et al. Factors that influence the willingness of private primary care pediatricians to accept more Medicaid patients. Pediatrics110(2 Pt 1):239–48.
39. American Academy of Pediatrics, Medical Home Initiatives for Children with Special Needs Project Advisory Committee. The medical home. Pediatrics 2002;110:184–6.
40. Bethell CD, Read D, Brockwood K, American Academy of Pediatrics. Using existing population-based data sets to measure the American Academy of Pediatrics definition of medical home for all children and children with special health care needs. Pediatrics 2004;113(5 Suppl):1529–37.
41. Seid M, Varni JW, Cummings L, et al. The impact of realized access to care on health-related quality of life: a two-year prospective cohort study of children in the California State Children's Health Insurance Program. J Pediatr 2006; 149(3):354–61.
42. Flores G, Laws MB, Mayo SJ, et al. Errors in medical interpretation and their potential clinical consequences in pediatric encounters. Pediatrics 2003;111: 6–14.
43. Wilson-Stronks A, Galvez E. Hospitals, language, and culture: a snapshot of the nation; exploring cultural and linguistic services in the nation's hospitals: a report of findings. Joint Commission and the California Endowment; 2007.
44. Youdelman M. 2007 Presentation at the Pediatric Academic Societies Meeting, 2007.
45. Wood D, Winterbauer N, Sloyer P, et al. A longitudinal study of a pediatric practice-based versus an agency-based model of care coordination for children and youth with special health care needs. Matern Child Health J 2008 Sep 3; [Epub ahead of print].
46. Antonelli RC, Stille CJ, Antonelli DM. Care coordination for children and youth with special health care needs: a descriptive, multisite study of activities, personnel costs, and outcomes. Pediatrics 2008;122(1):e209–16.

47. Forrest C, Simpson L, Clancy C. Child health services research: challenges and opportunities. JAMA 1997;277(22):1787–93.
48. Schuster MA, Asch SM, McGlynn EA, et al. Development of a quality of care measurement system for children and adolescents. Methodological considerations and comparisons with a system for adult women. Arch Pediatr Adolesc Med 1997;151(11):1085–92.
49. Committee on Clinical Research Involving Children. In: Field MJ, Berman RE, editors. The ethical conduct of clinical research involving children. Washington, DC: Institute of Medicine, National Academies of Sciences. National Academies Press; 2004.
50. Gitterman DP, Greenwood RS, Kocis KC, et al. Did a rising tide lift all boats? The NIH budget and pediatric research portfolio. Health Aff (Millwood) 2004;23(5): 113–24.
51. Closing the quality gap: a critical analysis of quality improvement strategies: volume 1—series overview and methodology, structured abstract. Rockville (MD): Agency for Healthcare Research and Quality; August 2004. Available at: http://www.ahrq.gov/clinic/tp/qgap1tp.htm. Accessed July 16, 2009.
52. Shojania KG, Grimshaw JS. Evidence-based quality improvement: the state of the science quality improvement strategies, just like medical interventions, need to rest on a strong evidence base. Health Aff (Millwood) 2005;24(1):138–50.
53. Ferris TG. Improving quality improvement research. Eff Clin Pract 2000;3(1):40–4.
54. Ferris TG, Dougherty D, Blumenthal D, et al. A report card on quality improvement for children's health care. Pediatrics 2001;107(1):143–55 [review].
55. National initiative for children's healthcare quality. Available at: www.nichq.org. Accessed March 11, 2009.
56. Partridge L. Review of access and quality of care using standardized nation performance measures. Washington, DC: National Health Policy Forum; 2007.
57. Dougherty D, Simpson L. Measuring the quality of children's health care: a prerequisite to action. Pediatrics 2004;113(Suppl 1):185–96.
58. Beal AC, Co JPT, Dougherty D, et al. Quality measures for children's health care. Pediatrics 2004;113(1 Pt 2):199–209.
59. Miller MR, Gergen P, Honour M, et al. Burden of illness for children and where we stand in measuring the quality of healthcare. Ambul Pediatrs 2005;5(5):268–78.
60. Simpson L, Lawless S. Quality measurement: is the glass half full yet? Ambul Pediatrs 2005;5(5):279–80.
61. For a complete list of HIT terms, refer to the Certification Commission for HIT. Available at: http://www.cchit.org/about/resources/glossary.htm. Accessed on April 25, 2007.
62. Marchibroda calls stimulus law 'game changing' for health IT. March 18, 2009. iHealthbeat. Available at: http://www.ihealthbeat.org/Articles/2009/3/18/Marchibroda-Calls-Stimulus-Law-Game-Changing-for-Health-IT.aspx. Accessed April 11, 2009.
63. Summary of health information technology provisions of the American Recovery and Reinvestment Act of 2009. Alexandria (VA): National Association of Children's Hospitals and Related Institutions; 2009.

Index

Note: Page numbers of article titles are in **boldface** type.

Pediatr Clin N Am 56 (2009) 1023–1034
doi:10.1016/S0031-3955(09)00106-0
0031-3955/09/$ – see front matter

M

Q

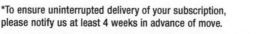

Printed and bound by CPI Group (UK) Ltd, Croydon, CR0 4YY
03/10/2024
01040452-0014